Concepts of Physical Fitness

ACTIVE LIFESTYLES FOR WELLNESS

eleventh edition

Concepts of Physical Fitness

ACTIVE LIFESTYLES FOR WELLNESS

eleventh edition

Charles B. Corbin
Arizona State University—East

Gregory J. Welk
Iowa State University

Ruth Lindsey
California State University—Long Beach

William R. Corbin
University of Texas—Austin

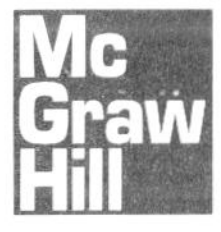

Boston Burr Ridge, IL Dubuque, IA Madison, WI New York San Francisco St. Louis
Bangkok Bogotá Caracas Kuala Lumpur Lisbon London Madrid Mexico City
Milan Montreal New Delhi Santiago Seoul Singapore Sydney Taipei Toronto

McGraw-Hill Higher Education

A Division of The **McGraw-Hill** *Companies*

CONCEPTS OF PHYSICAL FITNESS: ACTIVE LIFESTYLES FOR WELLNESS
ELEVENTH EDITION

Published by McGraw-Hill, a business unit of The McGraw-Hill Companies, Inc., 1221 Avenue of the Americas, New York, NY 10020.

2 3 4 5 6 7 8 9 0 QPD/QPD 0 9 8 7 6 5 4 3

ISBN 0-07-246191-8

Vice president and editor-in-chief: *Thalia Dorwick*
Publisher: *Jane E. Karpacz*
Executive editor: *Vicki Malinee*
Senior developmental editor: *Michelle Turenne*
Senior marketing manager: *Pamela S. Cooper*
Project manager: *Richard H. Hecker*
Production supervisor: *Enboge Chong*
Coordinator of freelance design: *Michelle D. Whitaker*
Cover designer: *Elsie Lansdon*
Interior designer: *Rebecca Lloyd Lemna*
[illegible]
Senior photo research coordinator: *John C. Leland*
Photo research: *Connie Gardner Picture Research*
Senior supplement producer: *Tammy Juran*
Media technology producer: *Lance Gerhart*
Compositor: *Precision Graphics*
Typeface: *10/12 Times*
Printer: *Quebecor World Dubuque, IA*

The credits section for this book begins on page C-1 and is considered an extension of the copyright page.

Library of Congress Cataloging-in-Publication Data

Concepts of physical fitness: active lifestyles for wellness / Charles B. Corbin . . . [et al.]. —11th ed.
p. cm.
Includes index.
Tenth ed. cataloged under the m.e. Corbin.
ISBN 0-07-246191-8
1. Exercise. 2. Physical fitness. 3. Physical fitness—Problems, exercises, etc. I. Corbin, Charles B.

RA781 .C58 2003
613.7–dc21 2001056233
CIP

Contents

Section IV

Physical Activity: Special Considerations

Section V
Nutrition and Body Composition

Section VI
Stress Management

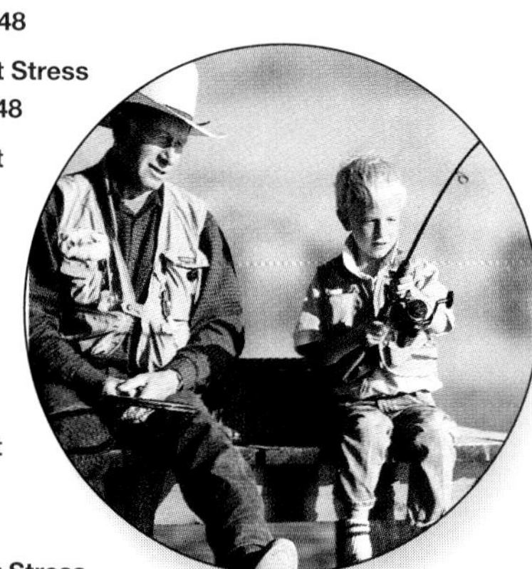

Section VII

Making Informed Choices

Appendices

Preface for the Instructor

Active Lifestyles for Fitness and Wellness: Facing the Future

With this eleventh edition of *Concepts of Physical Fitness: Active Lifestyles for Wellness,* Will Corbin, a clinical psychologist from the University of Texas, joins the author team. He is well published in the areas of behavioral medicine and addictive behaviors with an expertise in high-risk behaviors. He is an experienced teacher who works to promote healthy lifestyles of college students. Will, and Greg Welk who joined the author team with the third edition, add expertise not only in fitness and wellness but also in computer technology. We think that this combination of young energetic authors with older experienced authors (Chuck Corbin and Ruth Lindsey) brings a unique mix that will help us produce the best possible books in the future.

As we pioneered the development of fitness and wellness classes over thirty years ago, we focused on trying to get people fit and well. To be sure, fitness is an important product, as is wellness, another product of healthy lifestyle change. But scientific advances have shown that health, fitness, and wellness (all products) are not things you can "do" to people. You have to help people help themselves. Educating them and giving them the self-management skills that help them adopt healthy lifestyles can do this.

The focus of the new millennium is on the *process.* Healthy lifestyles, or what a person does, rather than what a person can do, constitutes process. If a person does the process (i.e., adopting a healthy lifestyle), positive changes will occur to the extent that change is possible for that specific person. As noted in the first concept of the book, lifestyles are the most important factors, influencing health, fitness, and wellness. Healthy lifestyles (the processes) are also within a person's individual control. *Any person* can benefit from lifestyle change, and any person can change a lifestyle. These lifestyle changes will make a difference in health, fitness, and wellness for all people.

The emphasis on lifestyle change in the eleventh edition is consistent with the focus of national health objectives for the new millennium. Though the principal national health goals are to increase years and quality of life (products) for all people, the methods of accomplishing these goals focus on changing lifestyles. As we move into the new century, we must adopt a new way of thinking to help all people change their lifestyles to promote health, fitness, and wellness.

Our Basic Philosophy

The HELP Philosophy

The "new way of thinking" for the new millennium is based on the HELP philosophy, which is outlined and emphasized in the text. **H** is for *health.* Health and its positive component—wellness—are central to the philosophy. Health, fitness, and wellness are for all people. **E** is for *everyone.* **L** is for *lifetime lifestyle* change, and **P** is for *personal.* The goal is to HELP all people to make personal lifetime lifestyle changes that promote health, fitness, and wellness.

The book adheres to this HELP philosophy. To assure that it is useful to everyone, we include discussions to adapt healthy lifestyles based on personal needs. Instead of including separate sections for specific groups such as older people, women, ethnic groups, or those with special needs, we focus on healthy lifestyles *for all people* throughout the book.

Meeting Higher-Order Objectives

The "new way of thinking" based on the HELP philosophy suggests that each person must make decisions about healthy lifetime lifestyles if the goals of longevity and quality of life are to be achieved. What one person chooses may be quite different from what another chooses. Accordingly, our goal in preparing this edition is to help readers become good problem solvers and decision makers. Rather than focusing on telling them what to do, we offer information to help readers make informed choices about lifestyles. The stairway to lifetime fitness and wellness that we present helps readers understand the importance of "higher-order objectives" devoted to problem solving and decision making.

New Features

Some of the features introduced in this eleventh edition are listed below.

- **Fitness and Wellness News Updates.** The new Update features appear at the end of selected concepts and include the most recent information about newsworthy fitness and wellness topics. In this edition there are twelve new

Update features on topics such as recent good news about health, adherence strategies, new exercise guidelines, new methods of self-monitoring physical activity, and new information about overtraining, nutrition, stress management, and consumer issues.

- **Internet Consumer Information.** The concept on "Becoming an Informed Consumer" includes new information on how to use the Internet to obtain accurate fitness, wellness, and health information. The lab has been revised to help students evaluate information obtained on the Internet.
- **Updated Exercise and Physical Activity Guidelines.** All FIT formula information for exercise and physical activity has been updated to be consistent with the new American College of Sports Medicine Guidelines published in 2000.
- ***Healthy People 2010* Update.** The national health goals that appear at the beginning of each concept have been updated to be consistent with the latest version of the *Healthy People 2010* objectives. Objectives in the tenth edition were based on draft objectives.
- **Nutrition Guidelines for the Year 2000.** Every five years the Department of Agriculture updates its nutrition guidelines. This edition includes materials from the recent year 2000 guidelines.
- **New Assessment Information.** A new chart for interpreting the results of the bicycle test has been added at the request of users. The authors wish to thank the users for their valuable input.
- **New Information on Coping with Stress.** Information concerning changing your way of thinking (untwisting distorted thinking) has been added to help users cope with stress.
- **New Lab and Lab Content.** A new lab has been added on "overtraining." In addition, one of the cardiovascular fitness labs was modified to include ratings of perceived exertion. The consumer lab was modified to help students evaluate Internet fitness, wellness, and health information.
- **New Web URLs.** In the tenth edition we introduced web icons that lead students to additional topical information on fitness, wellness, and health. In this new, eleventh edition we have modified the URLs to allow students to easily access information from the Web corresponding with that section of the book.
- **Other New Information.** New information concerning blood lipid standards, windchill factor, apparent temperature, maximal heart rate, osteoporosis, and the dose-response relationship has been added.

Popular Continuing Features

This new, eleventh edition retains many of the popular features that made the tenth edition so successful. Some of these features are as follows:

- **Pedagogically Sound Organization.** Planning and self-management strategies are presented early to familiarize students with basic principles and guidelines that will be used in later planning. Preparation strategies and basic activity principles follow. Each type of health-related fitness and the type of activity that promotes each component of fitness are included in the next section. This section is organized around the Physical Activity Pyramid. Special considerations—including safe exercise, care of the back and neck, posture, and performance—are included in the next section. Other priority healthy lifestyles are the focus of nutrition, body composition, and stress management sections. The final section is designed to help students become good fitness, wellness, and health consumers.
- **Strategies for Action.** At the end of each concept, *strategies for action* are provided. These are suggestions for putting content into action. Many of these strategies require readers to perform or practice self-assessment or other self-management techniques.
- **Magazine Format.** The attractive format supports student reading and studying with an appealing magazine format. This format has been shown to be educationally effective and has been well received by users.
- **Activity Features with Activity Labs.** Each of the exercises described in the book is contained in activity features using the magazine format. This format allows students to get immediately involved in activity and to keep activity logs. "Basic 8" tables feature easy to use exercises.
- **Web Icons.** The Web icons unique to this book allow learners to locate (at point of use) additional pictures, tables, and figures that illustrate concepts presented in the book. Web addresses to supplemental resource materials (such as a self-study guide, sample exam questions, and definitions of terms, as well as other enrichment materials) are also provided on the Online Learning Center and in the Web Review at the end of each concept.
- **Attractive and Easy to Use Labs.** The attractive and popular labs are designed to get users involved in practicing self-management skills that will promote healthy lifestyle change. The labs are in a bright, attractive, and educationally effective format. They are easy to find and easy to use. In many cases, resource materials precede the labs. These resources are designed to aid the student in performing lab activities and should be retained in the book even when the labs are torn out. This allows future use of such materials as fitness self-assessments. The physical activity labs are designed to get people active early in the course and ultimately to allow each user to plan his or her own personal activity program.
- **Focus on Self-Management Skills.** The educational effectiveness of a book depends on more than just presenting information. If lifestyle changes are to be implemented, there must be opportunities to learn how to make these changes. Research suggests that learning self-

management skills is important to lifestyle change. A revised section on self-management skills is included early in the book, and information about how to practice and implement these skills is included throughout the book.

- **Health Goals for the Year 2010.** The health goals are based on the revised health goals for the new millennium (Health Goals for the Year 2010). These goals are provided at the beginning of each concept to help readers relate content to goals.
- **Student Preface/User's Guide.** This guide follows the Preface to the Instructor and is designed to help students use the book more effectively. Instructors are encouraged to urge students to read this section prior to using the book.
- **Terms at Point-of-Use.** It greatly pleased us that the *Surgeon General's Report on Physical Activity and Health* adopted our physical fitness definitions in their report. Just as we have led the way in defining fitness, we now include state-of-the-art definitions related to wellness and quality of life. These—and all other definitions—are now included at the first point-of-use to make them easier to locate.
- **Continued Use of Conceptual Format.** We use concepts rather than chapters, and each concept contains factual statements that follow concise informational paragraphs. This tried-and-true method has proven to be educationally sound and well received by students and instructors.

Pedagogical Aids

Suggested Readings

Because students want to know more about a particular topic, a list of readings is given at the end of each chapter. Most suggested readings are readily available at bookstores or public libraries.

Appendices

Concepts of Physical Fitness: Active Lifestyles for Wellness, eleventh edition, includes five appendices that are valuable resources for the student. The metric conversion chart; metric conversions of selected charts and tables; caloric guide to common foods; calories of protein, carbohydrates, and fats in food; and the Canadian food guide are included for your use.

Ancillaries

A Note for Instructors

As with past editions, you will see that we have updated this edition with the most recent scientific information. As noted earlier, we have included a new lab. We have designed experiences to promote higher-order thinking. There is another consideration we think to be important. As usual, we have worked to keep the price of the book low.

As always with our *Concepts* books, an extensive list of ancillary materials is available to help you provide the most effective instruction. Brief descriptions of these materials follow.

Instructor's Resource Materials

Course Integrator Guide

Formerly the Instructor's Manual, this guide includes all the features of a useful instructor's manual, including learning objectives, suggested lecture outlines, suggested activities, media resources, and web links. It also integrates the text with all the health resources McGraw-Hill offers, such as the HealthQuest CD, the Online Learning Center, the Visual Resource Library, the AIDS booklet, the video clips CD, and the Health and Human Performances Discipline Page. The guide also includes references to relevant print and broadcast media.

Test Bank

This printed manual includes multiple choice questions for each concept, providing more than 600 test items. All questions have been entered into the computerized test bank.

Micro Test III Computerized Test Bank

The latest version of our computerized testing software is available on CD (Windows and Macintosh). This allows you to custom design your own tests, use the expanded test bank, and add your own testing questions.

Visual Resource Library Update

The Visual Resource Library is a bank of images for use in the classroom and in the accompanying PowerPoint presentation. A slide editor tool allows the user to create customized slide shows.

Instructional Videos

Video 1: Introduction to Physical Fitness. This video includes a statement of fitness philosophy, a look at important fitness objectives, including the Stairway to Lifetime Fitness, and a description of the fitness tests included in the *Concepts* books. Test descriptions include estimated 1 RM for strength, the trunk rotation test for flexibility, and the curl-up test for muscular endurance. Other fitness test descriptions are also described. This video may be viewed by instructors or shown to students to help them understand the various tests. It has been proven popular with both students and instructors. The HELP philosophy is part of the flow of the video presentation of concepts.

Video 2: Introduction to Wellness. This second instructional video defines wellness and puts wellness, health, and fitness in perspective for both students and instructors. The video helps establish common ground for the study of wellness. This proven video has helped provide the basic foundation for the study of wellness that is needed by many students.

Concepts Transparencies

Fifty four-color acetate transparencies illustrate anatomical and physiological concepts, and help instructors to describe the scientific concepts of physical fitness and health-related fitness.

Student Self-Assessment Materials

Fitsolve II Software. Fitsolve is educational software designed to facilitate the teaching of high-order physical fitness objectives such as self-evaluation, diagnosis, and problem-solving skills, which in turn enable the achievement of fitness independence, and a state of self-sufficiency in which individuals can design and implement their own fitness programs. Available for Windows.

Dietary Analysis Software. Available for Windows and Macintosh computers, this user-friendly diet analysis software allows students to track their food intake over a period of days and generate a variety of easy-to-read reports and graphs. The program tracks over thirty nutrient categories. Students can choose from nearly 8,000 foods or add their own to the database. Other features include a weight management function and a website devoted to diet analysis-related resources.

Testwell *by the National Wellness Institute.* This is a self-scoring, pencil-and-paper wellness assessment booklet developed by the National Wellness Institute in Stevens Point, Wisconsin, and distributed exclusively by McGraw-Hill Publishers. It adds flexibility to any personal health or wellness course by allowing adopters to offer pre- and postassessments at the beginning and end of the course, or at any time during the course.

Internet Resources

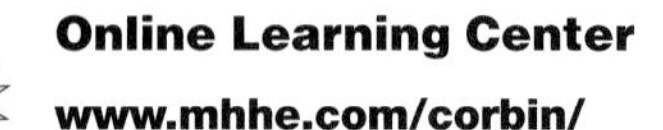

Online Learning Center

www.mhhe.com/corbin/

This website offers resources to students and instructors. It includes downloadable ancillaries, web links, student quizzes, additional information on topics of interest, and more. Resources for the instructor include:

- Downloadable PowerPoint Presentations
- Lecture outlines
- Discussion questions
- Concept summaries

Resources for the student include:

- Flashcards
- Online chapter reviews
- Interactive quizzes

Health and Human Performance Discipline Page

www.mhhe.com/hhp

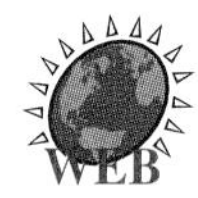

McGraw-Hill's Health and Human Performance Discipline Page provides a wide variety of information for instructors and students—including monthly articles that celebrate our diversity, text ancillaries, a "how to" guide to technology, study tips, and athletic training exam preparation materials. It includes professional organization, convention, and career information, and information on how to become a McGraw-Hill author. Additional features of the Discipline Page include:

- This Just In—This feature provides information on the latest hot topics, the best web resources, and more—all updated monthly.
- Faculty Support—Access online course supplements, such as lecture outlines and PowerPoint presentations, and create your own website with PageOut!
- Student Success Center—Find online study guides and other resources to improve your academic performance. Explore scholarship opportunities and learn how to launch your career!
- Author Arena—Interested in writing a textbook or supplement for the college market? Read the McGraw-Hill proposal guidelines and links to the Editorial Marketing teams, and meet and converse with our current authors!

PageOut: The Course Website Development Center

PageOut enables you to develop a website for your course. The site includes:

- A course home page
- An instructor home page
- A syllabus (interactive, customizable, and includes quizzing, instructor notes, and links to the Online Learning Center)
- Web links
- Discussions (multiple discussion areas per class)
- An online grade book
- Student web pages
- Design templates

This program is now available to registered adopters of McGraw-Hill textbooks.

Primis Online

www.mhhe.com/primis/online

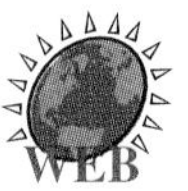

Create content-rich textbooks, lab manuals, or readers right from our website. Choose the material you would like to include in your own customized book. A Primis e-book is a digital version of the text you created (and is sold directly to your students as a downloadable file to their computer, or it may be accessed online by a password). And Primis Online customized books are affordable for your students. Visit our website for further information.

Interactive CD-ROMs

HealthQuest ***CD-ROM.*** *HealthQuest* is designed to help students explore the behavioral aspects of personal health and wellness through a state-of-the-art interactive CD-ROM. Your students will be able to assess their current health and wellness status, determine their health risks, and explore options and make decisions to improve the behaviors that impact their health.

Interactive Personal Trainer CD-ROM. The Interactive Personal Trainer CD-ROM provides users with a variety of features. First, self-assessments for all parts of health-related fitness are provided. Still pictures and QuickTime movies illustrate the assessments, and written statements describe each one. Second, a fitness profile allows users to input assessment results to get a rating profile. In many cases (e.g., skinfolds), calculations are made automatically. Third, physical activities and exercises are provided for each part of fitness and for care of the back and good posture. Users can select exercises for any part of fitness or for different body parts and get descriptions, still pictures, and real-time videos of each. Finally, pictures and descriptions of risky exercises are provided, followed by descriptions and real-time movies of appropriate alternatives. The CD-ROM is available in either Windows or Mac versions. Instructors may encourage use on a computer accessible to students.

Print Publications

The AIDS Booklet, sixth edition, **by Frank Cox.** This booklet provides current and accurate facts about AIDS and HIV: what it is, how the disease is transmitted, its prevalence among various population groups, symptoms of HIV infection, strategies for prevention, etc. Also included are various legal, social, medical, and ethical issues related to HIV and AIDS. This short booklet makes HIV and AIDS understandable to your students and insures that they get the most current information possible on HIV and AIDS. Additional updates are posted to the website at www.mhhe.com/hhp and click on the Student Success Center.

Diet and Fitness Log by McGraw-Hill. This logbook helps students keep track of their diet and exercise programs, and it serves as a diary to help students log their behaviors.

Acknowledgments

It is only fitting as we enter the new millennium that we acknowledge those people who have contributed to the development of this book over its more than thirty year history. For this edition an exceptionally large number of people contributed reviews and comments. At the risk of inadvertently failing to mention someone, we want to acknowledge the following people for their role in the development of this book.

First, we would like to acknowledge a few people who have made special contributions over the years. Linus Dowell, Carl Landiss, and Homer Tolson, all of Texas A & M University, were involved in the development of the first *Concepts* book, and their contributions were also important as we helped start the fitness movement in the 1960s. Other pioneers were Jimmy Jones of Henderson State University, who started one of the first *Concepts* classes in 1970 and has led the way in teaching fitness in the years that have followed; Charles Erickson, who started a quality program at Missouri Western; and Al Lesiter, a leader in the East at Mercer Community College in New Jersey. David Laurie and Barbara Gench (now at Texas Women's University) at Kansas State University, as well as others on that faculty, were instrumental in developing a prototype concepts program, which research has shown to be successful. A special thanks is extended to Andy Herrick and Jim Whitehead, who have contributed to much of the development of most recent editions of the book, including excellent suggestions for change. Mark Ahn, Keri Chesney, Chris MacCrate, Guy Mullin, Stephen Hustedde, Greg Nigh, Doreen Mauro, Marc vanHorne, along with other employees of the Consortium for Instructional Innovation and the Micro Computer Resource Facility at Arizona State University, and Betty Craft and Ken Rudich and other employees at the Distance Learning Technology Program at Arizona State University, deserve special recognition.

Second, we wish to extend thanks to the following people who provided comments for the current editions of our *Concepts* books: Craig Koppelman, University of Central Arkansas; Robert W. Rausch, Jr., Westfield State College; Amy P. Richardson, University of Central Arkansas; Terry R. Tabor, University of North Florida; Sharon Rifkin, Broward Community College; William B. Karper, University of North Carolina at Greensboro; Larry E. Knuth, Rio Hondo College; Maridy Troy, University of Alabama at Tuscaloosa; Kenneth L. Cameron, United States Military Academy at West Point; Thomas E. Temples, North Georgia College & State University; Bridget Cobb, Armstrong Atlantic State University; Tillman (Chuck) Williams, Southwest Missouri State University; Mary Jeanne Kuhar, Central Oregon Community College; Jennifer L. H. Lechner, St. Petersburg Junior College; Laura Switzer, Southwestern Oklahoma State University; Robert L. Slevin, Towson University; Karen (Pea) Poole, University of North Carolina at Greensboro; and Paul Downing, Towson University.

Third, we want to acknowledge the following people who have aided us in the preparation of past editions: David Horton, Liberty University; Lindy S. Pickard, Broward Community College; Laura L. Borsdorf, Ursinus College; Frederick C. Surgent, Frostburg State University; James A. Gemar, Moorhead State University; Vincent Angotti, Towson University; Judi Phillips, Del Mar College; Joseph Donnelly, Montclair State University; Harold L. Rainwater, Asbury College; Candi D. Ashley, University of South Florida; Dennis Docheff, United States Military Academy; Robin Hoppenworth, Wartburg College; Linda Farver, Liberty University; Peter Rehor, Montana State University; Martin W. Johnson, Mayville State University; Keri Lewis, North Carolina State University; J. D. Parsley, University of St. Thomas; Marika Botha, Lewis-Clark State College; Robert J. Mravetz, University of Akron; Debra A. Beal, Northern Essex Community College; Roger Bishop, Wartburg College; David S. Brewster, Indiana State University; Ronnie Carda, University of Wisconsin—Madison; Curt W. Cattau, Concordia University; Cindy Ekstedt Connelley, Catawaba College; J. Ellen Eason, Towson State University; Bridgit A. Finley, Oklahoma City Community College; Diane Sanders Flickner, Bethel College; Judy Fox, Indiana Wesleyan University; Earlene Hannah, Hendrix College; Carole J. Hanson, University of Northern Iowa; David Horton, Liberty University; John Merriman, Valdosta State College; Beverly F. Mitchell, Kennesaw State College; George Perkins, Northwestern State University; James J. Sheehan, Fitchburg State College; Mary Slaughter, University of Illinois; Paul H. Todd, Polk Community College; Susan M. Todd, Vancouver Community College—Langara Campus; Kenneth E. Weatherman, Floyd College; Newton Wilkes, Bridget Cobb, John Dippel, and Todd Kleinfelter of Northwestern State University of Louisiana and John R. Webster, Central Connecticut State University. A special thanks is extended to Patty Williams, Ann Woodard, Laurel Smith, Bill Carr (Polk Community College), James Angel, Jeanne Ashley, Stanley Brown, Ronnie Carda, Robert Clayton, Melvin Ezell Jr., Brigit Finley, Pay Floyd, Carole Hanson, James Harvey, John Hayes, David Horton, Sister Janice Iverson, Tony Jadin, Richard Krejei, Ron Lawman, James Marett, Pat McSwegin, Betty McVaigh, John Merriman, Beverly Mitchell, Sandra Morgan, Robert Pugh, Larry Reagan, Mary Rice, Roberts Stokes, Paul Tood, Susan Todd, Marjorie Avery Willard, Karen Cookson, Dawn Strout, Earlene Hannah, Ken Weatherman, J. Ellen Eason, William Podoll, John Webster, James Shebban, David Brewster, Kelly Adam, Lisa Hibbard, Roger Bishop, Mary Slaughter, Jack Clayton Stovall, Karen Watkins, Ruth Cohoon, Mark Bailey, Nena Amundson, Bruce Wilson, Sarah Collie, Carl Beal, George Perkins, Stan Rettew, Ragene Gwin, Judy Fox, Diane Flickner, Cindy Connelley, Curt Cattau, Don Torok, and Dennis Wilson.

Finally, we want to acknowledge others who have contributed, including Virginia Atkins, Charles Cicciarella, Donna Landers, Susan Miller, Robert Pangrazi, Karen Ward, Darl Waterman, and Weimo Zhu. Among other important contributors are former graduate students who have contributed ideas, made corrections, and contributed in other untold ways to the success of these books. We wish to acknowledge Jeff Boone, Laura Borsdorf, Lisa Chase, Tom Cuddihy, Darren Dale, Bo Fernhall, Ken Fox, Connie Fye, Louie Garcia, Steve Feyrer-Melk, Kirk Rose, Jack Rutherford, Cara Sidman, Scott Slava, Dave Thomas, Min Qui Wang, Jim Whitehead, Bridgette Wilde, and Ashley Woodcock.

Author Acknowledgments

A very special thanks goes to David E. Corbin of the University of Nebraska at Omaha and Karen Welk of Ames, Iowa. David is a health educator who has provided valuable assistance. Karen is a physical therapist who advised us concerning correct performance of the exercises in the book. We also want to thank Ron Hager and Lynda Ransdell for their assistance with the development of the web resources and the development of the test bank materials.

Finally, we would like to thank two excellent students—George Ritz, who provided excellent proofreading, and Tony Ericson, who assisted with locating valuable references. A special thanks goes to Jodi Hickman who spent many hours researching photos for this book.

Preface for the Student

This book is designed to help you—the reader—adopt behaviors that lead to lifelong fitness, health, and wellness. The focus on lifetime behaviors (lifestyle change) is consistent with national health goals for the new millennium (the year 2010).

First, you are given a brief introduction to lifestyles for health, wellness, and fitness. Information is then presented to advise you about the fundamental principles and health benefits of physical activity. A variety of self-management skills are discussed and opportunities to practice these skills are provided in laboratory activities. You are also provided with information concerning nutrition and body composition, stress management, and other healthy lifestyles. The emphasis is on making informed choices about active healthy living.

Before you begin reading this book, it is important that you become familiar with its special features, each of which is designed to help you use the book more effectively.

Features

Concept Statement. Chapters in the book are referred to as concepts. Each concept begins with a title and a conceptual statement that characterizes the nature of the material. Be sure to read the statement prior to reading the content of the concept.

Health Goals. The health goals that appear on the second page of each concept (green box) are adapted from the national health goals (*Healthy People 2010*). These health goals help the reader understand how the content of each concept relates to meeting national health objectives. They are meant to be realistic goals that can be accomplished by the year 2010. A more complete description of the health goals is included at the beginning of Concept 1.

Concept Introduction. After the health goals, an introduction to each concept is provided. This expands on the concept statement and is designed to set the stage for the materials that follow.

Fact Statements. Each concept includes "fact statements" followed by a discussion that expands on the fact statement. Fact statements are important points that are highlighted as much as you might emphasize material with a highlighter in other books. We have done this for you.

Definitions of Terms. As you read, you will come across terms that are **bold.** All terms in bold are defined in a light-blue definition box on the right page. Look for this box when you see a bold-faced term.

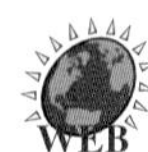

Web Icons. As you read, you will come across icons to indicate that supplemental materials are available on the Web. Look for the icons in the book. To access the information, type the web address (URL) and you will be taken directly to the supplementary information.

Exercise Features. In many of the concepts on physical activity, exercise features are included on specially tabbed pages. You can look at the side of the book and easily locate the dark blue tabs. The featured exercises are ones you can incorporate into your personal plan and record on an activity log.

Strategies for Action. Toward the end of each concept, you will find strategies for action, which provide a basis for action. You can find information about self-management skills that enhance adherence to healthy lifestyles. In many cases, the strategies refer you to labs that allow you to perform activities that lead to lifestyle changes.

Web Review. Web review at the end of each concept links you to study questions, sample test questions, supplemental pictures and tables, and the definitions of terms. You may get information about access to the Web at **www.mhhe.com/hper/physed/clw/student.** Also provided are web URLs that will take you to additional information sources.

Suggested Readings. The suggested readings are at the end of each concept. These readings are not original research articles but rather review articles that give easy-to-read, scientifically sound information on topics covered in the concept. The research articles that document concept content are included in the reference list at the end of the book.

Lab Resource Materials. Lab resource materials include information that you will need in order to complete the various lab activities in the book. They are on the yellow pages with dark red tabs that precede the labs. Unlike labs, lab resource materials are *not* meant to be torn from the book.

Tear-Out Labs. The tear-out labs are located at the end of each concept. The page is bright yellow with a blue tab. Read the Purpose and Procedures sections carefully before entering data or answering questions. In many cases, the labs are self-explanatory, though some require lab resource materials.

Physical Fitness News Updates. The "news updates" included at the end of selected concepts include "hot off the press" information on a variety of current fitness and wellness topics.

Concept 1

Health, Wellness, Fitness, and Healthy Lifestyles: An Introduction

Good health, wellness, fitness, and healthy lifestyles are important for all people.

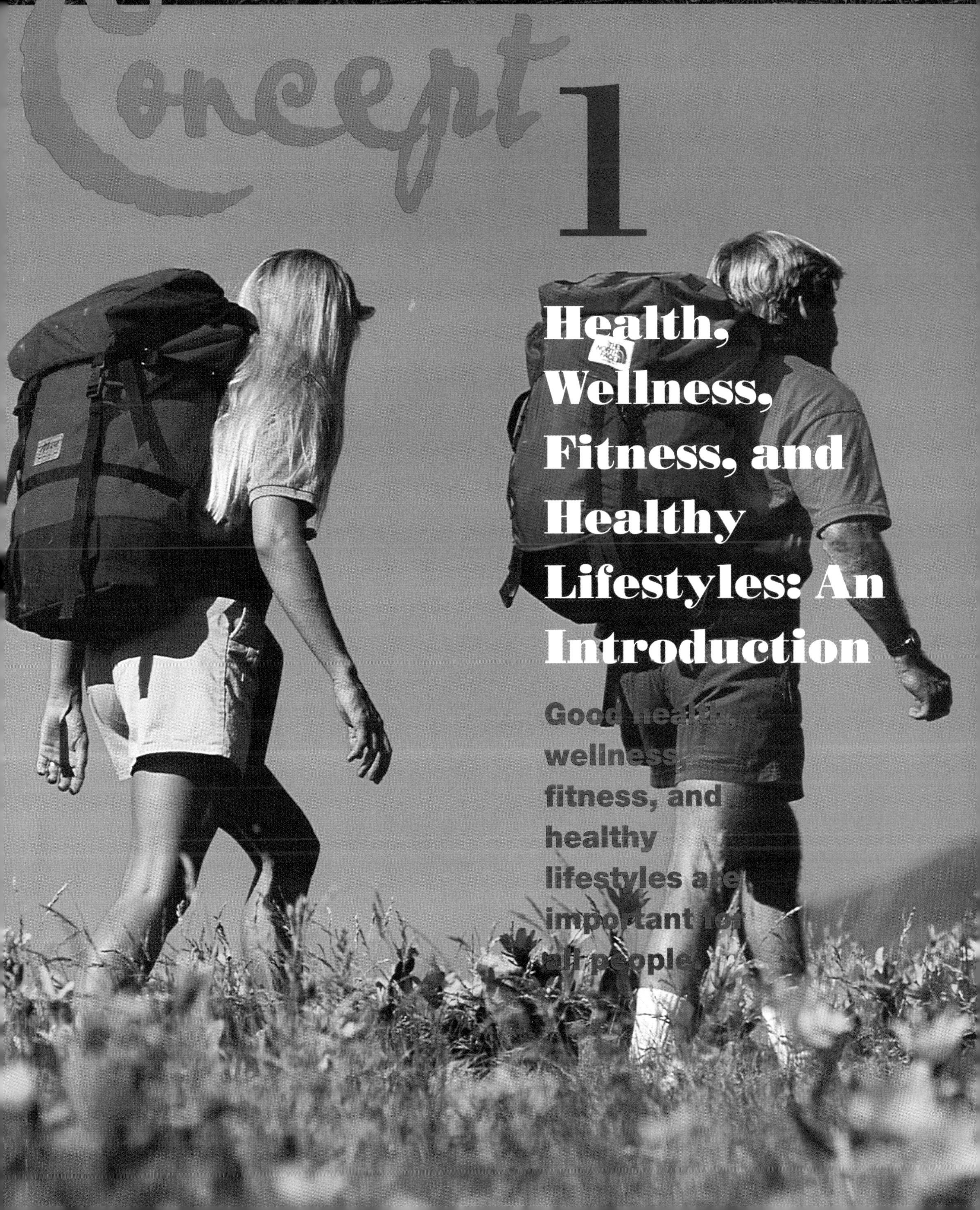

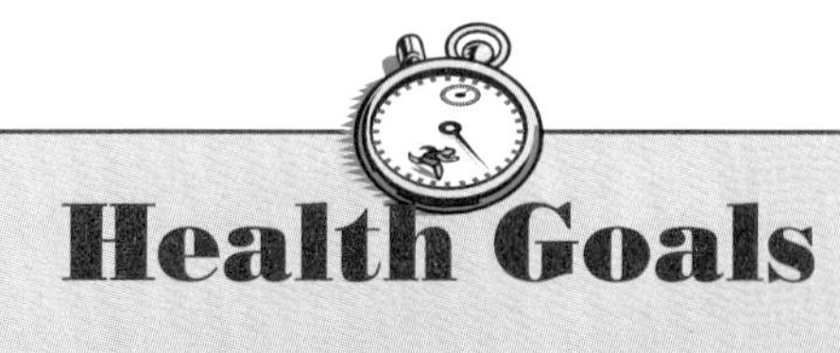

Health Goals

for year 2010

Increase quality and years of healthy life.

Eliminate health disparities.

Increase incidence of people reporting "healthy days."

Increase incidence of people reporting "active days."

Increase access to health information and services for all people.

A Statement about National Health Goals

At the beginning of each concept in this book is a section containing abbreviated statements of the new national health goals from the document *Healthy People 2010: National Health Promotion and Disease Prevention Objectives.* These statements, established by expert groups representing more than 350 national organizations, are intended as realistic national health goals to be achieved by the year 2010. These objectives for the first decade of the new millennium, are intended to improve the health of those in the United States, but they seem important for all people in North America and in other industrialized cultures throughout the world. The health objectives are designed to contribute to the current World Health Organization strategy of "Health for All." This book is written with the achievement of these important health goals in mind.

Introduction

www.mhhe.com/phys_fit/webreview01 Click 01

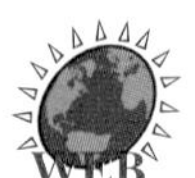

The first national health goals were developed in 1979 to be accomplished by the year 1990. The focus of those objectives was on reduction in the death rate among infants, children, adolescents, young adults, and adults. Except for reducing death rates among adolescents, those goals were met and the average life expectancy was increased by more than 2 years by the 1990s. Those first national health objectives gave way to the *Healthy People 2000* objectives designed to be accomplished by the turn of the century. The emphasis in these objectives shifted from reduction in premature death to disease prevention and health promotion. While many of these objectives have been achieved, others have yet to be accomplished.

For *Healthy People 2010,* achieving the vision of "healthy people in healthy communities" is paramount. Two central goals have been established. First, the goals emphasize quality of life, well-being, and functional capacity—all important wellness considerations. This emphasis is based on the World Health Organization statement that "It is counterproductive to evaluate development of programs without considering their impact on the quality of life of the community. We can no longer maintain strict, artificial divisions between physical and mental well-being (World Health Organization, 1995)." Second, the national health goals for 2010 take the "bold step" of trying to "eliminate" health disparities as opposed to reducing them. Consistent with national health goals for the new millennium, this book is designed to aid all people in adopting healthy lifestyles that will allow them to achieve lifetime health, fitness, and wellness.

The Facts about Health and Wellness

Good health is of primary importance to adults in our society.

When polled about important social values, 99 percent of adults in the United States identified "being in good **health**" as one of their major concerns. Two other concerns expressed most often were good family life and good self-image. The one percent who did not identify good health as an important concern had no opinion on any social issues. Among those polled, none felt that good health was unimportant. Results of surveys in Canada and other Western nations show similar commitments to good health.

Health varies greatly with income, gender, age, and family origin.

Reducing health disparities among adults over 18 is a major national health goal. We have some distance to go in accomplishing this goal because health varies widely depending on income, gender, age, and family origin. Self-ratings of health have been shown to be good general indicators of health status. When asked to rate health as excellent, good, fair, or poor, more than a few adults indicated that their health was only fair or poor (see Figure 1). It is evident that many more people in poor or near-poor income groups are considered to be fair or poor in health as opposed to good or excellent. African Americans and Hispanics are more often classified as fair or poor in health than white non-Hispanics. Minority women are also likely to be classified as fair or poor in health. Though not indicated in Figure 1, there is good evidence that older adults are especially likely to report poor health and wellness. An important national health goal is to increase the number of **healthy days** people have each month.

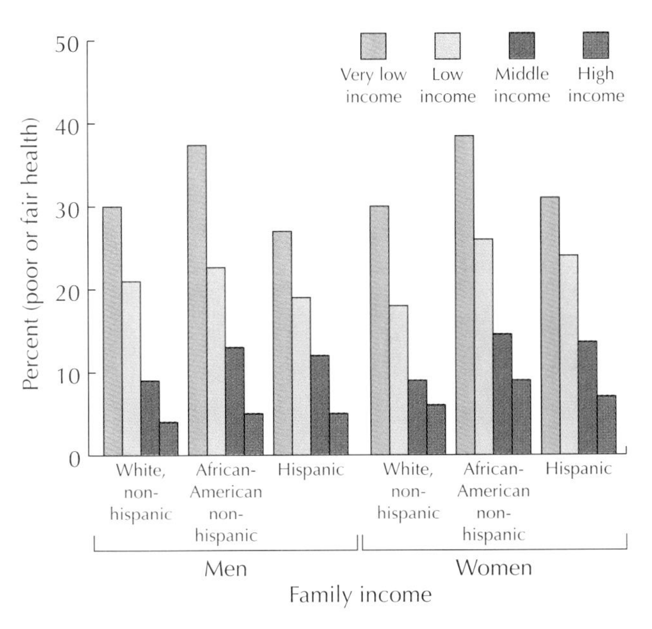

Figure 1

Fair or poor health among adults 18 and over by income, gender, and family origin.

Note: Percents are age adjusted.

Source: Centers for Disease Control and Prevention, National Center for Health Statistics, National Health Interview Survey. *Health United States, 1998.*

Increasing the span of healthy life is a principal health goal.

www.mhhe.com/phys_fit/webreview01 Click 02

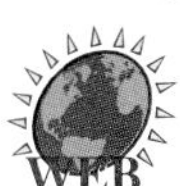

The principal public health goal of Western nations is to increase the healthy life span of all individuals. During this century, the life expectancy for the average person has increased by 60 percent. A child born in 1900 could expect to live only 47 years. By 1930, the life expectancy increased by more than 10 years. Currently, life expectancy is at a record high of nearly 77 years. As illustrated in Figure 2, women live longer than men, with the difference between men and women becoming more dramatic with each passing decade. Unfortunately, the average person can expect only about 64 years of healthy life. Approximately 12 years are characterized as dysfunctional or lacking in quality of life (see Figure 3). Disease and illness often associated with poor health limit length of life and contribute to the dysfunctional living.

Health is more than freedom from illness and disease.

Over 50 years ago, the World Health Organization defined *health* as being more than freedom from illness, disease, and debilitating conditions. In recent years, public health experts

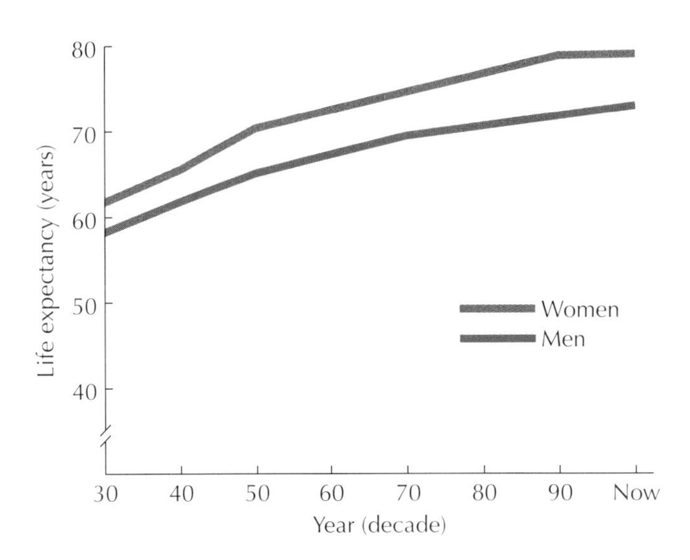

Figure 2

Life expectancy.

Source: National Center for Health Statistics.

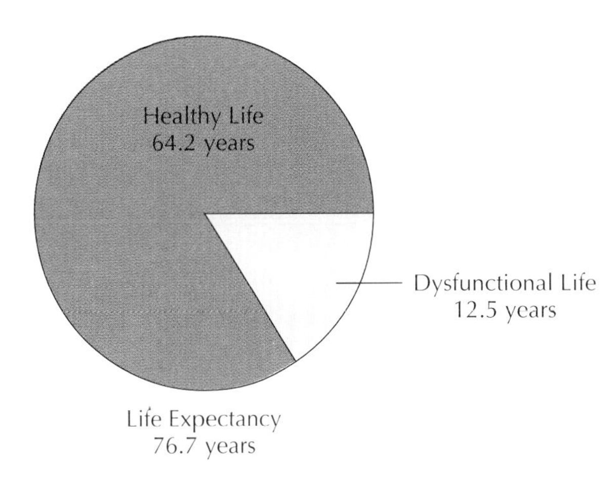

Figure 3

Years of healthy life as a proportion of life expectancy (U.S. population).

Source: Data from *National Vital Statistics System* and *National Health Interview Survey*. Centers for Disease Control and Prevention, Atlanta, GA.

Health Health is optimal well-being that contributes to quality of life. It is more than freedom from disease and illness, though freedom from disease is important to good health. Optimal health includes high-level mental, social, emotional, spiritual, and physical wellness within the limits of one's heredity and personal abilities.

Healthy Days A self-rating of the number of days (per week or month) a person considers himself or herself to be in good or better than good health.

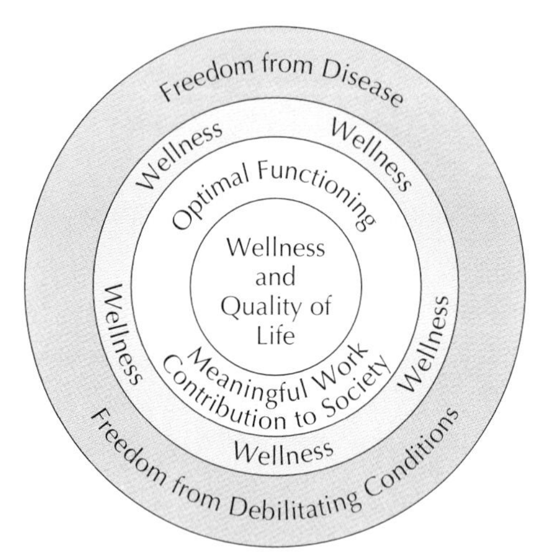

Figure 4
A model of optimal health including wellness.

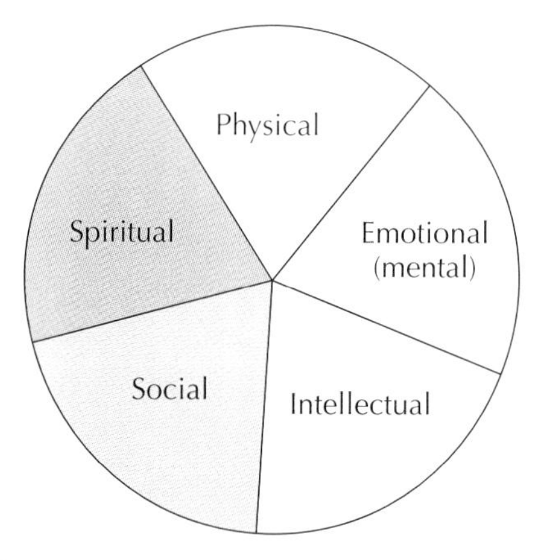

Figure 5
The dimensions of health and wellness.

have identified **wellness** as "a sense of well-being" and **"quality of life."** *Healthy People 2010* objectives use the number of **"activity days"** as one indicator of wellness.

Many illnesses are manageable and have only limited effect on total health.

Many **illnesses** are curable and may have only a temporary effect on health. Others, such as diabetes, are not curable but can be managed with proper eating, physical activity, and sound medical supervision. It should be noted that those possessing manageable conditions may be more at risk for other health problems, so proper management is essential. For example, unmanaged diabetes is associated with high risk for heart disease and other health problems.

Wellness is the positive component of optimal health.

Death, disease, illness, and debilitating conditions are negative components that detract from optimal health. Death is the ultimate opposite of optimal health. Disease, illness, and debilitating conditions obviously detract from optimal health. Wellness has been recognized as the positive component of optimal health as evidenced by a sense of well-being reflected in optimal functioning, a good quality of life, meaningful work, and a contribution to society (see Figure 4). Wellness allows the expansion of one's potential to live and work effectively and to make a significant contribution to society.

Health and wellness are multidimensional.

The dimensions of health and wellness include the emotional (mental), intellectual, physical, social, and spiritual. Figure 5 illustrates the importance of each dimension to total wellness. Throughout this book, references will be made to these wellness dimensions (see Table 1) to help reinforce their importance.

Wellness reflects how one feels about life as well as one's ability to function effectively.

A positive total outlook on life is essential to wellness and each of the wellness dimensions. A "well" person is satisfied in his/her work, is spiritually fulfilled, enjoys leisure time, is physically fit, is socially involved, and has a positive emotional-mental outlook. This person is happy and fulfilled. Many experts believe that a positive total outlook is a key to wellness (see Table 2).

The way one perceives each of the dimensions of wellness affects total outlook. Researchers use the term *self-perceptions* to describe these feelings. Many researchers believe that self-perceptions about wellness are more important than actual ability. For example, a person who has an important job may find less meaning and job satisfaction than another person with a much less important job. Apparently, one of the important factors for a person who has achieved high-level wellness and a positive life's outlook is the ability to reward himself/herself. Some people, however, seem unable to give themselves credit for their life's experiences. The development of a system that allows a person to positively perceive the self is important. Of course, the adoption of positive **lifestyles** that encourage improved self-perceptions is also important. The questionnaire in the Lab 1A will help you assess your self-perceptions of the various wellness dimensions. For optimal wellness, it would be important to find positive feelings about each dimension.

Table 1 Health and Wellness Definitions

Emotional health—A person with emotional health is (1) free from emotional-mental illnesses or debilitating conditions such as clinical depression and (2) possesses emotional wellness. The goals for the nation's health refer to mental rather than emotional health and wellness. In this book, mental health and wellness are considered to be the same as emotional health and wellness.

Emotional wellness—Emotional wellness is a person's ability to cope with daily circumstances and to deal with personal feelings in a positive, optimistic, and constructive manner. A person with emotional wellness is generally characterized as happy, as opposed to depressed.

Intellectual health—A person with intellectual health is free from illnesses that invade the brain and other systems that allow learning. A person with intellectual health also possesses intellectual wellness.

Intellectual wellness—Intellectual wellness is a person's ability to learn and to use information to enhance the quality of daily living and optimal functioning. A person with intellectual wellness is generally characterized as informed, as opposed to ignorant.

Physical health—A person with physical health is free from illnesses that affect the physiological systems of the body such as the heart, the nervous system, etc. A person with physical health possesses an adequate level of physical fitness and physical wellness.

Physical wellness—Physical wellness is a person's ability to function effectively in meeting the demands of the day's work and to use free time effectively. Physical wellness includes good physical fitness and the possession of useful motor skills. A person with physical wellness is generally characterized as fit versus unfit.

Social health—A person with social health is free from illnesses or conditions that severely limit functioning in society, including antisocial pathologies.

Social wellness—Social wellness is a person's ability to successfully interact with others and to establish meaningful relationships that enhance the quality of life for all people involved in the interaction (including self). A person with social wellness is generally characterized as involved as opposed to lonely.

Spiritual health—Spiritual health is the one component of health that is totally comprised of the wellness dimension; for this reason, spiritual health is considered to be synonymous with spiritual wellness.

Spiritual wellness—A person's ability to establish a values system and act on the system of beliefs, as well as to establish and carry out meaningful and constructive lifetime goals. Spiritual wellness is often based on a belief in a force greater than the individual that helps one contribute to an improved quality of life for all people. A person with spiritual wellness is generally characterized as fulfilled as opposed to unfulfilled.

Table 2 The Dimensions of Wellness

–	Wellness Dimensions	+
Depressed	Emotional-mental	Happy
Ignorant	Intellectual	Informed
Unfit	Physical	Fit
Lonely	Social	Involved
Unfulfilled	Spiritual	Fulfilled
Negative	Total outlook	Positive

Health and wellness are integrated states of being.

The segmented pictures of health and wellness shown in Figure 5 and Table 2 are used only to illustrate the multidimensional nature of health and wellness. In reality, health,

Wellness Wellness is the integration of many different components (mental, social, emotional, spiritual, and physical) that expand one's potential to live (quality of life) and work effectively and to make a significant contribution to society. Wellness reflects how one feels (a sense of well-being) about life as well as one's ability to function effectively. Wellness, as opposed to illness (a negative), is sometimes described as the positive component of good health.

Quality of Life A term used to describe wellness. An individual with quality of life can enjoyably do the activities of life with little or no limitation and can function independently. Individual quality of life requires a pleasant and supportive community.

Activity Days A self-rating of the number of days (per week or month) a person feels that he/she can perform usual daily activities successfully and in good health.

Illness Illness is the ill feeling and/or symptoms associated with a disease or circumstances that upset homeostasis.

Lifestyles Lifestyles are patterns of behavior or ways an individual typically lives.

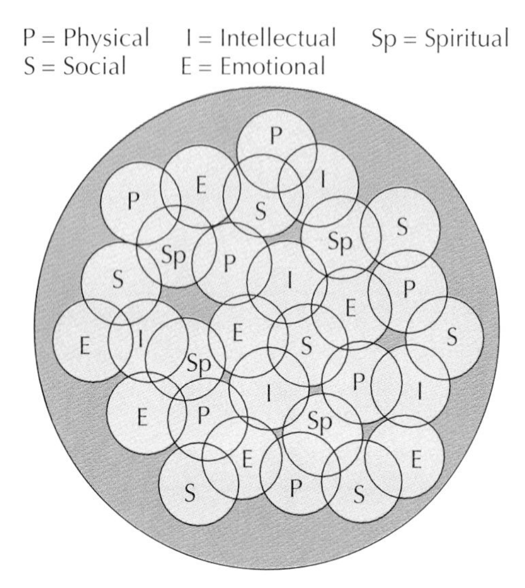

Figure 6
The integration of wellness dimensions.

and its positive component (wellness), is an integrated state of being that is best depicted as many threads that can be woven together to produce a larger, integrated fabric. Each specific dimension relates to each of the others and overlaps all others. The overlap is so frequent and so great that the specific contribution of each thread is almost indistinguishable when looking at the total (Figure 6). The total is clearly greater than the sum of the parts.

Health and wellness are individual in nature.

Each individual is different from all others. Health and wellness depend on each person's individual characteristics. Making comparisons to other people on specific individual characteristics may produce feelings of inadequacy that detract from one's profile of total health and wellness. Each of us has personal limitations and personal strengths. Focusing on strengths and learning to accommodate weaknesses are essential keys to optimal health and wellness.

It is possible to possess wellness while being ill or possessing a debilitating condition.

All people can benefit from enhanced wellness. Wellness and an improved quality of life are possible for everyone, regardless of disease states. Evidence is accumulating to indicate that people with a positive outlook are better able to resist the progress of disease and illness than those with a negative outlook. Thinking positive thoughts has been associated with enhanced results from various medical treatments and better results from surgical procedures.

Because self-perceptions are important to wellness, positive perceptions of self are especially important to the wellness

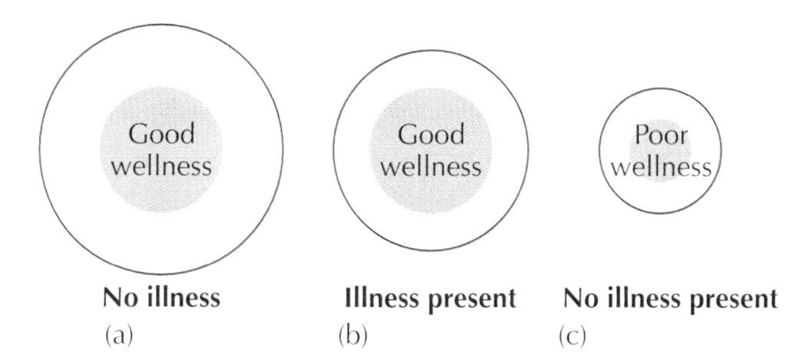

Figure 7
Wellness need not be limited by illness.

of people with disease, illness, and disability. The concepts of wellness and optimal health must be considered in light of one's heredity and personal disabilities and disease states.

Figure 7 illustrates the fact that the most desirable condition is buoyant health (*a*) including freedom from illness and a high level of wellness. However, a person with a physical illness but who possesses a good wellness (*b*) has a better overall health status than a person with no illness but poor wellness (*c*).

Wellness is a useful term that may be used by quacks as well as experts.

Unfortunately, some individuals and groups have tried to identify wellness with products and services that promise benefits that cannot be documented. Because "well-being" is a subjective feeling that is hard to document, it is easy for quacks to make claims of improved wellness for their product or service without facts to back them up.

Holistic health is a term that is similarly abused. Optimal health includes many areas, thus the term *holistic* (total) is appropriate. In fact, the word *health* originates from a root word meaning "wholeness." Unfortunately, many quacks include their questionable health practices under this guise of "holistic health." Care should be used when considering services and products that make claims of wellness and/or holistic health to be sure that they are legitimate.

Facts about Physical Fitness

Physical fitness is a multidimensional state of being.

Physical fitness is the body's ability to function efficiently and effectively. It is a state of being that consists of at least five health-related and six skill-related, physical fitness components, each of which contributes to total quality of life. Physical fitness is associated with a person's ability to work effectively, enjoy leisure time, be healthy, resist **hypokinetic diseases,** and meet emergency situations. It is related to, but

Table 3 Health-Related Physical Fitness Terms

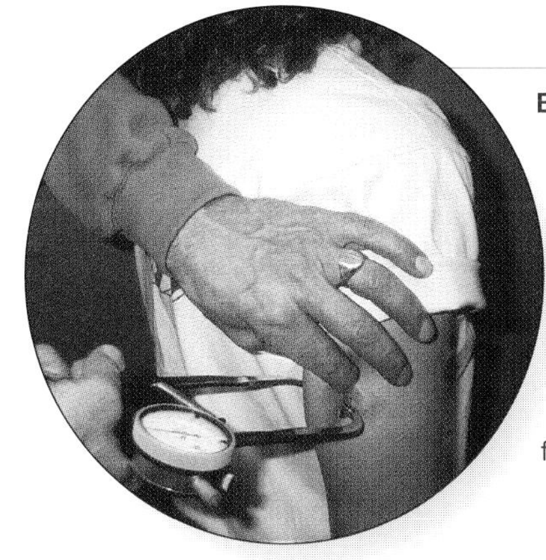

Body composition—The relative percentage of muscle, fat, bone, and other tissues that comprise the body. A fit person has a relatively low, but not too low, percentage of body fat (body fatness).

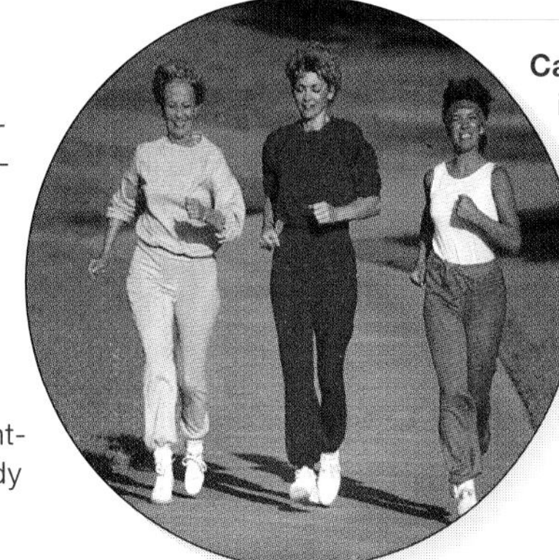

Cardiovascular fitness—The ability of the heart, blood vessels, blood, and respiratory system to supply fuel and oxygen to the muscles and the ability of the muscles to utilize fuel to allow sustained exercise. A fit person can persist in physical activity for relatively long periods without undue stress.

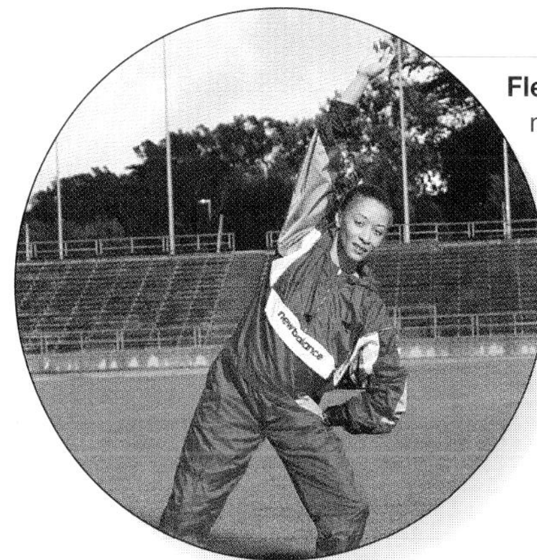

Flexibility—The range of motion available in a joint. It is affected by muscle length, joint structure, and other factors. A fit person can move the body joints through a full range of motion in work and in play.

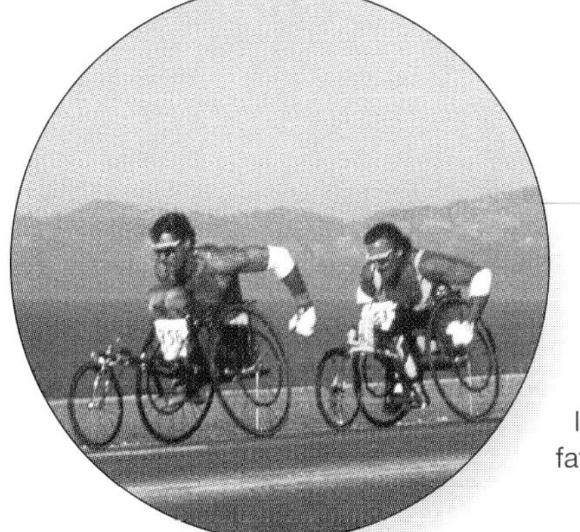

Muscular Endurance—The ability of the muscles to repeatedly exert themselves. A fit person can repeat movements for a long period without undue fatigue.

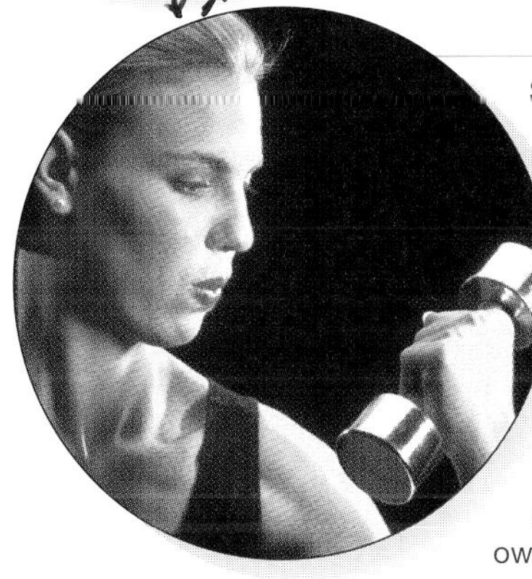

Strength—The ability of the muscles to exert an external force or to lift a heavy weight. A fit person can do work or play that involves exerting force, such as lifting or controlling one's own body weight.

different from, health and wellness. Although the development of physical fitness is the result of many things, optimal physical fitness is not possible without regular physical activity.

> The health-related components of physical fitness are directly associated with good health.

The five components of health-related physical fitness are body composition, cardiovascular fitness, flexibility, muscular endurance, and strength (see Table 3). Each health-related fitness characteristic has a direct relationship to good health and reduced risk of hypokinetic disease.

Physical Fitness Physical fitness is the body's ability to function efficiently and effectively. It consists of health-related physical fitness and skill-related physical fitness, which have at least 11 different components, each of which contributes to total quality of life. Physical fitness also includes metabolic fitness (see page 9). Physical fitness is associated with a person's ability to work effectively, enjoy leisure time, be healthy, resist hypokinetic diseases, and meet emergency situations. It is related to, but different from health, wellness, and the psychological, sociological, emotional, and spiritual components of fitness. Although the development of physical fitness is the result of many things, optimal physical fitness is not possible without regular exercise.

Hypokinetic Diseases or Conditions *Hypo-* means "under" or "too little," and *-kinetic* means "movement" or "activity." Thus, *hypokinetic* means "too little activity." A hypokinetic disease or condition is one associated with lack of physical activity or too little regular exercise. Examples of such conditions include heart disease, low back pain, adult-onset diabetes, and obesity.

Table 4 Skill-Related Physical Fitness Terms

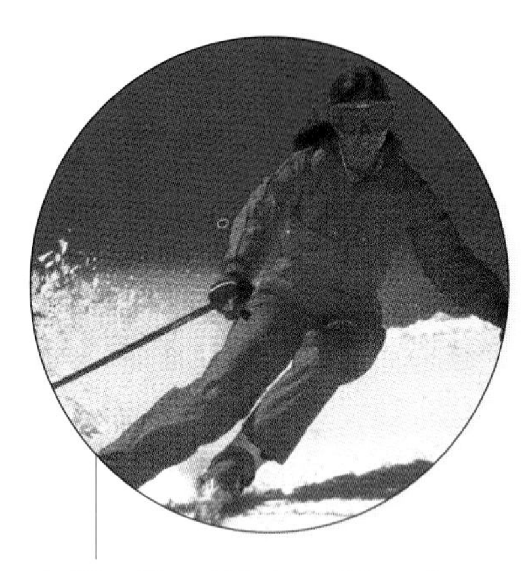

Agility—The ability to rapidly and accurately change the direction of the movement of the entire body in space. Skiing and wrestling are examples of activities that require exceptional agility.

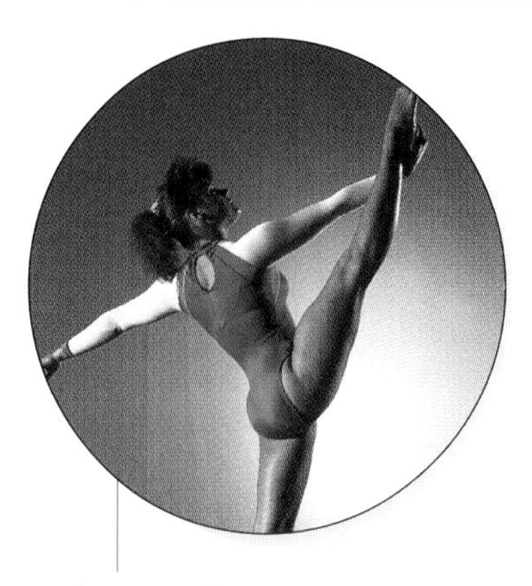

Balance—The maintenance of equilibrium while stationary or while moving. Water skiing, performing on the balance beam, or working as a riveter on a high-rise building are activities that require exceptional balance.

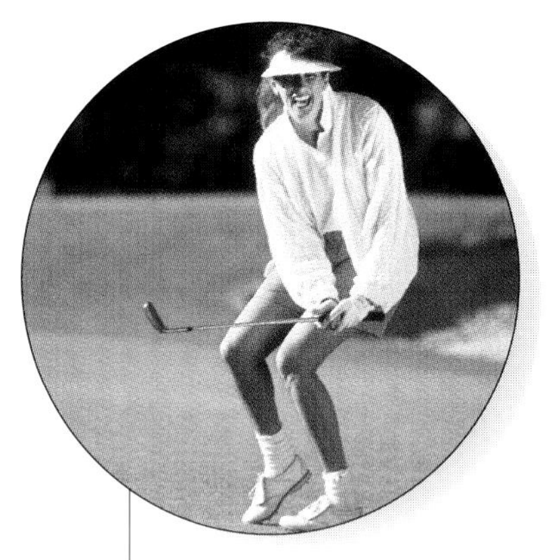

Coordination—The ability to use the senses with the body parts to perform motor tasks smoothly and accurately. Juggling, hitting a golf ball, batting a baseball, or kicking a ball are examples of activities requiring good coordination.

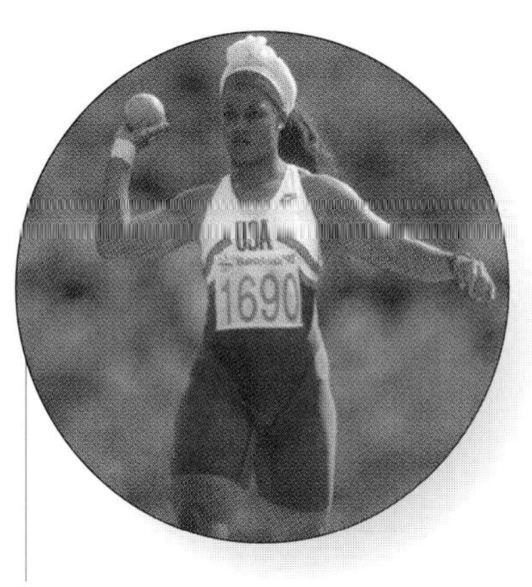

Power—The ability to transfer energy into force at a fast rate. Throwing the discus and putting the shot are activities that require considerable power.

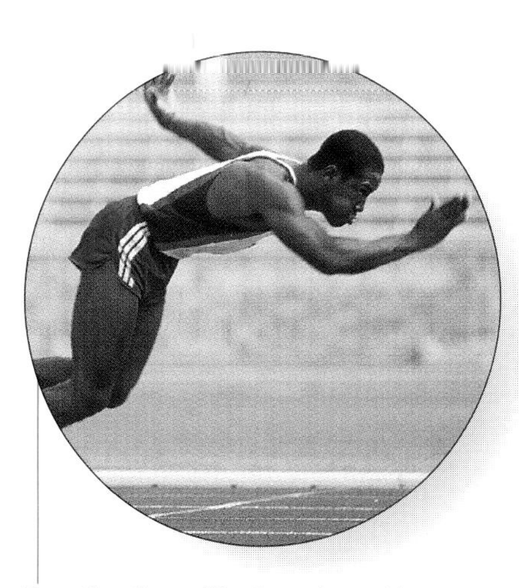

Reaction time—The time elapsed between stimulation and the beginning of reaction to that stimulation. Driving a racing car and starting a sprint race require good reaction time.

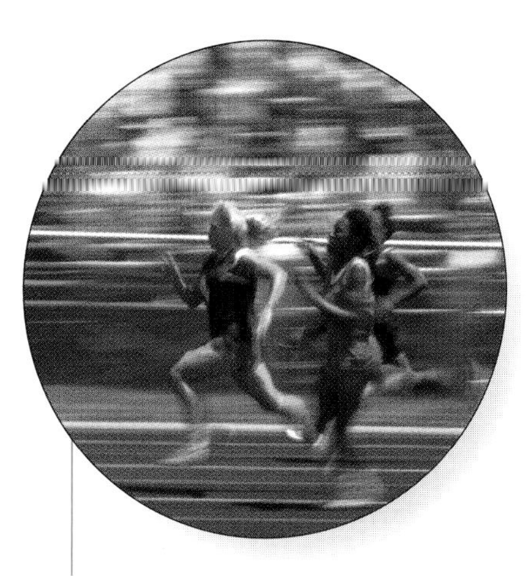

Speed—The ability to perform a movement in a short period of time. A runner on a track team or a wide receiver on a football team needs good foot and leg speed.

Possessing a moderate amount of each component of health-related fitness is essential to disease prevention and health promotion, but it is not essential to have exceptionally high levels of fitness to achieve health benefits. High levels of health-related fitness relate more to performance than health benefits. For example, moderate amounts of strength are necessary to prevent back and posture problems, whereas high levels of strength contribute most to improved performance in activities such as football and jobs involving heavy lifting.

> The skill-related components of physical fitness are more associated with performance than good health.

The components of skill-related physical fitness are agility, balance, coordination, power, reaction time, and speed (see Table 4). They are called skill-related because people who possess them find it easy to achieve high levels of performance in motor skills, such as those required in sports and in specific types of jobs. Skill-related fitness is sometimes called sports fitness or motor fitness.

There is little doubt that there are other abilities that could be classified as skill-related fitness components. Also, each part of skill-related fitness is multidimensional. For example, coordination could be hand-eye coordination such as batting a ball, foot-eye coordination such as kicking a ball, or any of many other possibilities. The six parts of skill-related fitness identified here are those that are commonly associated with successful sports and work performance. It should be noted that each could be measured in ways other than those presented in this book. Measurements are provided to help the reader understand the nature of total physical fitness and to help the reader make important decisions about lifetime physical activity.

Metabolic fitness is a nonperformance component of total fitness.

Research studies show that health benefits often occur even without dramatic improvements in traditional health-related physical fitness measures. **Metabolic fitness** is a state of being associated with lower risk of many chronic health problems, but not necessarily associated with high performance levels of health-related physical fitness. Examples of nonperformance indicators of reduced risk are lowered blood pressure, lowered fat levels in the blood, and better regulation of blood sugar. Moderate physical activity has been shown to enhance metabolic fitness. Conventional wisdom classifies body composition as a component of health-related physical fitness, but some consider it to be a part of metabolic fitness because it is a nonperformance measure, and it is highly related to nutrition as well as physical activity. You will learn how to assess your metabolic fitness in subsequent concepts.

Bone integrity is often considered to be a nonperformance measure of fitness.

Traditional definitions do not include **bone integrity** as a part of physical fitness, but some experts feel that it should be. Like metabolic fitness, bone integrity cannot be assessed with performance measures as can most health-related fitness parts. Regardless of whether it is considered as a part of fitness or a component of health, there is little doubt that strong, healthy bones are important to optimal health and are associated with regular physical activity and sound diet.

The many components of physical fitness are specific in nature, but are also interrelated.

Physical fitness is a combination of several aspects rather than a single characteristic. A fit person possesses at least adequate levels of each of the health-related, skill-related, and metabolic fitness components. People who possess one aspect of physical fitness do not necessarily possess the other aspects.

Some relationships exist among different fitness characteristics, but each of the components of physical fitness is separate and different from the others. For example, people who possess exceptional strength do not necessarily have good cardiovascular fitness, and those who have good coordination do not necessarily possess good flexibility. Lab 1B is designed to help you distinguish among the different parts of health-related and skill-related physical fitness. A separate questionnaire helps you estimate your current fitness levels.

Good physical fitness is important too, but it is not the same as physical health and wellness.

Good physical fitness contributes directly to the physical component of good health and wellness, and indirectly to the other four components. Good fitness has been shown to be associated with reduced risk of chronic diseases such as coronary heart disease and has been shown to reduce the

Metabolic Fitness Metabolic fitness is a positive state of the physiological systems commonly associated with reduced risk of chronic diseases such as diabetes and heart disease. Metabolic fitness is evidenced by healthy blood fat (lipid) profiles, healthy blood pressure, healthy blood sugar and insulin levels, and other nonperformance measures. This type of fitness shows positive responses to moderate physical activity.

Bone Integrity Soundness of the bones associated with high density and absence of symptoms of deterioration.

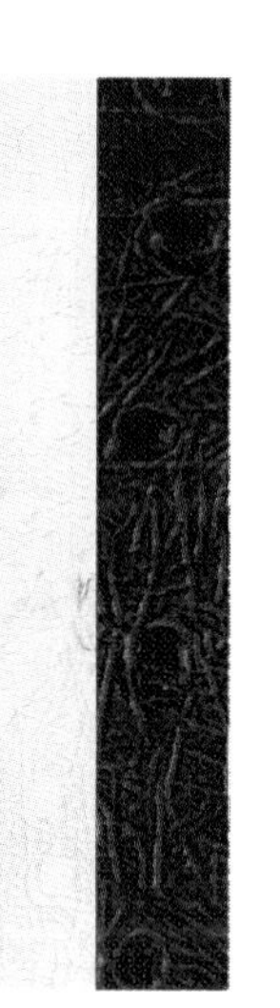

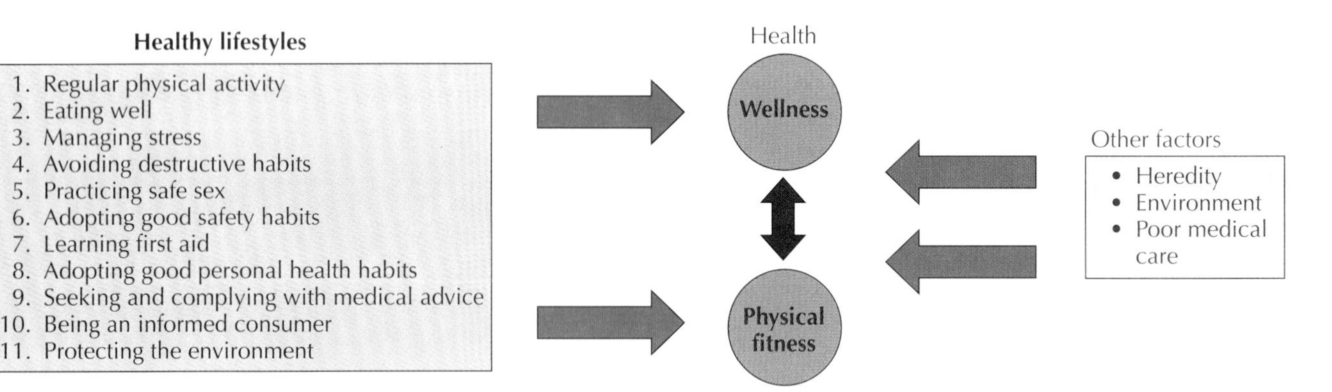

Figure 8
Factors influencing health, wellness, and physical fitness.

consequences of many debilitating conditions. In addition, good fitness contributes to wellness by helping us look our best, feel good, and enjoy life. Other physical factors can also influence health and wellness. For example, having good physical skills enhances quality of life by allowing us to participate in enjoyable activities such as tennis, golf, and bowling. While fitness can assist in performing these activities, regular practice is also necessary. Another example is the ability to fight off viral and bacterial infections. While fitness can promote a strong immune system, other physical factors can influence our susceptibility to these and other conditions.

For optimal health and wellness it is important to have good physical fitness *and* physical wellness. It is also important to strive for good emotional (mental), social, spiritual, and intellectual health and wellness.

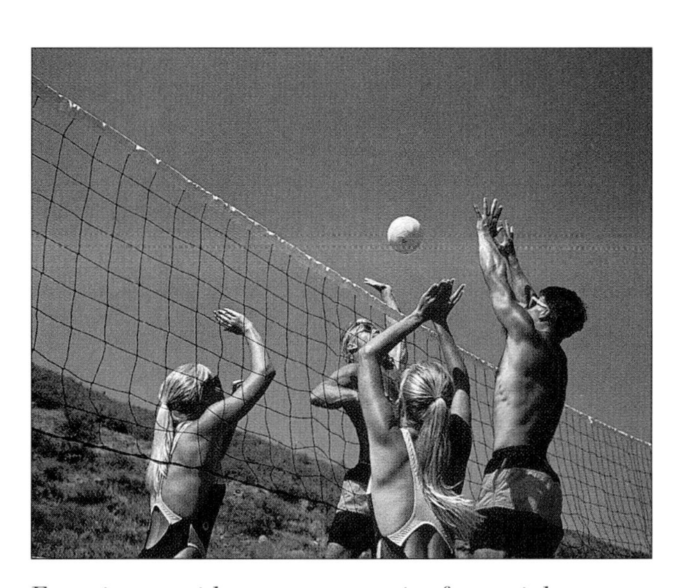

Exercise provides an opportunity for social involvement.

The Facts about Healthy Lifestyles

> Lifestyle change, more than any other factor, is considered to be the best way of preventing illness and early death in our society.

When people in Western society die before the age of 65, it is considered to be early or premature death. The most important factors contributing to early death are unhealthy lifestyles. Based on the "leading health indicators" in *Healthy People 2010,* eleven healthy lifestyles have been identified that are associated with reduced disease risk and increased wellness. As shown in Figure 8, these lifestyles affect health, wellness, and physical fitness. The double-headed arrow between health and wellness and physical fitness illustrate the interaction between these factors. Physical fitness is important to health and wellness development, and vice versa. Others factors, some not as much in your control as healthy lifestyles, also affect your health, fitness, and wellness. These factors include environmental factors (e.g., pollution, contaminants in the workplace), human biology (inherited conditions), and inadequacies in the health-care system, to name but a few.

Table 5 Major Causes of Death

1900 Rank	Cause	Current Rank	Cause
1.	Pneumonia	1.	Heart disease
2.	Tuberculosis	2.	Cancer
3.	Diarrhea/enteritis	3.	Stroke
4.	Heart disease	4.	Bronchitis/emphysema
5.	Stroke	5.	Injuries
6.	Liver disease	6.	Pneumonia/influenza
7.	Injuries	7.	Diabetes
8.	Cancer	8.	Suicide
9.	Senility	9.	Kidney disease
10.	Diphtheria	10.	Chronic liver disease

SOURCE: National Center for Health Statistics.

The major causes of early death have shifted from infectious diseases to chronic lifestyle-related conditions.

www.mhhe.com/phys_fit/webreview01 Click 03

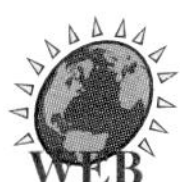

Scientific advances and improvements in medicine and health care have dramatically reduced the incidence of infectious diseases over the past 100 years (see Table 5). For example, new drugs have dramatically reduced deaths from pneumonia and influenza. Small pox, a major cause of death less than a century ago, was globally eradicated in 1977 because of the advent of immunizations. Other examples are the virtual elimination of diphtheria and polio in the United States and Canada.

As infectious diseases have been eliminated, other illnesses have replaced them as the leading causes of early death in Western culture. HIV/AIDS, formerly eighth on the list, has dropped from the top fifteen, not because of fewer new cases, but because of new treatments that increase length of life among those who are infected. Many among the top ten are referred to as chronic lifestyle-related conditions because alteration of lifestyles can result in reduced risk for these conditions.

Healthy lifestyles are critical to wellness.

Just as unhealthy lifestyles are the principal causes of modern-day illnesses such as heart disease, cancer, and diabetes, healthy lifestyles can result in an improved feeling of wellness that is critical to optimal health. In recognizing the importance of "years of healthy life," the Public Health Service also recognizes what it calls "measures of well-being." This well-being or wellness is associated with social, mental, spiritual, and physical functioning. Being physically active and eating well are two examples of healthy lifestyles that can improve well-being and add years of quality living. Many of the healthy lifestyles associated with good physical fitness and optimal wellness will be discussed in detail later in this book. The Healthy Lifestyle Questionnaire at the end if this concept gives you the opportunity to assess your current lifestyles.

Regular physical activity, sound nutrition, and stress management are considered to be priority healthy lifestyles.

Three of the healthy lifestyles listed in Figure 8 are considered to be priority healthy lifestyles. These are regular **physical activity (exercise)**, eating well, and managing stress. There are several reasons for placing priority on these lifestyles. First, they are behaviors that affect the lives of all people. Second, they are lifestyles in which large numbers of people can make improvement. Finally, modest changes in these behaviors can make dramatic improvements in individual and public health.

To be sure, the other healthy lifestyles listed in Figure 8 are important. For example people who use tobacco, abuse drugs (including alcohol), or practice unsafe sex can have immediate and dramatic health benefits by changing these behaviors. On the other hand, large segments of the population do not have problems in these areas. Obviously, these people cannot benefit from lifestyle changes in these areas. However, the majority of the population can benefit from

Exercise Exercise is defined as physical activity done for the purpose of getting physically fit.

Physical Activity Generally considered to be a broad term used to describe all forms of large muscle movements including sports, dance, games, work, lifestyle activities, and exercise for fitness. In this book, exercise and physical activity will often be used interchangeably to make reading less repetitive and more interesting.

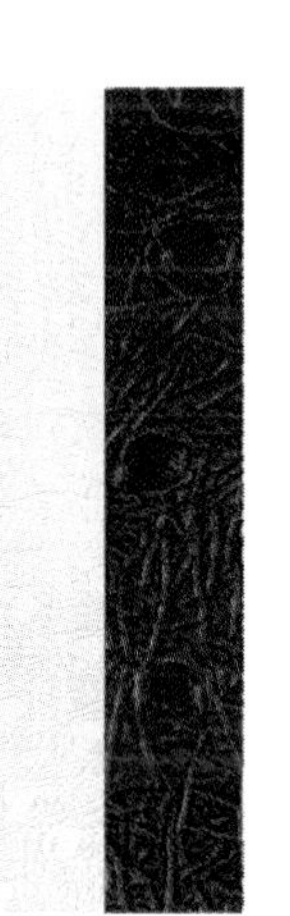

increasing their activity level, eating a better diet, and managing personal stress. For example, statistics suggest that modest changes in physical activity patterns and nutrition can prevent more than 200,000 premature deaths annually. Similarly, learning to manage stresses that all of us face on a daily basis can result in significant reductions in more than a few health problems. Stress has a major impact on drug, alcohol, and smoking behavior so managing stress can help individuals minimize or avoid these behaviors. Many healthy lifestyles will be discussed in this book, but the focus is on the priority healthy lifestyles because virtually all people can achieve positive wellness benefits if they adopt them.

The change in causes of illness and the new emphasis on fitness, wellness, and healthy lifestyles have resulted in a shift toward prevention and promotion.

Early medicine focused on treatment of disease. Physicians were scarce and were consulted only when illness occurred. A shift toward prevention began with advancements in medical science (e.g., immunizations, antibiotics) and the development of public health efforts (e.g., safe water supplies). Now more than at any other time in history, efforts are being made to promote healthy lifestyles that lead to fitness and wellness. In this text, the emphasis will be on strategies for preventing chronic diseases and promoting fitness and wellness.

The HELP Philosophy: The Facts

The HELP philosophy can provide a basis for making healthy lifestyle change possible.

The four-letter acronym illustrated in Table 6 provides a basis for a philosophy that has helped thousands of people adopt healthy lifestyles. Each letter in the word *HELP* characterizes an important part of the philosophy. The twenty-one concepts in this book are based on the *HELP* philosophy. The forty-two lab experiences are designed to help all people (everyone) to develop personal programs for lifetime health, fitness, and wellness.

Table 6 The HELP Philosophy

H	=	Health
E	=	Everyone
L	=	Lifetime
P	=	Personal

A personal philosophy that emphasizes **H**ealth can lead to behaviors that promote it.

The **H** in HELP stands for "health." One theory that has been extensively tested indicates that people who believe in the benefits of healthy lifestyles are more likely to engage in healthy behaviors. The theory also suggests that people who state intentions to put their beliefs in action are likely to adopt behaviors that lead to health, wellness, and fitness.

Everyone can benefit from healthy lifestyles.

The **E** in HELP stands for "everyone." Accepting the fact that anyone can change a behavior or lifestyle means that *YOU* are included. Nevertheless, many adults feel ineffective in making lifestyle changes. Physical activity is not just for athletes—it is for all people. Eating well is not just for other people—you can do it too. All people can learn stress-management techniques. Healthy lifestyles can be practiced by everyone. As noted earlier in this concept, important health goals include eliminating health disparities and promoting "Health for All."

Healthy behaviors are most effective when practiced for a **L**ifetime.

The **L** in HELP stands for "lifetime." Young people sometimes feel immortal because the harmful effects of unhealthy lifestyles are often not immediate. As we grow older, we begin to realize that we are not immortal and that unhealthy lifestyles have cumulative negative effects. Starting early in life to emphasize healthy behaviors results in long-term

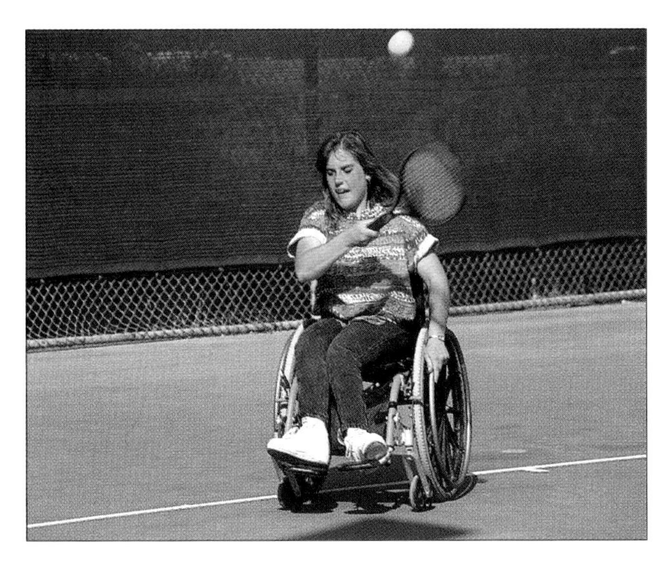

Physical activity is for everyone.

health, wellness, and fitness benefits. One recent study shows that the longer healthy lifestyles are practiced, the greater the beneficial effects. This study also demonstrated that long-term healthy lifestyles can even overcome hereditary predisposition to illness and disease.

Healthy lifestyles should be based on **P**ersonal needs.

The **P** in HELP stands for "personal." No two people are exactly alike. Just as there is no single pill that will cure all illnesses, there is no single lifestyle prescription for good health, wellness, and fitness. It is important for each person to assess personal needs and make lifestyle changes based on those needs.

Strategies for Action: The Facts

Self-assessments of lifestyles will help you determine areas in which you may need changes to promote optimal health, wellness, and fitness.

As you begin your study of health, wellness, fitness, and healthy lifestyles, it is wise to make a self-assessment of your current behaviors. The Healthy Lifestyle Questionnaire in the lab resource materials will allow you to assess your current lifestyle behaviors to determine if they are contributing positively to your health, wellness, and fitness. Because this questionnaire contains some very personal information, answering all questions honestly will help you get an accurate assessment. As you continue your study, you may want to refer back to this questionnaire to see if your lifestyles have changed.

Initial self-assessments of wellness and fitness will provide information for self-comparison.

www.mhhe.com/phys_fit/webreview01 Click 04

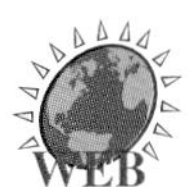

The Healthy Lifestyle Questionnaire allows you to assess your lifestyles or behaviors. It is also important to assess your wellness and fitness at an early stage. These early assessments will only be estimates. As you continue your study, you will have the opportunity to do more comprehensive self-assessments that will allow you to see how accurate your early estimates were.

In Lab 1A you will estimate your wellness using a Wellness Self-Perceptions Questionnaire, which assesses five wellness dimensions. Remember, wellness is a state of being that is influenced by healthy lifestyles. Because other factors such as heredity, environment, and health care affect wellness, it is possible to have good wellness scores even if you do not do well on the lifestyle questionnaire. However, over a lifetime, unhealthy lifestyles will catch up with you and have an influence on your wellness and fitness.

Lab 1B allows you to get a better understanding of the different components of health-related and skill-related physical fitness. You will perform some simple stunts to help you distinguish among the different fitness parts. You can use these as a basis for estimating your current fitness levels. Later, you will use more accurate tests to get a good assessment of your fitness. Like wellness, fitness is a state of being that is influenced by healthy lifestyles, especially regular physical activity. Young people sometimes have relatively good fitness—especially skill-related fitness—even if they have not been doing regular activity. Over a lifetime, inactivity greatly influences your fitness.

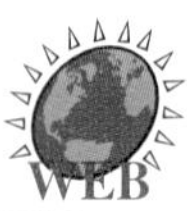

Web Review

Web review materials for Concept 1 are available at *www.mhhe.com/phys_fit/webreview01 Click 05.*

American Medical Association (AMA)
www.ama-assn.org

Centers for Disease Control and Prevention (CDC)
www.cdc.gov

Healthfinder
www.healthfinder.gov

Healthy People 2010
www.health.gov/healthypeople

Mayo Clinic Web Site
www.mayohealth.com

National Center for Chronic Disease Prevention and Health Promotion Publications
www.cdc.gov/nccdphp/publicat.htm

National Center for Health Statistics
www.cdc.gov/nchs/

WebMD.com
www.webMD.com

Suggested Readings

Armbruster, B., and Gladwin, L. A. "More than Fitness for Older Adults." A Whole-istic Approach to Wellness. *ACSM's Health and Fitness Journal.* 5(2)(2001): 6–10.

Blair, S. N. et al. *Active Living Every Day.* Champaign, IL: Human Kinetics, 2001.

Centers for Disease Control and Prevention. "Ten Great Public Health Accomplishments—United States." *Morbidity and Mortality Weekly Reports.* 48(12)(2000): 241–243. Also available at www.cdc.gov.

Corbin, C. B., and Pangrazi, R. P. (Editors), *Towards a Better Understanding of Physical Fitness and Activity.* Scottsdale, AZ: Holcomb-Hathaway, 1999.

Corbin, C. B., Pangrazi, R. P., and Franks, B. D. "Definitions: Health, Fitness, and Physical Activity." *President's Council on Physical Fitness and Sports Research Digest.* 3(9)(2000): 1–8. Also available at www.fitness.gov.

Payne, W. A., and Hahn, D. B. *Understanding Your Health.* (6th ed.) St. Louis: McGraw-Hill, 2000.

Spain, C. G., and Franks, B. D. "Healthy People 2010: Physical Activity and Fitness." *President's Council on Physical Fitness and Sports Research Digest.* 3(13)(2001):1–16.

USA Today/Gallup. "American Opinion in the 20th Century." *USA Today,* 31 December 1999, 11A and 29A.

U.S. Department of Health and Human Services. *Physical Activity and Health: A Report of the Surgeon General.* Atlanta: U.S. Department of Health and Human Services, 1996.

U.S. Department of Health and Human Services. *Healthy People 2010.* 2nd. ed. With *Understanding and Improving Health* and *Objectives for Improving Health.* 2 vols. Washington, DC: U.S. Government Printing Office, November 2000.

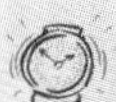

Physical Fitness News Update

Though many of us are appropriately concerned about problems associated with unhealthy lifestyles in our society, much progress has been made in the past century in regard to health, fitness, and wellness.

Good news from a national health agency

The Centers for Disease Control and Prevention recently identified ten great public health achievements for the 20th century. The achievements have greatly increased years of healthy living in our society. Included among the achievements are vaccinations, safer workplaces, safer and healthier foods, improved motor-vehicle safety, control of infectious diseases, decline in deaths from heart disease, family planning, recognition of tobacco use as a health hazard, healthier mothers and babies, and fluoridation of drinking water. These achievements are largely responsible for the increase in life expectancy and the improved quality of life over the last century.

Good news concerning public opinion

Recent public opinion polls indicate that most adults are optimistic about the future and satisfied with their current situation. Important findings include the following:

- Eighty-one percent of adults rate their personal health as good or excellent.
- More than 78 percent are satisfied with their standard of living.
- We work fewer hours than in 1900 (though there is an upward trend in work hours in recent years).
- We have more vacation time.
- Nearly 6 times more people graduate from high school.
- We enjoy many new conveniences (e.g., telephones, refrigerators, televisions, cars, computers).
- Nearly two times as many adults are satisfied with their income now as compared to 1948.
- The number of smokers is nearly half what it was in 1949.
- Over half of adults own home exercise equipment.
- The number of health and fitness clubs has increased by more than 100 percent since 1982.

The "good news" provides optimism that we can continue to make progress in meeting national health goals outlined in this book. We have placed a special emphasis on the *Healthy People 2010* vision of helping "each individual to make healthy lifestyle choices for themselves and their families."

Lab Resource Materials: The Healthy Lifestyle Questionnaire

The purpose of this questionnaire is to help you analyze your lifestyle behaviors and to help you in making decisions concerning good health and wellness for the future. Information on this Healthy Lifestyle Questionnaire is of a very personal nature. For this reason, this questionnaire is not designed to be submitted to your instructor. It is for your information only. Answer each question as honestly as possible and use the scoring information to help you assess your lifestyle.

Directions: Place an X over the "yes" circle to answer yes. If you answer "no," make no mark. Score the questionnaire using the procedures that follow.

yes	1. I accumulate 30 minutes of moderate physical activity most days of the week (brisk walking, climbing the stairs, yard work, or home chores).	17. I abstain from sex or limit sexual activity to a safe partner.	yes
yes	2. I do vigorous activity that elevates my heart rate for 20 minutes at least three days a week.	18. I practice safe procedures for avoiding STDs.	yes
yes	3. I do exercises for flexibility at least three days a week.	19. I use seat belts and adhere to the speed limit when I drive.	yes
yes	4. I do exercises for muscle fitness at least two days a week.	20. I have a smoke detector in my home and check it regularly to see that it is working.	yes
yes	5. I eat three regular meals each day.	21. I have had training to perform CPR if called on in an emergency.	yes
yes	6. I select appropriate servings from the food guide pyramid each day.	22. I can perform the Heimlich maneuver effectively if called on in an emergency.	yes
yes	7. I restrict the amount of fat in my diet.	23. I brush my teeth at least two times a day and floss at least once a day.	yes
yes	8. I consume only as many calories as I expend each day.	24. I get an adequate amount of sleep each night.	yes
yes	9. I am able to identify situations in daily life that cause stress.	25. I do regular self-exams, have regular medical check-ups, and seek medical advice when symptoms are present.	yes
yes	10. I take time out during the day to relax and recover from daily stress.	26. When I receive advice and/or medication from a physician, I follow the advice and take the medication as prescribed.	yes
yes	11. I find time for family, friends, and things I especially enjoy doing.	27. I read product labels and investigate their effectiveness before I buy them.	yes
yes	12. I regularly perform exercises designed to relieve tension.	28. I avoid using products that have not been shown by research to be effective.	yes
yes	13. I do not smoke or use other tobacco products.	29. I recycle paper, glass, or aluminum.	yes
yes	14. I do not abuse alcohol.	30. I practice environmental protection such as car pooling and conserving energy.	yes
yes	15. I do not abuse drugs (prescription or illegal).		
yes	16. I take over-the-counter drugs sparingly and use them only according to directions.	**Overall Score—Total Yes Answers**	

Scoring: Give yourself one point for each yes answer. Add your scores for each of the lifestyle behaviors. To calculate your overall score, sum the totals for all lifestyles.

Physical Activity		Nutrition		Managing Stress		Avoiding Destructive Habits		Practicing Safe Sex		Adopting Safety Habits
——— 1		——— 5		——— 9		——— 13		——— 17		——— 19
——— 2		——— 6		——— 10		——— 14		——— 18		——— 20
——— 3		——— 7		——— 11		——— 15				
——— 4		——— 8		——— 12		——— 16				
——— Total	+	——— Total	+	——— Total	+	——— Total	+	——— Total	+	——— Total +

Knowing First Aid		Personal Health Habits		Using Medical Advice		Being an Informed Consumer		Protecting the Environment		Sum All Totals for Overall Score
——— 21		——— 23		——— 25		——— 27		——— 29		
——— 22		——— 24		——— 26		——— 28		——— 30		
——— Total	+	——— Total	+	——— Total	+	——— Total	+	——— Total	=	[ ]

Interpreting Scores: Scores of 3 or 4 on the four-item scales are indicative of generally positive lifestyles. For the two-item scales, a score of 2 would indicate the presence of positive lifestyles. An overall score of 26 or more would be a good indicator of healthy lifestyle behaviors. It is important to consider the following special note when interpreting scores.

Special Note: Your scores on the Healthy Lifestyle Questionnaire should be interpreted with caution. There are several reasons for this. First, all lifestyle behaviors do not pose the same risks. For example, using tobacco or abusing drugs has immediate negative affects on health and wellness, while others, such as knowing first aid, may have only occasional use. Second, you may score well on one item in a scale, but not on another. If one item indicates an unhealthy lifestyle in an area that poses a serious health risk, your lifestyle may appear to be healthier than it really is. For example, you could get a score of 3 on the destructive habits scale and be a regular smoker. For this reason, the overall score can be particularly deceiving.

Strategies for Change: In the space below, you may want to make some notes concerning the healthy lifestyle areas in which you could make some changes. You can refer to these notes later to see if you have made progress.

Lab 1A: Wellness Self-Perception

Name	Section	Date

Purpose: To assess self-perceptions of wellness.

Procedures:

1. Place an X over the appropriate circle for each question (4 = strongly agree, 3 = agree, 2 = disagree, 1 = strongly disagree).
2. Write the number found in that circle in the box to the right.
3. Sum the three boxes for each wellness dimension to get your wellness dimension totals.
4. Sum all wellness dimension totals to get your comprehensive wellness total.
5. Use the rating chart to rate each wellness area.
6. Complete the Results and Conclusions and Implications sections.

Question	Strongly Agree	Agree	Disagree	Strongly Disagree	Score
1. I am happy most of the time.	4	3	2	1	
2. I have good self-esteem.	4	3	2	1	
3. I do not generally feel stressed.	4	3	2	1	
		Emotional Wellness Total		=	
4. I am well informed about current events.	4	3	2	1	
5. I am comfortable expressing my views and opinions.	4	3	2	1	
6. I am interested in my career development.	4	3	2	1	
		Intellectual Wellness Total		=	
7. I am physically fit.	4	3	2	1	
8. I am able to perform the physical tasks of my work.	4	3	2	1	
9. I am physically able to perform leisure activities.	4	3	2	1	
		Physical Wellness Total		=	
10. I have many friends and am involved socially.	4	3	2	1	
11. I have close ties with my family.	4	3	2	1	
12. I am confident in social situations.	4	3	2	1	
		Social Wellness Total		=	
13. I am fulfilled spiritually.	4	3	2	1	
14. I feel connected to the world around me.	4	3	2	1	
15. I have a sense of purpose in my life.	4	3	2	1	
		Spiritual Wellness Total		=	
		Comprehensive Wellness (Sum of 5 wellness scores)			

Wellness Rating Chart:

Rating	Wellness Dimension Scores	Comprehensive Wellness Score
High-level wellness	10–12	50–60
Good wellness	8–9	40–49
Marginal wellness	6–7	30–39
Low wellness	below 6	below 30

Results:

Wellness Dimension	Score	Rating
Emotional		
Intellectual		
Physical		
Social		
Spiritual		
Comprehensive		

Conclusions and Implications: In the space provided below, use several paragraphs to describe your current state of wellness. Do you think the ratings are indicative of your true state of wellness? Are there areas in which there is room for improvement?

Concept 2

Using Self-Management Skills to Adhere to Healthy Lifestyle Behaviors

Learning and regularly using self-management skills can help you to adopt and maintain healthy lifestyles throughout life.

Prochaska, J. O., and Markus, B. H. "The Transtheoretical Model: Applications to Exercise." In *Advances in Exercise Adherence*, Dishman, R. K. (ed.). Champaign, IL: Human Kinetics (1994).

Roberts, G. *Advances in Motivation in Sport and Exercise*. Champaign, IL: Human Kinetics, 2001.

Rosenstock, I. M. *The Health Belief Model: Explaining Health Behavior Through Expectancies*. In Glantz, K., Lewis, F. M., and Riner, B. K. *Health Behavior and Education*. San Francisco: Jossey-Bass, 1990.

Sallis, J. F. "Influences of Physical Activity on Children, Adolescents, and Adults or Determinants of Physical Activity." In Corbin, C. B., and Pangrazi, R. P. (eds.), *Towards a Better Understanding of Physical Fitness and Activity*. Scottsdale, AZ: Holcomb-Hathaway, 1999, Chapter 4.

Sallis, J. F., and Owen N. "Determinants of Physical Activity." Chap. 7 in *Physical Activity and Behavioral Medicine*. Thousand Oaks, CA: Sage, 1999.

Surgeon General's Office. *Surgeon General's Report on Physical Activity and Health*. Washington D.C.: U.S. Government Printing Office, 1996, Chapter 6.

Welk, G. J. "The Youth Physical Activity Promotion Model: A Conceptual Bridge Between Theory and Practice." *Quest*. 51 (1999):5–23.

Whitehead, J. R. "Physical Activity and Intrinsic Motivation." In Corbin, C. B., and Pangrazi, R. P. (eds.), *Towards a Better Understanding of Physical Fitness and Activity*. Scottsdale, AZ: Holcomb-Hathaway, 1999, Chapter 5.

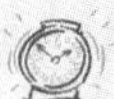

Physical Fitness News Update

Balancing your feelings about physical activity and other healthy lifestyle behaviors is important to lifetime adherence. As part of its new guidelines for exercise testing and prescription, The American College of Sports Medicine uses a scale to illustrate how more negative than positive factors results in poor adherence (see Figure 3). Many of the predisposing, enabling, and reinforcing factors described previously in this concept are included in this illustration. Ideally, a person would have more positive than negative factors, resulting in good adherence. You will have an opportunity to learn about your own personal feelings about physical activity (lab 2A) and how the factors balance for you (lab 5A).

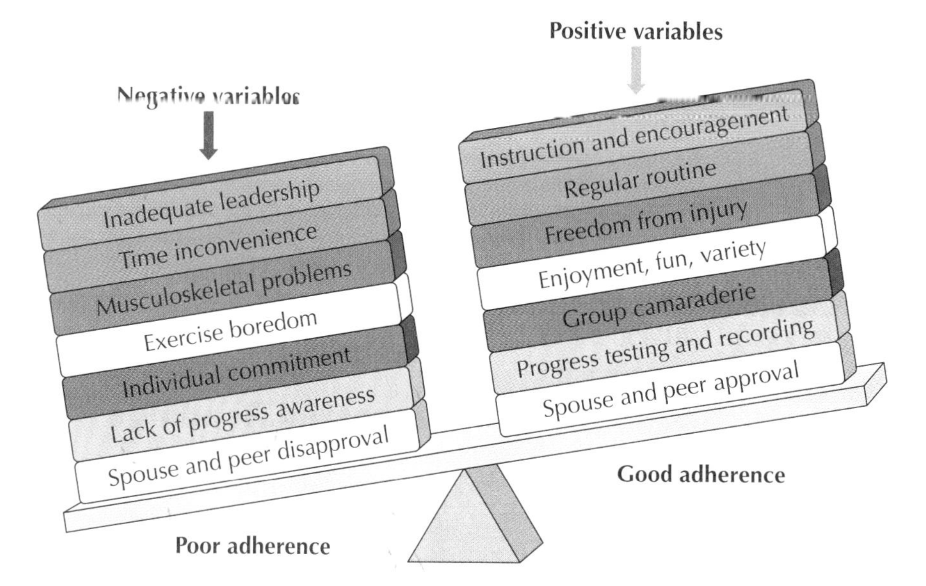

Figure 3

Factors affecting adherence to physical activity participation.

SOURCE: Adapted from American College of Sports Medicine. "Methods for Changing Exercise Behaviors." Chap. 12 in *ACSM's Guidelines for Exercise Testing and Prescription*. 6th ed. Philadelphia, PA: Lippincott, Williams, and Wilkins, 2000.

Table 5 Theories and Models Associated with Healthy Lifestyle Adoption

Theory	Brief Description
Transtheoretical model	This model is also referred to as the stages of change model. As described earlier in this concept, this model suggests five stages of change that characterize various health behaviors. The model suggests that doing the correct things (processes) at the right time (stage of change) is important to self-change in health behaviors.
Health beliefs model	This model suggests that a person's health behavior is related to the following five factors: the belief that a health problem will have harmful effects, the belief that a person is susceptible to the problem, the perceived benefits of changing a lifestyle to prevent the problem, the perceived barriers to overcoming the problem, and the confidence that he/she can do what is necessary to prevent it.
Social cognitive theory	Social cognitive theory is also referred to as social learning theory. Central to this theory are self-efficacy and positive expectations about behavior change. Also, the theory suggests that a person must value the outcomes of a behavior if he or she is likely to do that behavior.
Theory of reasoned action	This theory suggests that a person's behavior is most associated with the person's intention to do the behavior. The two factors most likely to influence a person's intentions are attitudes (beliefs) and the social environment (opinions of others).
Theory of planned behavior	This theory is often combined with the theory for reasoned action. It has the same basic tenets but adds the concept of "perceived control" over the environment. The person must believe that he or she has some control over the factors that allow performance of that behavior. Perceived control is in many ways similar to self-efficacy in social cognitive theory.
Self-determination theory	Central to self-determination theory is the importance of choice in a person's life (autonomy). Perceptions of competence at mastering life's tasks are also critical to the theory. Making personal choices in attempt to master the tasks of daily living are emphasized rather than making choices based on external pressures to comply. Self-determination theory, and its subtheory cognitive evaluation theory, emphasize intrinsic motivation. The intrinsic motivation inherent in behaviors that are exciting and/or fulfilling to do, is very important in making activity choices.

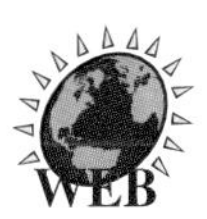

Web Review

Web review materials for Concept 2 are available at *www.mhhe.com/phys_fit/webreview02 Click 04.*

ACSM's Health and Fitness Journal

www.acsm-healthfitness.org

Journal of Sport and Exercise Psychology

www.humankinetics.com/products/journals/journal.cfm?id=JSEP

Medicine and Science in Sports and Exercise

www.acsm-msse.org

The Sport Psychologist

www.humankinetics.com/products/journals/journal.cfm?id=TSP

Suggested Readings

American College of Sports Medicine. "Methods for Changing Exercise Behaviors." In *ACSM's Guidelines for Exercise Testing and Prescription.* 6th ed. Philadelphia: Lippincott, Williams, and Wilkins, 2000, Chapter 12.

Bandura, A. *Social Foundations of Thought and Action: A Social-Cognitive Theory.* Englewood Cliffs, NJ: Prentice-Hall, 1986.

Duda, J. L. (ed.) *Advances in Sport and Exercise Psychology Measurement.* Morgantown, WV: Fitness Information Technology Inc., 1998.

Epstein, L. H., and Roemmich, J. N. "Reducing Sedentary Behavior: Role in Modifying Physical Activity." *Exercise and Sport Sciences Reviews.* 29(3)(2001):103–108.

Gill, D. L. *Psychological Dynamics of Sport and Exercise.* 2nd ed. Champaign, IL: Human Kinetics, 2000.

Haussenblas, H. A. et al. "Applications of the Theories of Reasoned Action and Planned Behaviors: A Meta Analysis." *The Journal of Sport and Exercise Psychology.* 19 (1997): 36.

McAuley, E., and Blissmer, B. "Self-Efficacy Determinants and Consequences of Physical Activity." *Exercise and Sport Sciences Reviews.* 28 (2000): 85–88.

Prochaska, J. O. "Strong and Weak Principles for Progressing From Precontemplation to Action on the Basis of Twelve Problem Behaviors." *Health Psychology.* 13 (1994): 47–51.

Prochaska, J. O., and Markus, B. H. "The Transtheoretical Model: Applications to Exercise." In *Advances in Exercise Adherence,* Dishman, R. K. (ed.). Champaign, IL: Human Kinetics (1994).

Roberts, G. *Advances in Motivation in Sport and Exercise.* Champaign, IL: Human Kinetics, 2001.

Rosenstock, I. M. *The Health Belief Model: Explaining Health Behavior Through Expectancies.* In Glantz, K., Lewis, F. M., and Riner, B. K. *Health Behavior and Education.* San Francisco: Jossey–Bass, 1990.

Sallis, J. F. "Influences of Physical Activity on Children, Adolescents, and Adults or Determinants of Physical Activity." In Corbin, C. B., and Pangrazi, R. P. (eds.), *Towards a Better Understanding of Physical Fitness and Activity.* Scottsdale, AZ: Holcomb-Hathaway, 1999, Chapter 4.

Sallis, J. F., and Owen N. "Determinants of Physical Activity." Chap. 7 in *Physical Activity and Behavioral Medicine.* Thousand Oaks, CA: Sage, 1999.

Surgeon General's Office. *Surgeon General's Report on Physical Activity and Health.* Washington D.C.: U.S. Government Printing Office, 1996, Chapter 6.

Welk, G. J. "The Youth Physical Activity Promotion Model: A Conceptual Bridge Between Theory and Practice." *Quest.* 51 (1999):5–23.

Whitehead, J. R. "Physical Activity and Intrinsic Motivation." In Corbin, C. B., and Pangrazi, R. P. (eds.), *Towards a Better Understanding of Physical Fitness and Activity.* Scottsdale, AZ: Holcomb-Hathaway, 1999, Chapter 5.

Physical Fitness News Update

Balancing your feelings about physical activity and other healthy lifestyle behaviors is important to lifetime adherence. As part of its new guidelines for exercise testing and prescription, The American College of Sports Medicine uses a scale to illustrate how more negative than positive factors results in poor adherence (see Figure 3). Many of the predisposing, enabling, and reinforcing factors described previously in this concept are included in this illustration. Ideally, a person would have more positive than negative factors, resulting in good adherence. You will have an opportunity to learn about your own personal feelings about physical activity (lab 2A) and how the factors balance for you (lab 5A).

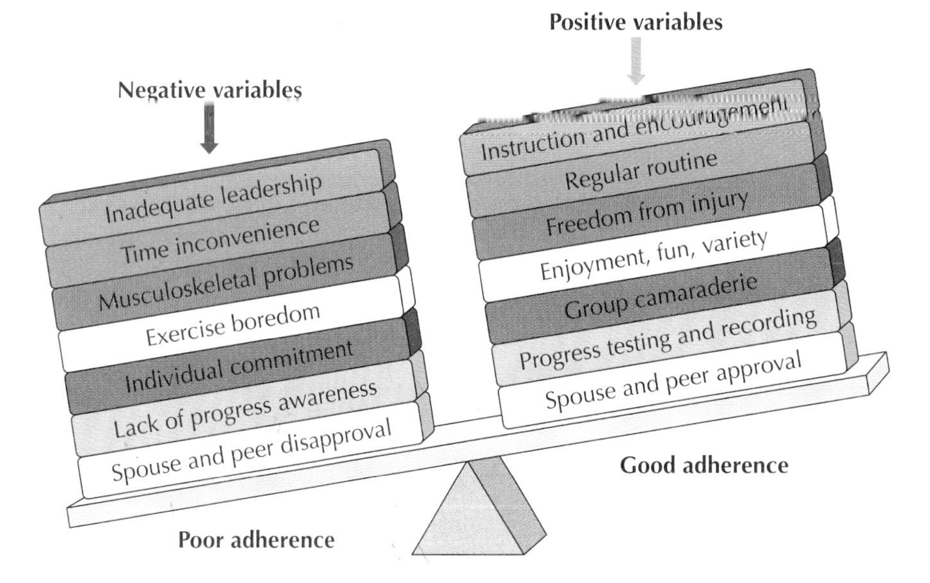

Figure 3

Factors affecting adherence to physical activity participation.

SOURCE: Adapted from American College of Sports Medicine. "Methods for Changing Exercise Behaviors." Chap. 12 in *ACSM's Guidelines for Exercise Testing and Prescription.* 6th ed. Philadelphia, PA: Lippincott, Williams, and Wilkins, 2000.

Section II

An Introduction to Physical Activity

Concept 3

Preparing for Physical Activity

Proper preparation can help make physical activity enjoyable, effective, and safe.

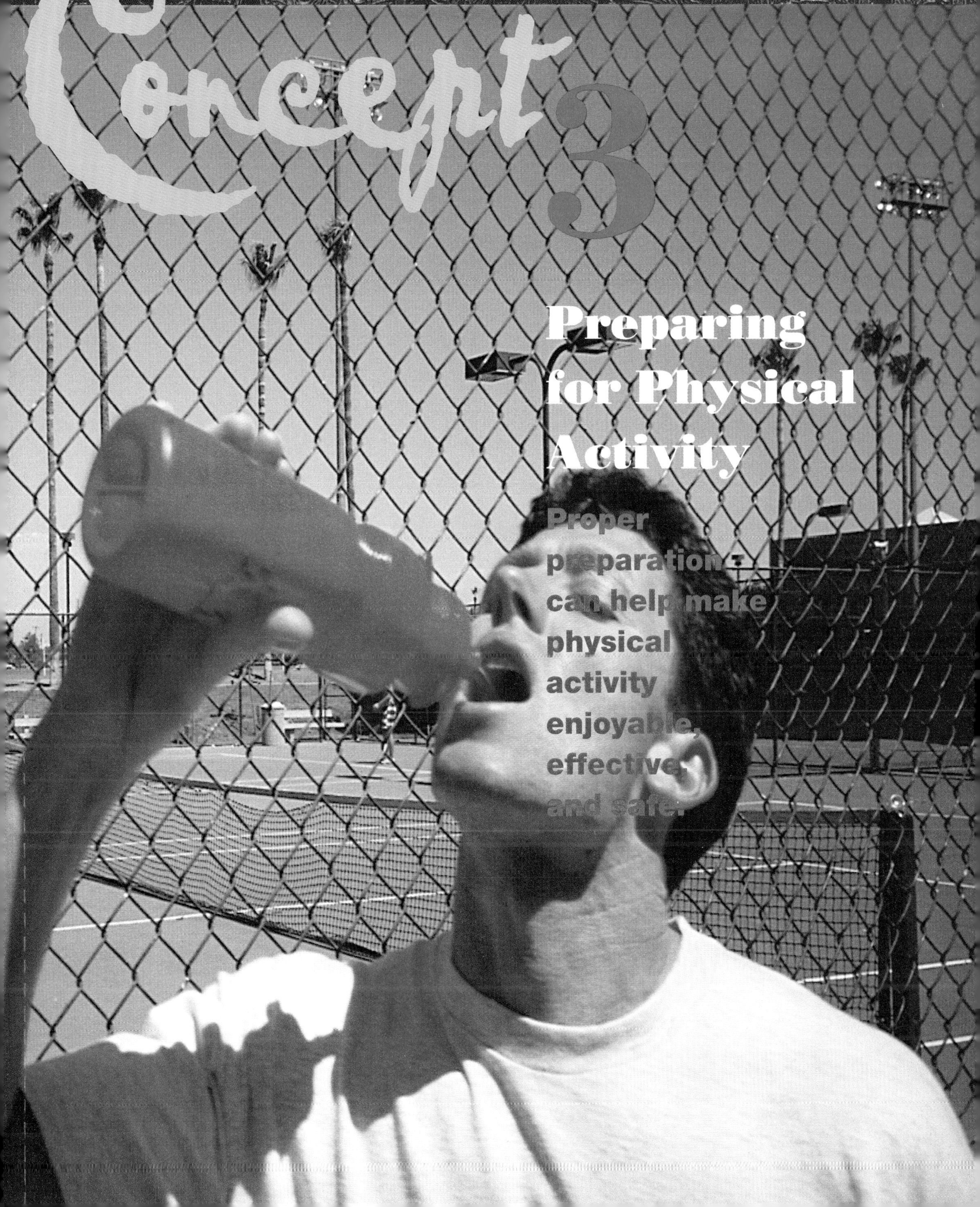

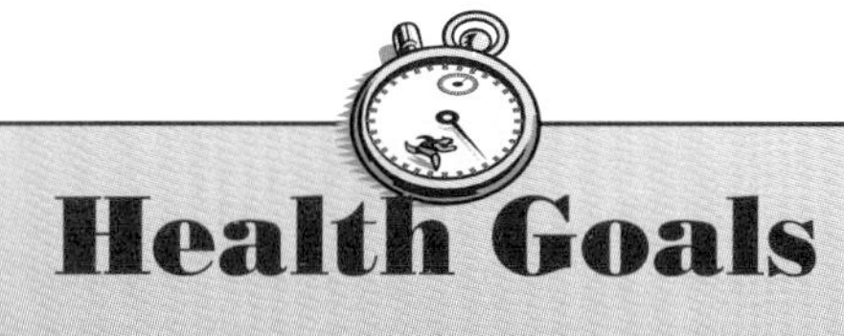

Health Goals

for year 2010

Improve the health, fitness, and quality of life of all people through the adoption and maintenance of regular, daily physical activity.

Increase leisure time physical activity.

Introduction

For people just beginning a physical activity program, adequate preparation may be the key to persistence. For those who have been regularly active for some time, sound preparation can help reduce risk of injury and make activity more enjoyable. It is hoped that a person armed with good information about preparation will become involved and stay involved in physical activity for a lifetime. For long-term maintenance, physical activity must be something that is a part of a person's normal lifestyle. Some facts that will help you prepare for and make physical activity a part of your normal routine are presented in this concept.

The Facts to Consider before Beginning Physical Activity

> Before beginning a regular physical activity program, it is important to establish your medical readiness to participate.

Physical activity requires the cardiovascular system to work harder. While this level of stress can promote positive adaptations, the stress on the heart can be unsafe and dangerous for certain individuals. The British Columbia (Canada) Ministry of Health conducted extensive research to devise a procedure that would help people know when it was advisable to seek medical consultation prior to beginning or altering an exercise program. The goal was to prevent unnecessary medical examinations, while at the same time helping people to be reasonably assured that regular exercise was appropriate. The research resulted in the development of the Physical Activity Readiness Questionnaire (**PAR-Q**). The most recent revision of the PAR-Q consists of seven simple questions you can ask yourself to determine if medical consultation is necessary prior to exercise involvement.

The American College of Sports Medicine (ACSM) has developed additional guidelines to help determine if medical consultation or if a **clinical exercise test** is necessary prior to participation in physical activity programs. The ACSM divides people into three general categories (see Table 1). Apparently healthy young adults classified with low risk and who give no yes answers to the PAR-Q are generally cleared for moderate and vigorous physical activity without a medical exam or clinical exercise testing. For those with moderate risk, moderate exercise is generally appropriate without a medical exam or an exercise test, but both are recommended prior to undertaking vigorous physical activity. For those in the high risk category, both a medical exam and exercise testing is recommended for both moderate and vigorous activity. When resuming physical activity after an injury or illness, consultation with a physician is always wise no matter what your age or medical condition.

There is no way to be absolutely sure that you are medically sound to begin a physical activity program. Even a thorough exam by a physician cannot guarantee that a person does not have some limitations that may cause a problem

Table 1 American College of Sports Medicine Risk Stratification Categories and Criteria

Stratification Category	Criteria
Low Risk	Younger people (less than 45 for men and 55 for women) are considered at low risk when they have no heart disease symptoms and have no more than one of the risk factors listed below.
Moderate Risk	People without heart disease symptoms but who are older (men 45 or more and women 55 and older) OR who have two or more of the risk factors listed below.
High Risk	People with one or more of the signs or symptoms listed below OR who have known cardiovascular, pulmonary, or metabolic disease.

Risk Factors

Family history of heart disease; smoker; high blood pressure (hypertension); high cholesterol; abnormal blood glucose levels; obesity (BMI of >30 or waist girth of >100 cm); sedentary lifestyle, low HDL cholesterol level.

Signs and Symptoms

Chest, neck, or jaw pain from lack of oxygen to the heart; shortness of breath at rest or in mild exercise; dizziness or fainting; difficult or labored breathing when lying, sitting, or standing; ankle swelling; fast heart beat or heart palpitations; pain in the legs from poor circulation; heart murmur; unusual fatigue or shortness of breath with usual activities.

SOURCE: Adapted from ACSM's Guidelines for Exercise Testing and Prescription, 2000. For more information on risk factors or signs and symptoms, consult this Suggested Reading.

during exercise. Use of the PAR-Q and adherence to the ACSM guidelines are advised to help minimize the risk while preventing unnecessary medical cost. However, if there is any doubt about your readiness for activity, a medical exam and a clinical exercise test are the surest ways to make certain that you are ready to participate.

Those who plan to do intensive training (particularly for sports) may want to answer some additional questions concerning whether a medical exam is necessary before beginning (see Lab 3A).

It is important to dress properly for physical activity.

The clothing you wear for exercise should be specifically for that exercise. It should be comfortable and not too tight or binding at the joints. Though appearance is important to everyone, comfort in exercise is more important than looks. Clothing should not restrict movement in any way. Preferably, the clothing that comes in direct contact with the body should be porous to allow for sweat evaporation. Some fabrics (e.g., Gortex) allow heat loss and sweat evaporation while protecting against wind and rain. Some women, especially those who need extra support, should consider using an exercise bra, and men may benefit from an athletic supporter. A warm-up suit over other exercise apparel is recommended because it can be removed during exercise if desired. Some exercise apparel marketed to promote weight loss resulting from increased sweating can be dangerous. Suits that are nonporous and trap sweat inside preventing the cooling effect that results from the normal evaporation of sweat should not be worn.

Absorbent socks that fit properly should be worn during exercise. Socks that are too short can cause ingrown toenails, and loose-fitting socks can cause blisters. Not wearing socks can result in blisters, abrasions, odor, and excess wear on shoes.

Some activities require special protective apparel. For example, helmets are recommended for bikers and inline skaters. Statistics indicate a 75 percent decrease in risk of injury when wearing a helmet. Gloves, pads, and padded clothing can also help reduce risk of injury. These may be especially important for beginning rollerbladers since there is a high rate of falling for novices. Bikers, joggers, and walkers should consider reflective clothing and shoes, especially if activity takes place when light is restricted. Some experts now recommend water shoes to protect the feet for those who do extensive water aerobic exercise. It would be wise to investigate proper apparel and equipment needs for new activities in your activity program.

Proper footwear is important for safe and effective physical activity.

www.mhhe.com/phys_fit/webreview03 Click 01

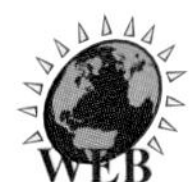

Most manufacturers now produce athletic shoes in six categories: running/jogging, walking, tennis, court, aerobic/fitness, and **cross-training.** Many produce even more specialized shoes within each category. For example, many manufacturers have separate court shoes for basketball and volleyball. For people who are highly dedicated to a specific activity, a specialized pair of shoes should be purchased. For those who do not specialize in one activity, the cross trainer is a good choice.

The essential characteristics of all athletic shoes are described below (see Figure 1):

- **Support.** The heel counter and the heel stabilizer provide stability and control foot movement. The heel protects the Achilles tendon from trauma. The heel in running shoes should not be too narrow. Adequate width in the heel provides stability and protects against ankle turns. For court games such as basketball, a high-top shoe is recommended for additional ankle support.
- **Cushioning.** It is generally agreed that good cushioning is important, especially in the heel and midsole. However, excessive cushioning is not recommended. Too much cushioning may increase risk of injury by inhibiting the reflexes that help the body protect itself against the impact of the foot with the ground.
- **Performance.** A lightweight shoe requires less energy output over lengthy exercise periods. Good traction for a given sport is also important. For lengthy performances, a shoe that is at least partially made from a material that can breathe, such as nylon mesh, helps sweat evaporation and inhibits shoe weight gain.

PAR-Q An acronym for Physical Activity Readiness Questionnaire; designed to help you determine if you are medically suited to begin an exercise program.

Clinical Exercise Test A test typically administered on a treadmill in which exercise is gradually increased in intensity while the heart is monitored by an EKG. Symptoms not present at rest, such as an abnormal EKG, may be present in an exercise test.

Moderate Physical Activity Physical activity that is equal in intensity to brisk walking.

Vigorous Physical Activity Physical activity that is more intense than brisk walking; usually associated with elevated heart rate, increased breathing rates, and increased sweating.

Cross-Training A term commonly used to indicate participation in a variety of activities (e.g., running, tennis, resistance training).

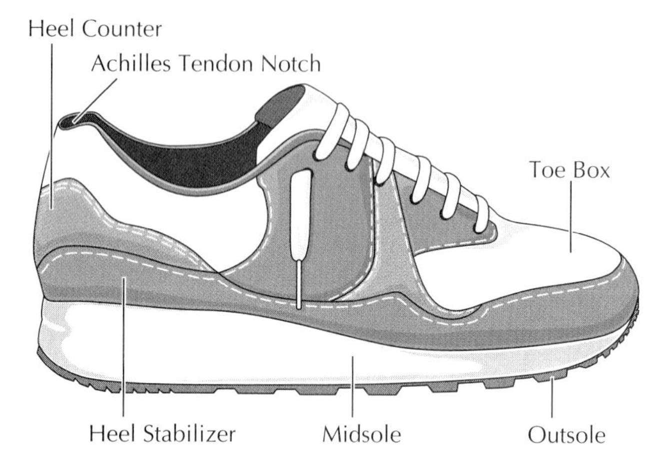

Figure 1
Characteristics of a good activity shoe.

- **Fit.** The toe box should be roomy enough so that you can wiggle your toes. Regardless of the type of shoe, exercise shoes should generally be one-half size larger than your regular shoes. If you wear two pairs of socks while exercising, you should wear two pairs when trying on the shoes. It is important to try on the shoes and move around in them before making a purchase. Make sure they feel good to you.

Probably the biggest mistake made regarding footwear is not replacing them when they wear out. The important cushioning areas of the shoe (heel and midsole) typically wear out before the sole or the fabric. Thus, it may be necessary to replace shoes before they appear worn out.

The Facts to Consider during Daily Physical Activity

There are three key components of the daily activity program: the warm-up exercise, the workout, and the cool-down exercise.

The key component of a fitness program is the daily workout. Experts agree, however, that the workout should be preceded by a **warm-up** and followed by a **cool-down.** The warm-up prepares the body for physical activity, and the cool-down returns the body to rest and promotes effective recovery.

The cardiovascular warm-up prior to the workout is recommended to prepare the muscles and heart for the workout.

www.mhhe.com/phys_fit/webreview03 Click 02

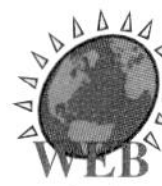

There are two good reasons for warming up prior to activity. The first is to prepare the heart muscle and circulatory system. When you start physical activity, blood flow is not immediately available to the heart and muscles. A proper warm-up decreases the risk of irregular heart beats associated with poor coronary circulation. A proper warm-up can also improve performance since it minimizes the premature formation of **lactic acid** at the start of physical activity. Research suggests that two minutes of walking, jogging, or mild exercise is adequate for moderate activities; however, some experts recommend five minutes or more of moderate activity as a warm-up for vigorous activity.

The second reason for a warm-up is to stretch the skeletal muscles. When you begin exercise, muscles and joints are usually cold and stiff. By gradually warming up the body, the muscles become more elastic and extensible. The skeletal muscle warm-up should include static stretching of the major muscle groups involved in the exercise that is to follow. It should be emphasized that even though warming up prior to an activity may help reduce the chance of muscle injury, it is not a substitute for a regular program of exercise designed to improve flexibility.

A warm-up that is suitable for walking, jogging, running, cycling, and even basketball is illustrated in Figure 2. This warm-up can be used for other activities provided stretching exercises for the major muscle groups involved in the activities are added. Additional exercises that are appropriate for inclusion in a stretching warm-up are illustrated in the flexibility concept. The cardiovascular warm-up is suitable for most activities, but other mild exercise (such as a slow swim for swimmers or a slow ride for cyclists) can be substituted.

Many experts recommend that the stretching portion of the warm-up be done after the cardiovascular portion.

Some experts believe that the cardiovascular portion of the warm-up should precede the stretching portion because warm muscles are less likely to be injured by the stretch. Warm muscles also stretch farther. Some experts are concerned that the stretch warm-up may be abandoned by people who feel that they do not have time to do both the cardiovascular and stretching warm-up before doing their activity program. In this case, it is better to do stretching without the cardiovascular warm-up than do nothing at all. If you choose to stretch before the warm-up, make certain it is a gentle, static stretch. This is not the time for a flexibility workout in which you try to increase your normal range of motion. Rather, it should be for the purpose of limbering up or loosening.

A cool-down after the workout is important to promote an effective recovery from physical activity.

Figure 2
Sample warm-up and cool-down exercises.

The exercises shown here can be used before a moderate workout as a warm-up, or after a workout as a cool-down. Perform these exercises slowly, preferably after completing a cardiovascular warm-up. Do not bounce or jerk against the muscle. Hold each stretch for at least 15 seconds. Perform each exercise at least once and up to three times. Other stretching exercises are presented in the concept on flexibility that can be used in a warm-up or cool-down.

Cardiovascular Exercise
Before you perform a vigorous workout, walk or jog slowly for 2 minutes or more. After exercise, do the same. If possible do this portion of the warm-up prior to muscle stretching.

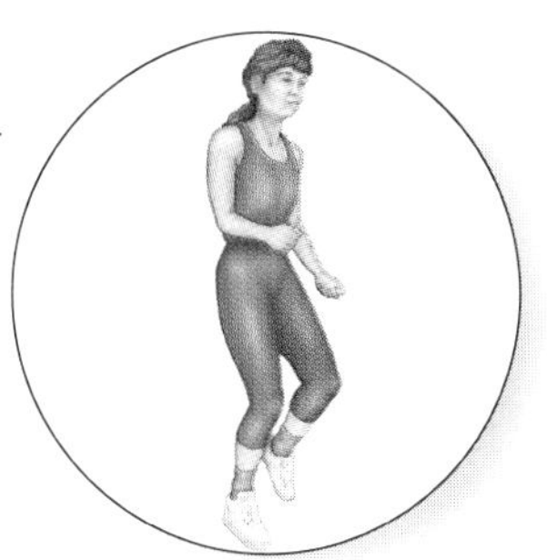

Calf Stretcher
This exercise stretches the calf muscles (gastrocnemius and soleus). Face a wall with your feet 2 or 3 feet away. Step forward on left foot to allow both hands to touch the wall. Keep the heel of your right foot on the ground, toe turned in slightly, knee straight, and buttocks tucked in. Lean forward by bending your front knee and arms and allowing your head to move nearer the wall. Hold. Repeat with the other leg.

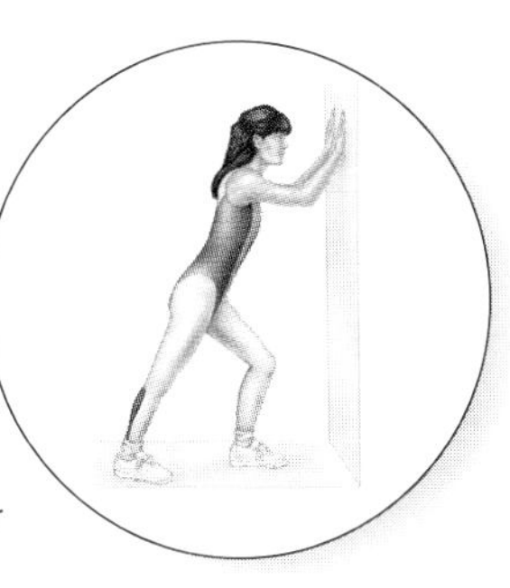

Hamstring Stretcher
This exercise stretches the muscles of the back of the upper leg (hamstrings) as well as those of the hip, knee, and ankle. Lie on your back. Bring the right knee to your chest and grasp the toes with the right hand. Place the left hand on the back of the right thigh. Pull the knee toward the chest, push the heel toward the ceiling, and pull the toes toward the shin. Attempt to straighten the knee. Stretch and hold. Repeat with the other leg.

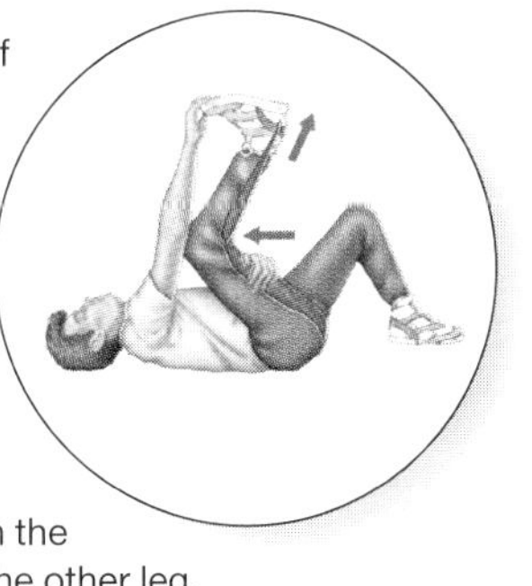

Leg Hug
This exercise stretches the hip and back extensor muscles. Lie on your back. Bend one leg and grasp your thigh under the knee. Hug it to your chest. Keep the other leg straight and on the floor. Hold. Repeat with the opposite leg.

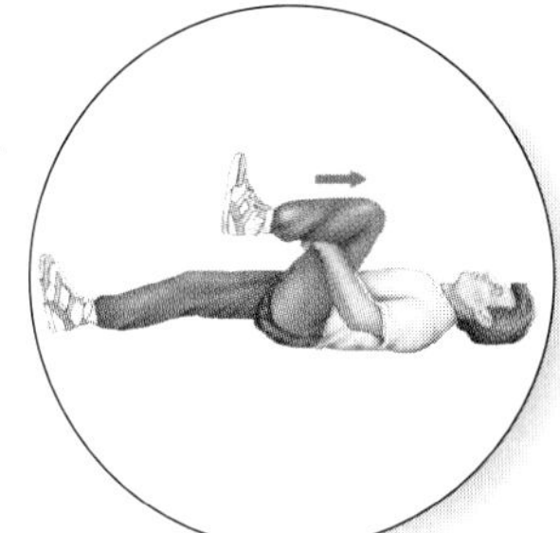

Seated Side Stretch
This exercise stretches the muscles of the trunk. Begin in a seated position with the legs crossed. Stretch the left arm over the head to the right. Bend at the waist (to right), reaching as far as possible to the left with the right arm. Hold. Do not let the trunk rotate. Repeat to the opposite side. For less stretch the overhead arm may be bent. This exercise can be done in the standing position but is less effective.

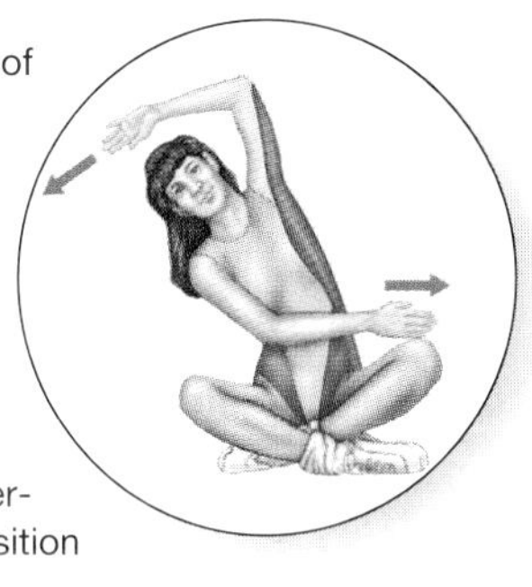

Zipper
This exercise stretches the muscle on the back of the arm (triceps) and the lower chest muscles (pecs). Lift right arm and reach behind head and down the spine (as if pulling up a zipper). With the left hand, push down on right elbow and hold. Reverse arm position and repeat.

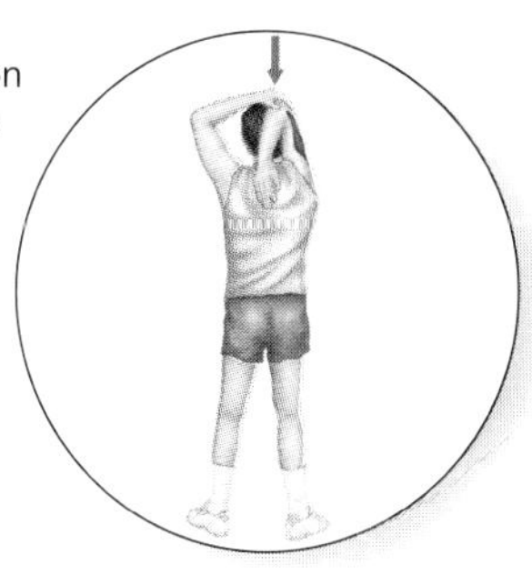

The cool-down is done immediately after the workout. Like the warm-up, there are two principal components of a cool-down: static muscle stretching and an activity for the cardiovascular system. Although not all experts agree, some believe that static muscle stretching *after* the workout is more important than stretching before because it may help relieve spasms in fatigued muscles. Stretching as part of the cool-down may be more effective for lengthening the muscles than stretching at other times because the muscle temperature is elevated and therefore the stretching is more likely to produce optimal flexibility improvements.

A cardiovascular portion of the cool-down is also important. During physical activity, the heart pumps a large amount of blood to supply the working muscles with the oxygen necessary to keep moving. The muscles squeeze the

Warm-Up Light to moderate activity done prior to the workout. Its purpose is to reduce the risk of injury and soreness and possibly to improve performance in a physical activity.

Cool-Down Light to moderate activity done after a workout to help the body recover; often consisting of the same exercises used in the warm-up.

Lactic Acid A byproduct of the metabolic processes that occurs during vigorous physical activity; a cause of muscle fatigue.

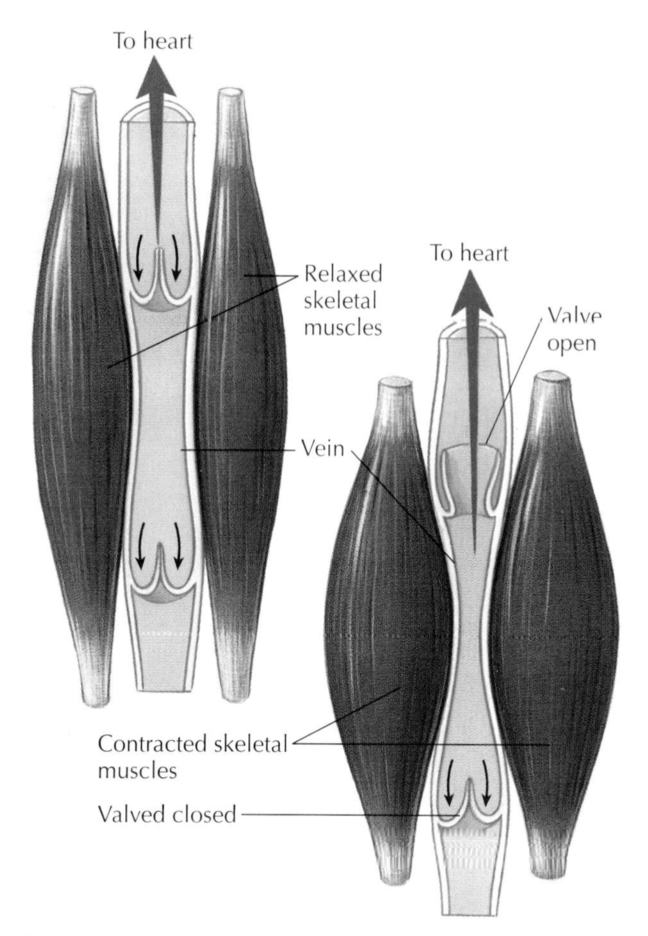

Figure 3
The pumping action of the muscles.

veins (see Figure 3), which forces the blood back to the heart. Valves in the veins prevent the blood from flowing backward. As long as exercise continues, the blood is moved by the muscles back to the heart, where it is once again pumped to the body. If exercise is stopped abruptly, the blood is left in the area of the working muscles and has no way to get back to the heart. In the case of the runner, the blood pools in the legs. Because the heart has less blood to pump, blood pressure may drop. This can result in dizziness, and can even cause a person to pass out. The best way to prevent this problem is to taper off or slow down gradually after exercise. A cardiovascular cool-down should include approximately 2 minutes of walking, slow jogging, or any nonvigorous activity that uses the muscles involved in the workout.

The Facts about Physical Activity in the Heat

Physical activity in hot and humid environments challenges the body's heat loss mechanisms.

www.mhhe.com/phys_fit/webreview03 Click 03

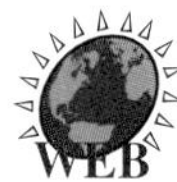

The normal human body temperature is 98.6°F. During vigorous activity, the body produces large amounts of heat, which must be dissipated to keep the body temperature regulated. The body has several ways to dissipate heat. Conduction is the transfer of heat from a hot body to a cold body. Convection is the transfer of heat through the air or other medium. Fans and wind can facilitate heat loss by convection and help regulate temperature. The primary method of cooling is through evaporation of sweat. The chemical process involved in evaporation transfers heat from the body and reduces the body temperature. When conditions are humid, the effectiveness of evaporation is reduced since the air is already saturated with moisture. This is why it is difficult to regulate body temperature when conditions are both hot and humid.

Heat-related illness can occur if proper hydration is not maintained.

Maximum sweat rates during physical activity in the heat can approach 1–2 liters per hour. If this fluid is not replaced, **dehydration** can occur. If dehydration is not corrected with water or other fluid-replacement drinks, it becomes increasingly more difficult for the body to maintain normal body temperatures. At some point, the rate of sweating decreases as the body begins to try to conserve its remaining water. It attempts to shunt blood to the skin to transfer excess heat directly to the environment, but this is less effective than evaporation, and various heat-related problems including heat stroke and **hyperthermia** can result (see Table 3).

One way to monitor the amount of fluid loss is to monitor the color of your urine. The American College of Sports Medicine indicates that clear (almost colorless) urine produced in large volumes indicates that you are hydrated and ready for activity. Dark yellow urine produced in small volume is a good indicator of dehydration and need for fluid replacement.

Acclimatization improves the body's tolerance in the heat.

Individuals with good fitness will respond better to activity in the heat than individuals with poor fitness. This is because the ability to sweat improves with training. With regular exposure to the heat, the body becomes conditioned to sweat earlier, to sweat more profusely, and to distribute sweat more effectively around the body. This process of acclimatization makes it easier for the body to maintain a safe body temperature.

When doing physical activity in hot and humid environments, special precautions should be taken to prevent heat-related problems.

Table 2 Exercise in the Heat (Apparent Temperatures)

To read the table, find air temperature on the top, then find the humidity on the left.
Find the apparent temperature where the columns meet.

Relative Humidity (%)	Air Temperature (Degrees F) 70	75	80	85	90	95	100	105	110	115	120
100	72	80	91	108	132						
95	71	79	89	105	128						
90	71	79	88	102	122						
85	71	78	87	99	117	141					
80	71	78	86	97	113	136					
75	70	77	86	95	109	130					
70	70	77	85	93	106	124	144				
65	70	76	83	91	102	119	138				
60	70	76	82	90	100	114	132	149			
55	69	75	81	89	98	110	126	142			
50	69	75	81	88	96	107	120	135	150		
45	68	74	80	87	95	104	115	129	143		
40	68	74	79	86	93	101	110	123	137	151	
35	67	73	79	85	91	98	107	118	130	143	
30	67	73	78	84	90	96	104	113	123	135	148
25	66	72	77	83	88	94	101	109	117	127	139
20	66	72	77	82	87	93	99	105	112	120	130
15	65	71	76	81	86	91	97	102	108	115	123
10	65	70	75	80	85	90	95	100	105	111	116
5	64	69	74	79	84	88	93	97	102	107	111
0	64	69	73	78	83	87	91	95	99	103	107

"Apparent Temperatures" (Heat Index)

- = Exreme Danger Zone
- = Danger Zone
- = Extreme Caution Zone
- = Caution Zone
- = Safe

SOURCE: Data from National Oceanic and Atmospheric Administration.

www.mhhe.com/phys_fit/webreview03 Click 04

- WEB Limit or avoid physical activity in hot or humid environments. The **apparent temperature** (also referred to as the heat index) is an index that combines temperature and humidity. Physical activity is safe when the apparent temperature is below 80°F (26.7°C). Above this apparent temperature there are four zones (see Table 2) that illustrate the danger of doing physical activity when the apparent temperature is high. When apparent temperatures reach the Danger Zones, activity should be limited or canceled. With extreme care, experienced exercisers who have become acclimatized to the heat may be able to perform at higher apparent temperatures than those who are less experienced. However, care should be used by all people who perform physical activity in hot and humid environments.
- Replace fluids regularly. Drink water before (2 cups or 16 ounces) and during activity (1 cup or 5–10 ounces every 15 to 20 minutes). After activity, replacing 16 ounces of fluid for each pound of weight lost is a good rule. For exercise lasting more than 1 hour, fluid-replacement drinks containing simple carbohydrates (glucose, fructose, or sucrose) and electrolytes are considered beneficial to performance and body cooling. If the concentration of sugars is no more than 4–8 percent, they can replace fluids as quickly as water.
- Gradually expose yourself to physical activity in hot and humid environments. Too much at once is especially dangerous.

Table 3 Types of Heat-Related Problems

Problem	Symptoms	Severity
Heat cramps	Muscle cramps, especially in muscles most used in exercise	Least severe
Heat exhaustion	Muscle cramps; weakness; dizziness; headache; nausea; clammy skin; paleness	Moderate severity
Heat stroke	Hot, flushed skin; dry skin (lack of sweating); dizziness; fast pulse; unconsciousness; high temperature	Extremely severe

Dehydration Excessive loss of water from the body, usually through perspiration, urination, or evaporation.

Hyperthermia Excessively high body temperature caused by excessive heat production or impaired heat loss capacity. Heat stroke is an example of a hyperthermic condition.

Apparent Temperature A combination of temperature and humidity used to determine if it is dangerous to perform physical activity (also called Heat Index).

- When possible, do your activity in the morning or evening.
- Dress properly for exercise in the heat and humidity. Wear white or light colors that reflect rather than absorb heat. Porous clothing allows the passage of air to cool the body. Rubber, plastic, or other nonporous clothing is especially dangerous. A porous hat or cap can help when exercising in direct sunlight.
- Do not change your wet shirt for a dry one. A wet shirt cools the body better.
- Rest at regular intervals, preferably in the shade.
- Watch for signs of heat stress. If signs are present, stop immediately.

If overheating occurs, take immediate steps to cool the body.

Take these steps: stop physical activity; get out of the heat and into the shade; remove excess clothing; drink cool water; immerse the body in cool water; if symptoms of heat stroke are present, seek immediate medical attention; and statically stretch cramped muscles.

Facts about Physical Activity in Other Environments

Physical activity in exceptionally cold and windy weather can be dangerous.

www.mhhe.com/phys_fit/webreview03 Click 05

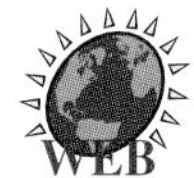

Physical activity in the cold presents the opposite problem of exercise in the heat. In the cold the primary goal is to retain the body's heat and avoid **hypothermia** or frostbite. A combination of cold and wind (windchill) poses the greatest danger. Consider the following guidelines for performing physical activity in cold and windy environments.

- Limit or cancel activity if the time to frostbite is 30 minutes or less. Table 4 includes new information from the National Weather Service concerning windchill and the time of exposure necessary to get frostbite.
- Dress properly in the wind and cold. Wear light clothing in several layers rather than one heavy garment. The layer of clothing closest to the body should ideally help to transfer (wick) moisture away from the skin and transfer it to a second, more absorbent layer. Fabric such as polypropylene and capilene are examples of wickable fabrics. A porous windbreaker will keep wind from cooling the body and will allow the release of body heat. The hands, feet, nose, and ears are most susceptible to frostbite so they should be covered. Wear a hat or cap, mask, and mittens. Mittens are warmer than gloves. A light coating of petroleum jelly on exposed body parts can be helpful.
- Try to keep from getting wet in cold weather.

High altitude and/or air pollution may limit performance and require adaptation of normal physical activity.

The ability to do vigorous physical tasks is diminished as altitude increases. Breathing rate and heart rates are more elevated at high altitude. With proper acclimation (gradual exposure), the body adjusts to the lower oxygen pressure found at high altitude, and performance improves. Nevertheless, performance ability at high altitudes, especially for activities requiring cardiovascular fitness, is usually less than would be expected at sea level. At extremely high altitudes, the ability to perform vigorous physical activity may be impossible without an extra oxygen supply. When moving to a high altitude from sea level, vigorous exercise should be done with caution. Acclimation to high altitudes requires a minimum of two weeks and may not be complete for several months. Care should be taken to drink adequate water at high altitude.

www.mhhe.com/phys_fit/webreview03 Click 06

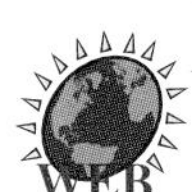

Various pollutants such as ozone, carbon monoxide, pollens, and particulates can also cause poor physical performance, and in some cases, health problems. Ozone, a pollutant produced primarily by the sun's reaction to car exhaust, can cause symptoms including headache, wheezing, and eye irritation. Similar symptoms result from exposure to carbon monoxide, a tasteless and odorless gas, caused by combustion of oil, gasoline, and cigarette smoke. Most news media in metropolitan areas now provide updates on ozone and carbon monoxide levels in their weather reports. When levels of these pollutants reach moderate levels, exercise may need to be modified for some people. When levels are high, exercise may need to be postponed. Exercisers wishing to avoid ozone and carbon monoxide may want to exercise indoors early in the morning, or later in the evening. It is wise to avoid areas with a high concentration of motor vehicles.

Pollens from certain plants may cause allergic reactions for certain people. Some people are allergic to dust or other particulates in the air. Weather reports of pollens and particulates may help exercisers determine the best times for their activities and when to avoid vigorous activities.

The Facts about Soreness and Injury

Understanding soreness can help you persist in physical activity and avoid problems.

www.mhhe.com/phys_fit/webreview03 Click 07

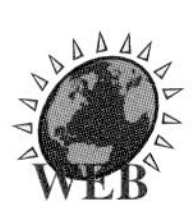

Some people avoid physical activity because they remember earlier experiences such as team practices or training for special events that led to

Table 4 Windchill Factor Chart

Actual Temperature Reading (Degrees F)	Estimated Wind Speed (mph)									Minutes to frostbite
	Calm	5	10	15	20	25	30	35	40	
40	40	36	34	32	30	29	28	27	27	
30	30	25	21	19	17	16	15	14	13	
20	20	13	9	6	4	3	1	0	-1	
10	10	1	-4	-7	-9	-11	-12	-14	-15	
0	0	-11	-16	-19	-22	-24	-26	-27	-29	30
-10	-10	-22	-28	-32	-35	-37	-39	-41	-43	10
-20	-20	-34	-41	-45	-48	-51	-53	-55	-57	5
-30	-30	-46	-53	-58	-61	-64	-67	-69	-71	
-40	-40	-57	-66	-71	-74	-78	-80	-82	-84	

Source: National Weather Service, 2001.

soreness 24 to 48 hours after the intense exercise. They feel that all activity will make them sore, and they want to avoid this unpleasant experience. It is true that intense exercise, especially to muscle groups that are not normally exercised, can cause what is called delayed-onset muscle soreness (**DOMS**). Some people mistakenly believe that lactic acid is the cause of muscle soreness. Lactic acid, however, returns to normal levels 30 minutes after exercise, whereas DOMS occurs at least 24 hours following exercise. We now know that DOMS results from microscopic muscle tears. In some cases, DOMS is accompanied by swelling and pain, but in general the condition has no long-term consequences.

There are several steps that can be taken to avoid DOMS and to make activity more enjoyable. Starting gradually is perhaps the most important thing you can do. It is known that lengthening contractions (eccentric) are more likely to cause DOMS than shortening muscle contractions (concentric contractions). For this reason, walking or running downhill or downstairs should be gradually phased into your program. Of course, a regular warm-up is also advised. Fortunately, DOMS lasts only a day or so. Doing moderate exercise when you have soreness does not seem to put you at risk of muscle injury. DOMS is only temporary and not a common occurrence for those who exercise regularly and consistently.

> Being able to treat minor injuries will help reduce their negative effects.

Minor injuries such as muscle sprains and strains are not uncommon to those who are persistent in their exercise. If a serious injury should occur, it is important to get immediate medical attention. However, for minor injuries, following the **"RICE"** formula will help you reduce the pain or the injury and will speed recovery. In this acronym, **R** stands for "rest." Muscle sprains and strains heal best if rested, and rest also helps you avoid further damage to the muscle. **I** stands for "ice." The quick application of cold (ice or ice water) to a minor injury minimizes swelling and speeds recovery. Cold should be applied to as large a surface area as possible (soaking is best). If ice is used, it should be wrapped to avoid direct contact with the skin. Apply cold for 20–30 minutes, three times a day for several days. **C** stands for "compression." Wrapping or compressing the injured area also helps minimize swelling and speeds recovery. Elastic bandages are good for applying compression. For a sprained ankle, wearing a tied high-top shoe

Hypothermia Excessively low body temperature (less than 95°F) characterized by uncontrollable shivering, loss of coordination, and mental confusion.

Windchill Factor An index that uses air temperature and wind speed to determine the chilling effect of the environment on humans.

DOMS An acronym for delayed-onset muscle soreness; a common malady that follows relatively vigorous activity especially among beginners.

RICE An acronym for rest, ice, compression and elevation; a method of treating minor injuries.

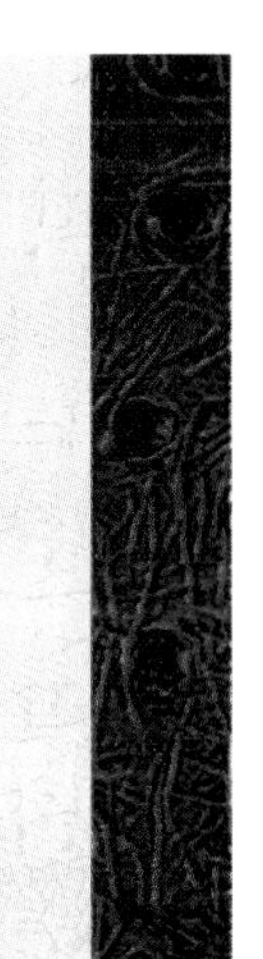

until a bandage can be located provides good compression. Elastic socks may also be useful. Care should be taken to avoid wrapping an injury too tightly because this can result in loss of circulation to the area. E stands for "elevation." Keeping the injured area elevated (above the level of the heart) is effective in minimizing swelling. If pain or swelling persists, or if there is any doubt about the seriousness of an injury, seek medical help.

Taking over-the-counter pain remedies can help reduce the pain of muscle strains and sprains. Aspirin and ibuprofen (e.g., Motrin, Excedrin) have anti-inflammatory properties. However, acetaminophen (e.g., Tylenol) does not have anti-inflammatory properties, so it may reduce the pain but it will not reduce the inflammation. Any over-the-counter remedy should be taken only as directed unless otherwise indicated by a physician.

The most common injuries incurred in physical activity are sprains and strains.

www.mhhe.com/phys_fit/webreview03 Click 08

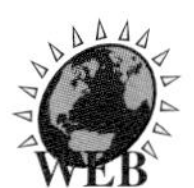

A strain occurs when the fibers in a muscle are injured. A sprain is an injury to a ligament—the connective tissue that connects bones to bones. Common activity related injuries are hamstring strains that occur after a vigorous sprint. A good example would be the occasional athlete who sprints to first base without warming up and after not playing in a long time. Other commonly strained muscles include the muscles in the front of the thigh, the low back, and the calf muscles. The most common sprain is to the ankle. It frequently occurs when the ankle is rolled to the outside when jumping or running. Evidence suggests that lace-up ankle braces made of non-elastic material are effective in reducing ankle sprains. Other common sprains are to the knee, the shoulder, and the wrist. Sprains and strains respond well to RICE.

Tendonitis is an inflammation of the tendon and is most often a result of overuse rather than trauma. Tendonitis can be painful but often does not swell to the extent that sprains do. For this reason, elevation and compression are not especially effective, but ice, and especially rest, are useful.

Muscle cramps can be relieved by statically stretching a muscle.

Muscle cramps are pains in the large muscles of the body that result when the muscle contracts vigorously for a continued period of time. A muscle cramp is usually not considered to be an injury, but they are painful and may seem like an injury. They are usually short in duration and can often be relieved with proper treatment. Cramps can result from lack of fluid replacement (dehydration), from fatigue, and from a blow directly to a muscle. A true cramp is not the same as a muscle tear, sprain, or strain. A cramp can be relieved by statically stretching the cramped muscle. For example, the calf muscle, which often cramps among runners, football players, and other sports participants, can be relieved using the calf stretcher exercise, which is part of the warm-up in this concept. Other stretching exercises from the concept on flexibility can be used to relieve cramps to other muscles or muscle groups. If stretching causes persistent pain, stop the stretching—you may have a muscle injury rather than a cramp. Of course, replacing fluids regularly during exercise helps avoid cramps, as does the development of flexibility.

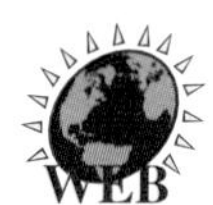

Web Review

Web review materials for Concept 3 are available at *www.mhhe.com/phys_fit/webreview03 Click 09.*

ACSM's Health and Fitness Journal
www.acsm-healthfitness.org

American Alliance for Health, Physical Education, Recreation and Dance
www.aahperd.org

American College of Sports Medicine
www.acsm.org

National Athletic Trainers Association
www.nata.org

The Physician and Sports Medicine
www.physsportsmed.com

Suggested Readings

Agostini, R. "Reduce Risks of Activity-Induced Injury." *ACSM's Health and Fitness Journal.* 2(2)(1998): S29.

American College of Sports Medicine. *ACSM's Guidelines for Exercise Testing and Prescription,* 6th ed. Philadelphia: Lippincott, Williams and Wilkins, 2000.

American College of Sports Medicine. "Position Stand on Exercise and Fluid Replacement." *Medicine and Science in Sports and Exercise.* 28 (1)(1996): i.

American College of Sports Medicine. "Position Stand on Heat and Cold Illness During Distance Running." *Medicine and Science in Sports and Exercise.* 28(12)(1996):i.

Hockenburry, R., and Sammarco, G. "Evaluation and Treatment of Ankle Sprains." *The Physician and Sports Medicine.* 29(2)(2001): 57–64.

Martin, D. R. "Athletic Shoes: Finding a Good Match." *The Physician and Sports Medicine.* 25(9)(1997):138.

Schwellnus, M. P. "Skeletal Muscle Cramps during Exercise." *The Physician and Sports Medicine.* 27(12)(1999): 109–115.

Shephard, R. J. "Preparing for Physical Activity." In Corbin, C. B., and Pangrazi, R. P. (ed.), *Towards a Better Understanding of Physical Fitness and Activity.* Scottsdale, AZ: Holcomb-Hathaway, 1999, Chapter 1.

Shirreffs, S. M., and Maughan, R. J. "Rehydration and Recovery of Fluid Balance after Exercise." *Exercise and Sport Sciences Reviews.* 28(1)(2000): 27–32.

Sparling, P. B., and Millard-Stafford, M. "Keeping Sports Participants Safe in Hot Weather." *The Physician and Sports Medicine.* 27(7)(1999): 27–40.

Concept 4

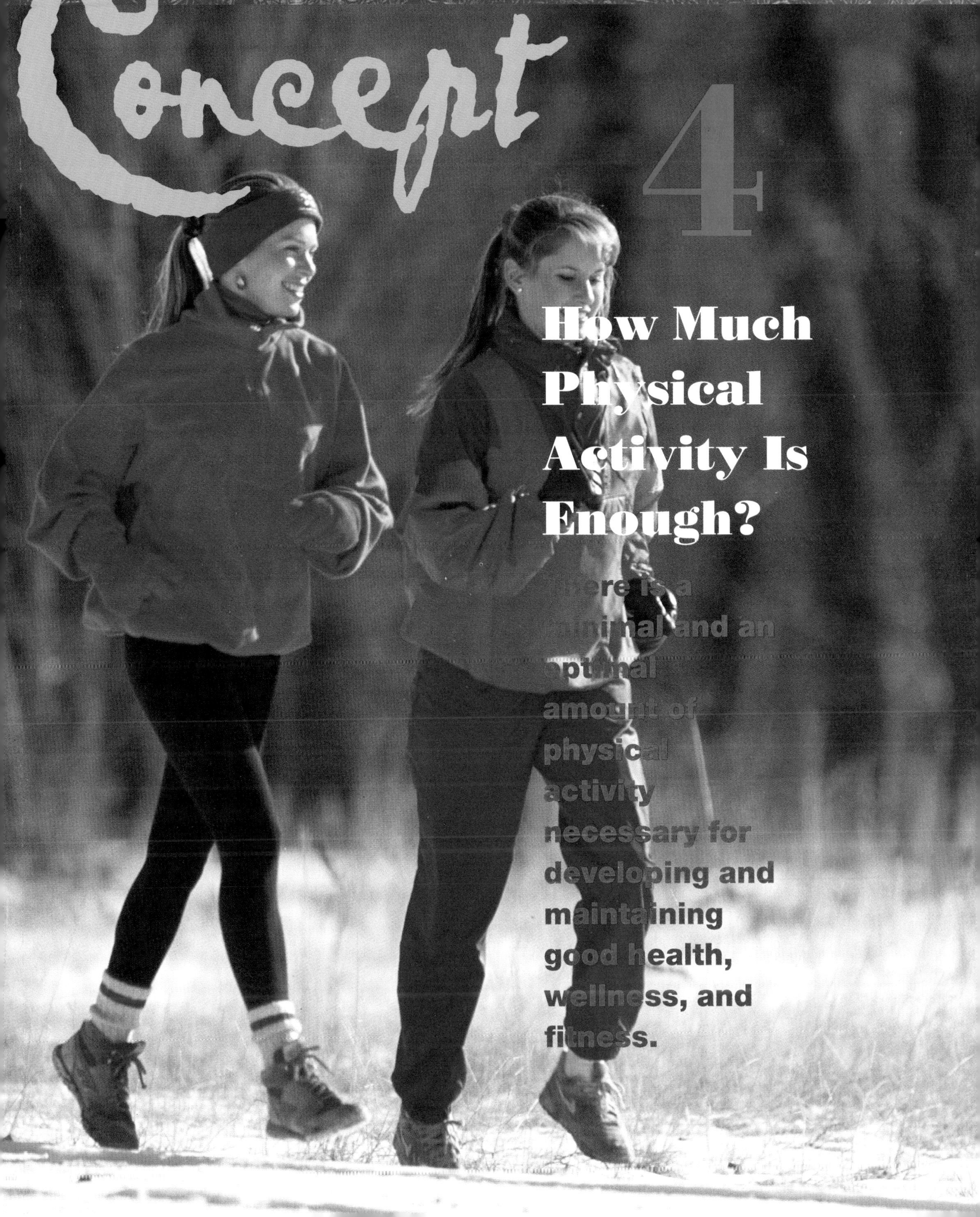

How Much Physical Activity Is Enough?

There is a minimal and an optimal amount of physical activity necessary for developing and maintaining good health, wellness, and fitness.

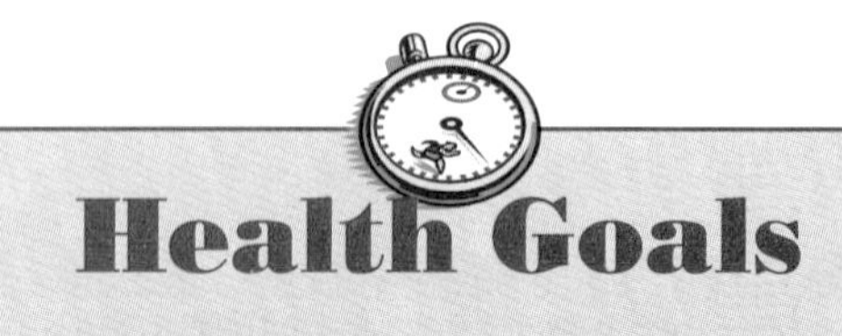

Health Goals

for year 2010

Improve the health, fitness, and quality of life of all people through the adoption and maintenance of regular, daily physical activity.

Increase the proportion of people who do moderate daily activity for 30 minutes.

Increase the proportion of people who do vigorous physical activity three days a week.

Increase the proportion of people who do regular exercises for muscle fitness.

Increase the proportion of people who do regular exercise for flexibility.

Introduction

Just as there is a correct dosage of medicine for healing an illness, there is a correct dosage of physical activity for promoting health benefits and developing physical fitness. Several important principles of physical activity provide the basis for determining the correct dose or amount of physical activity. In this concept, a formula for implementing the important physical activity principles will be presented. This formula and the concepts of "threshold of training" and "target zones" will be described to help you determine how much physical activity is enough. New evidence indicates that the amount of physical activity necessary for developing metabolic fitness, and its associated health benefits, is different from the amount of physical activity necessary for developing health-related fitness and other performance benefits. Research also shows that the amount of activity or exercise necessary for maintaining fitness may differ from the amount needed to develop it.

The Principles of Physical Activity: The Facts

Overload is necessary to achieve health, wellness, and fitness benefits of physical activity.

The **overload principle** is the most basic of all physical activity principles. This principle indicates that doing "more than normal" is necessary if benefits are to occur. In order for a muscle (including the heart muscle) to get stronger, it must be overloaded, or worked against a load greater than normal. To increase flexibility, a muscle must be stretched longer than is normal. To increase muscular endurance, muscles must be exposed to sustained exercise for a longer than normal period. The health benefits associated with metabolic fitness seems to require less overload than for health-related fitness improvement, but overload is required just the same.

Physical activity should be increased progressively for safe and effective results.

The **principle of progression** indicates that overload should not be increased too slowly or too rapidly if benefits are to result. A simple example relates to working with your hands. If you have not done anything for a while and you do too much work with your hands, you develop blisters. You are less able to work the next day. A day or more of recovery may be necessary before you are back to normal. If, however, you begin gradually and increase the work you do each day, you develop calluses. The calluses make your hands tougher, and you are able to work long, or longer without injury or soreness. The benefits of all forms of physical activity are best when you gradually increase overload. Doing too much too soon is counterproductive.

The benefits of physical activity are specific to the form of activity performed.

The **principle of specificity** states that to benefit from physical activity, you must overload specifically for that benefit. For example, strength-building exercises may do little for developing cardiovascular fitness, and stretching exercises may do little for altering body composition or metabolic fitness.

Overload is specific to each component of fitness and each health or wellness benefit desired. Overload is also specific to each body part. If you exercise the legs, you build fitness of the legs. If you exercise the arms, you build fitness of the arms. For this reason, it is not unusual to see some people with disproportionate fitness development. Some gymnasts, for example, have good upper body development but poor leg development, whereas some soccer players have well-developed legs but lack upper body development.

Specificity is important in designing your warm-up, workout, and cool-down programs for specific activities. Training is most effective when it closely resembles the activity for which you are preparing. For example, if your goal is to improve your skill in putting the shot, it is not enough to strengthen the arm muscles. You should perform a training activity requiring overload that closely resembles the motion you use in the actual sport.

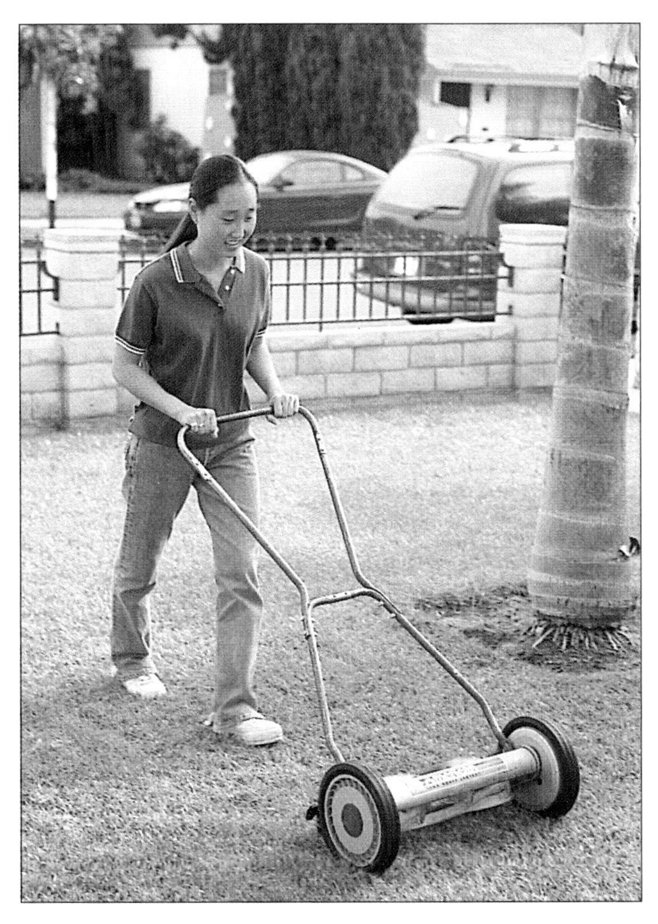

Doing lifestyle activities can benefit your health.

> The benefits achieved from overload last only as long as overload continues.

The **principle of reversibility** is basically the overload principle in reverse. To put it simply, if you don't use it, you will lose it. It is an important principle because some people have the mistaken impression that if they achieve a health or fitness benefit, it will last forever. This, of course, is not true. There is evidence that you can maintain health benefits with less physical activity than it took to achieve them. Still, if you do not adhere to regular physical activity, any benefits attained will gradually erode away.

> In general, the more physical activity you do the more benefits you receive. However, there are exceptions to this rule.

A recent report of an international symposium (see Exercise and Sports Sciences Reviews, suggested readings) provides evidence to suggest that the larger the dose of physical activity the greater the benefits (response). This is called the **dose-response** relationship. This relationship is illustrated by the fact that people who do moderate amounts of regular activity (a moderate dose) have a lower overall death rate compared to those who are sedentary (who do no doses of activity). People who do vigorous activity or moderate activity of longer duration (a bigger dose) have an even greater reduction in risk of early death.

In general, the evidence supports a dose-response relationship for physical activity. It is important, however, to recognize that more is not always better. As the principle of progression indicates, beginners will benefit most from small doses of activity. For them, doing too much too soon is not a good idea. Also, the **principle of diminishing returns** indicates that as you get fitter and fitter you may not get as big a benefit for each additional amount of activity that you perform. Typically improvement plateaus and for those interested in health, fitness, and wellness, maintenance may become most important. In some cases, excessive amounts of activity can be counter-productive.

Overload Principle A basic principle that specifies that you must perform physical activity in greater than normal amounts (overload) to get an improvement in physical fitness or health benefits.

Principle of Progression A corollary of the overload principle that indicates the need to gradually increase overload to achieve optimal benefits.

Principle of Specificity A corollary of the overload principle that indicates a need for a specific type of exercise to improve each fitness component or fitness of a specific part of the body.

Principle of Reversibility A corollary of the overload principle that indicates that disuse or inactivity results in loss of benefits achieved as a result of overload.

Principle of Diminishing Returns A corollary of the overload principle indicating that the more benefits you gain as a result of activity, the harder additional benefits are to achieve.

Dose-Response A term adopted from medicine. With medicine it is important to know what response (benefit) will occur from taking a specific dose. When studying physical activity it is important to know what dose provides the best response (most benefits). The contents of this book are designed to help you choose the best doses of activity for the responses (benefits) you desire.

Health, wellness, and fitness benefits increase your amount of physical activity. But it is important to understand that if you keep increasing physical activity by equal increments, each additional amount of activity will yield less benefit. At some point, improvements will plateau and if activity is overdone, may actually decrease.

The Facts about the FIT Formula

The acronym FIT can help you remember the three important variables for applying the overload principle and its corollaries.

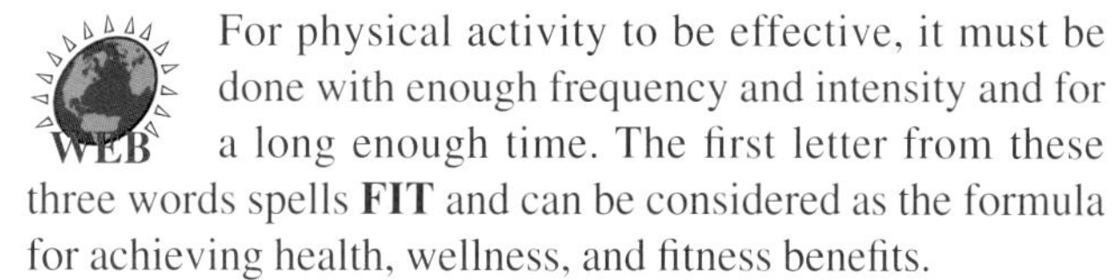

www.mhhe.com/phys_fit/webreview04 Click 01

For physical activity to be effective, it must be done with enough frequency and intensity and for a long enough time. The first letter from these three words spells **FIT** and can be considered as the formula for achieving health, wellness, and fitness benefits.

Frequency (how often)—Physical activity must be performed regularly to be effective. The number of days a person does activity in a week is used to determine frequency. Most benefits require at least three days and up to six days of activity per week but frequency ultimately depends on the specific benefit desired.

Intensity (how hard)—Physical activity must be intense enough to require more exertion (overload) than normal to produce benefits. The method for determining appropriate intensity varies with the desired benefit. For example, metabolic fitness and associated health benefits require only moderate intensity; cardiovascular fitness for high-level performance requires vigorous activity that elevates the heart rate well above normal.

Time (how long)—Physical activity must be done for an adequate length of time to be effective. Generally, an exercise period must be at least 15 minutes in length to be effective, while longer times are recommended for optimal benefits. As the length of time increases, intensities of exercise may be decreased. Time of physical activity involvement is also referred to as duration.

The FIT formula provides a practical means of applying the overload principle progressively for each specific benefit expected.

The type of physical activity you do is often considered to be part of the FITT formula.

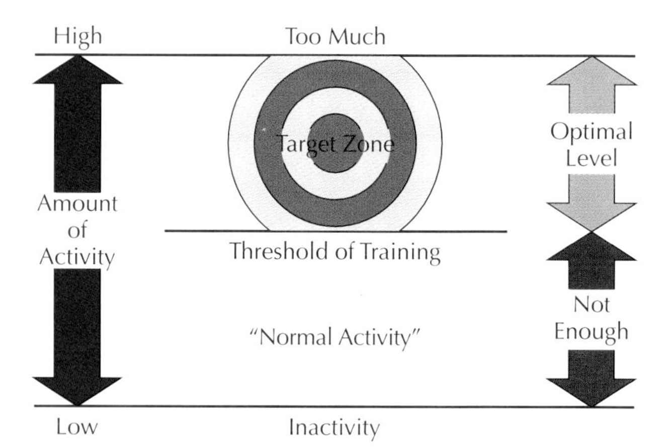

Figure 1
Physical activity target zone.

Sometimes a second *T* is added to the FIT formula to create the FITT formula, which indicates that the **T**ype of physical activity you perform is important. As the specificity principle indicates, different types of activity build different components of fitness and promote different health and wellness benefits. There is a FIT formula for each different benefit and each different type of physical activity. When the formula is applied to one specific type of activity, it is properly referred to as the FIT rather than the FITT formula.

The threshold of training and target zone concepts help you use the FIT formula.

The **threshold of training** is the minimum amount of activity (frequency, intensity, and time) necessary to produce benefits. Depending on the benefit expected, slightly more than normal activity may not be enough to promote health, wellness, or fitness benefits. The **target zone** begins at the threshold of training and stops at the point where the activity becomes counterproductive. Figure 1 illustrates the threshold of training and target zone concepts.

www.mhhe.com/phys_fit/webreview04 Click 02

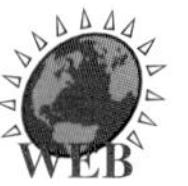

Some people incorrectly associate the concepts of threshold of training and target zones with only cardiovascular fitness. As the principle of specificity suggests, each component of fitness, including metabolic fitness, has its own FIT formula and its own threshold and target zone. The target and threshold levels for **health benefits** are different from those for achieving **performance benefits** associated with high levels of physical fitness. Details of the different FIT formula, threshold levels, and targets zones for the various benefits of activity are presented later in this book.

> It takes time for physical activity to produce health, wellness, and fitness benefits even when the FIT formula is properly applied.

www.mhhe.com/phys_fit/webreview04 Click 03

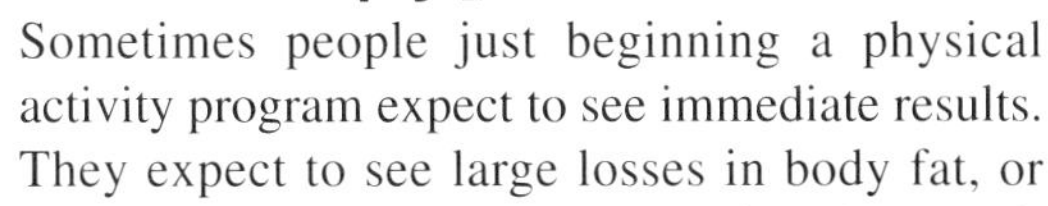

Sometimes people just beginning a physical activity program expect to see immediate results. They expect to see large losses in body fat, or great increases in muscle strength in just a few days. Evidence shows, however, that improvements in health-related physical fitness and the associated health benefits take several weeks to become apparent. Though some people report psychological benefits, such as "feeling better" and a "sense of personal accomplishment" almost immediately after beginning regular exercise, the physiological changes will take considerably longer to be realized. Proper preparation for physical activity includes learning not to expect too much too soon, and not to do too much too soon. Attempts to overdo it and to try to get fit fast will probably be counterproductive, resulting in soreness and even injury. The key is to start slowly, stay with it, and enjoy yourself. Benefits will come to those who persist.

The Physical Activity Pyramid: The Facts

> The physical activity pyramid classifies activities by type and associated benefits.

www.mhhe.com/phys_fit/webreview04 Click 04

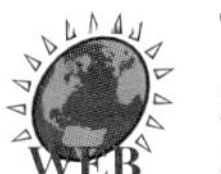

The **physical activity pyramid** (see Figure 2) is a good way to illustrate different types of activities and how each contributes to the development of health, wellness, and physical fitness. The pyramid evolved from a pyramid of activity emphasis developed more than 20 years ago and from the food guide pyramid developed by the U.S. Department of Agriculture to help people understand appropriate servings of foods. Like the food guide pyramid, the physical activity pyramid has four different levels. Each level includes one or two types of activity and characterizes the "portions" of physical activity necessary to produce different health, wellness, and fitness benefits.

The four levels of the pyramid are based on the beneficial health outcomes associated with regular physical activity. Activities having broad general health and wellness benefits for the largest number of people are placed at the base of the pyramid. The *Surgeon General's Report on Physical Activity and Health* points out that significant national health and economic benefits will occur if we can get inactive people, especially those who are totally sedentary, to do some type of activity. The activities at the lower levels can provide these benefits, and because they are relatively low in intensity, they may appeal to the large number of people who can most benefit from beginning an activity program. The activities at the lower levels of the pyramid typically require greater frequency than those at higher levels.

> Lifestyle activities are at the base of the physical activity pyramid.

Lifestyle physical activity is encouraged as a part of everyday living and can contribute significantly to good health, fitness, and wellness. Lifestyle activities include walking to or from work, climbing the stairs rather than taking an elevator, working in the yard, or doing any other type of exercise as part of your normal daily activities. The *Surgeon General's Report on Physical Activity and Health* suggests the accumulation of 30 minutes of physical activity equal to brisk walking on most, if not all, days of the week (see pyramid level 1).

Studies that track active versus inactive adults over long periods of time show that lifestyle activities provide many

FIT A formula used to describe the frequency, intensity, and length of time for physical activity to produce benefits. (When "FITT" is used, the second *T* refers to the type of physical activity you perform.)

Threshold of Training The minimum amount of physical activity that will produce benefits.

Target Zone Amounts of physical activity that produce optimal benefits.

Health Benefit A result of physical activity that provides protection from hypokinetic disease or early death.

Performance Benefit A result of physical activity that improves physical fitness and physical performance capabilities.

Physical Activity Pyramid This pyramid illustrates how different types of activities contribute to the development of health and physical fitness. Activities lower in the pyramid require more frequent participation, whereas activities higher in the pyramid require less frequency.

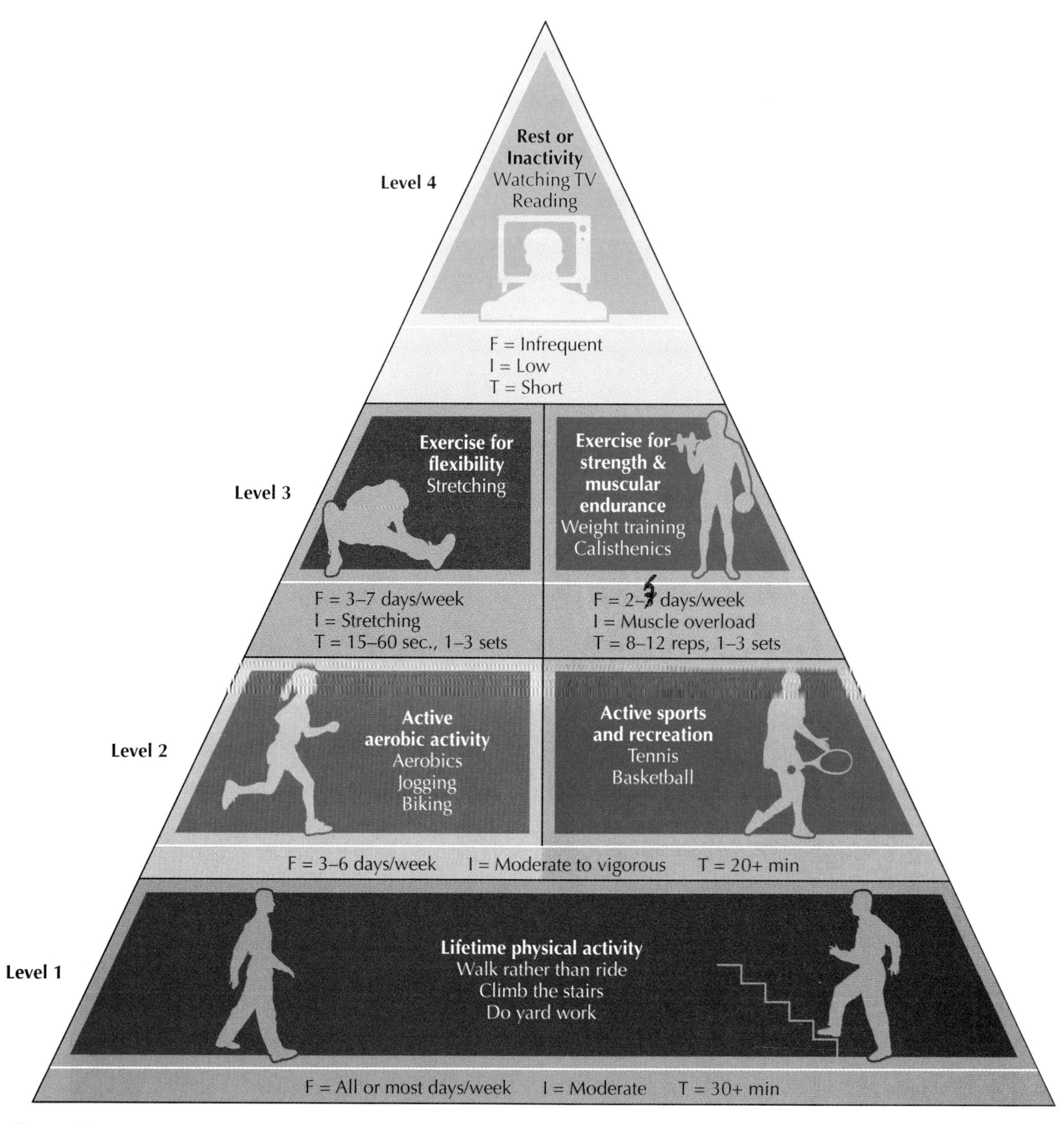

Figure 2
The physical activity pyramid.

health and wellness benefits. Metabolic fitness and modest gains in some parts of health-related physical fitness are associated with lifestyle activities. However, health-related fitness improvement as evidenced by high scores on performance tests are not generally considered to be a major benefit of this type of activity. The fact that lifestyles activities are moderate in intensity may encourage sedentary people to be more active. A summary of the FIT formula for this type of activity is illustrated in level one of Figure 2. While additional activity is encouraged, lifestyle activity is a baseline target that most people can achieve.

Active aerobics and sports and recreation are at the second level of the pyramid.

Aerobic activities (level 2) include those that are of such an intensity that they can be performed for relatively long periods of time without stopping but that also elevate the heart rate significantly. Lifestyle activities (level 1), also known as **moderate activity,** are technically aerobic in nature but are not especially vigorous and are therefore not considered to be "active aerobics." More **vigorous activities** such as jogging, biking, and aerobic dance are commonly classified as "active aerobic" activities. This type of activity is included in the second level of the pyramid because benefits can be accomplished in as few as three days a week and is especially good for building cardiovascular fitness and helping to control body fatness. This type of activity can provide metabolic fitness and health benefits similar to lifestyle activities.

Active sports and recreation are also included at level 2 of the pyramid. Examples of active sports include basketball, tennis, and racquetball, and active recreation includes hiking, backpacking, skiing, and rock climbing. Some active sports and recreational activities involve short bursts of physical activity followed by rests and therefore may not be considered to be aerobic in nature. If done for relatively long periods of time without stopping, active sports and recreation activities can have the same benefits of active aerobic activities. Sports such as golf and bowling may be classified as lifestyle activities rather than active sports since they are done at more moderate intensities. Activities at level 2 of the pyramid may substitute for activities at level 1 if done according to the FIT formula, but many experts encourage activities from both levels. They reason that people who develop active lifestyles from level 1 will be more likely to stay active later in life when they are less likely to participate in activities from level 2. Others argue that if you are active at level 2 you will be fit enough to continue active aerobics and sports as you grow older. A summary of the FIT formula for level 2 activities is included in Figure 2.

Flexibility and muscle fitness exercises are at level 3 of the pyramid.

Flexibility (stretching) exercises are a type of physical activity that is planned specifically to develop flexibility. This type of exercise is necessary because activities lower in the pyramid often do not contribute to flexibility development. The muscle fitness category includes exercises that are planned specifically to build strength and muscular endurance. This type of exercise is necessary because activities lower in the pyramid often do not contribute to these parts of fitness. A general description of the FIT formula for level 3 exercises is included in Figure 2.

Some rest is necessary, but with the exception of sleep, long periods of inactivity are discouraged.

Rest or inactivity can be important to good health. Some time off just to relax is important to us all, and of course proper amounts of rest and 8 hours of uninterrupted sleep help us recuperate. But, sedentary living (too much inactivity) results in low fitness as well as poor health and wellness. Rest and inactivity are placed at the top of the pyramid (see Figure 2) because they should be done sparingly compared to other types of activity in the pyramid.

There are some important guidelines that should be considered when using the physical activity pyramid.

The physical activity pyramid is a useful model for describing different types of activity and their benefits. The pyramid is also useful in summarizing the FIT formula for each of the different benefits of activity. But as the American College of Sports Medicine (2000, p. 139) pointed out, physical activity guidelines ". . . cannot be implemented in an overly rigid fashion . . . and . . . recommendations presented should be used with careful attention to the goals of the individual." This important point should be considered when using the pyramid. The following guidelines for using the pyramid should also be considered.

- *No single activity provides all of the benefits.* More than a few people have asked the question, "What is the perfect form of physical activity?" It is now evident that there is no single activity that can provide all of the health, wellness, and fitness benefits. For optimal benefits to occur, it is desirable to perform activities from all levels of the pyramid because each type of activity has quite different benefits. As other guidelines will indicate, care should be used not to overgeneralize this recommendation.
- *In some cases, one type of activity can substitute for another.* If a person does appropriate activity of either type at level 2 of the pyramid, similar benefits can result.

Moderate Activity For the purposes of this book, moderate activity refers to activity equal in intensity to a brisk walk. Level 1 activities from the activity pyramid are included in this category.

Vigorous Activity For the purposes of this book, vigorous activity refers to activities that elevate the heart rate and are greater in intensity than brisk walking. It is also referred to as moderate to vigorous activity. Those activities from level 2 of the pyramid are included in this category.

Both types are not required. Also, if a person does adequate activity of either type at level 2, it can provide similar benefits to those at level 1 of the pyramid. Selecting activities from more than one category does provide variety and may aid in adherence for some people.

- *Something is better than nothing.* Some people may look at the pyramid and say, "I just don't have time to do all of these activities." This could lead some to throw up their hands in despair, resulting in the conclusion "I just won't do anything at all." The best evidence indicates that something is better than nothing. If you do nothing or feel that you can't do it all, performing a lifestyle physical activity is a good start. Additional activities from different levels of the pyramid can be added as time allows.
- *Activities from Level 3 are useful even if you are limited in performing activities at other levels.* Though flexibility and muscle fitness exercises do not produce all of the benefits associated with regular physical activity, they will produce benefits even if you are unable to perform as much activity from other levels as you like.
- *Good planning will allow you to schedule activities from all levels in a reasonable amount of time.* In subsequent concepts, you will learn more about each level of the pyramid as well as more information about planning a total physical activity program.

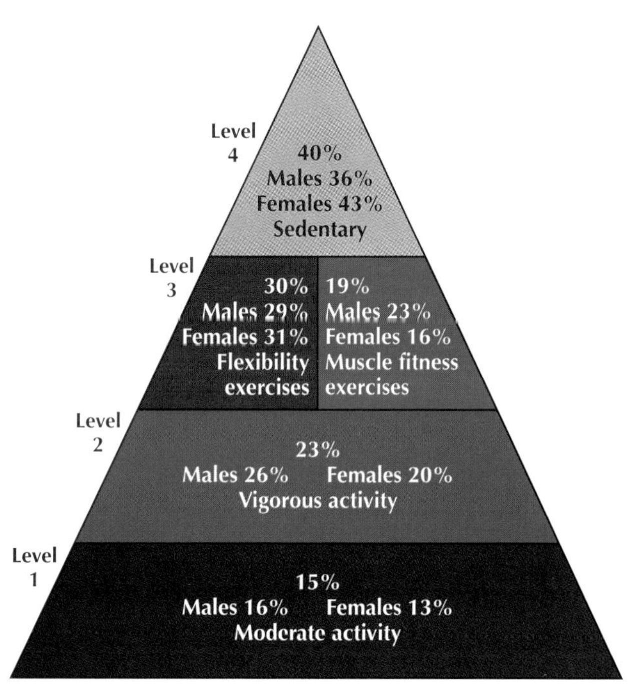

Figure 3

Proportion of adults meeting activity goals.

Based on data from *Healthy People 2010* (see Suggested Readings).

The Facts about Physical Activity Patterns

> The proportion of adults meeting national health goals varies with activity type and gender.

www.mhhe.com/phys_fit/webreview04 Click 05

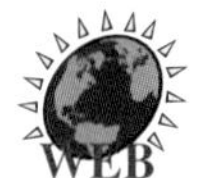

National health goals have been established for each of the different types of activity illustrated in the physical activity pyramid. The proportion of adults 18 years of age and older meeting these goals is shown in Figure 3. While lifestyle physical activities are recommended for 30+ minutes on most, if not all, days of the week, an adult is considered to be active if he or she does activity at least 5 days a week. The *Healthy People 2010* report shows that only 15 percent of adults meet this standard, with more men being active than women. The national goal is to increase this to 30 percent by the year 2010.

It is interesting that in recent years there has been a decrease in moderate activity and an increase in vigorous activity among adults (vigorous activity at least 3 days a week for 20 minutes). In the past more adults did moderate activity than vigorous activity, but the recent *Healthy People 2010* report indicates that more adults now do vigorous activity—mostly young adults—than moderate activity. The type of activity most practiced by adults is flexibility exercise (stretching), performed by 30 percent of all adults, though this statistic may be deceiving because of the frequency of doing the stretching exercises in days per week was not specified. Stretching is one form of exercise performed more frequently by women than men. Males are considerably more likely than females to do muscle fitness exercises at least two days per week. A total of 40 percent of adults do no regular leisure time physical activity, up considerably from previous years. Women are more likely than males to be sedentary (do no leisure time activity).

> The proportion of people meeting national health goals varies based on age.

Because it is difficult to measure physical activity among young children, the evidence concerning activity levels of children under age 12 is not as prevalent as for adolescents and adults. It is clear, however, that children are the most active group in western society, though they are active in different ways from adults. Young children are not likely to perform activity continuously but rather do intermittent bouts of activity followed by short rests. Recent guidelines indicate that this type of activity is very appropriate for children and attempts to get children to be active in ways similar to adults are inappropriate. For children, 60+ minutes and up to several hours of physical activity is recommended per day.

During adolescence, activity decreases with each year of schooling. Middle school students and freshmen in high school are much more active than seniors in high school. Though teens become less active with time, they still perform considerably more vigorous physical activity than adults in their 20s. Fifty-eight percent of high school seniors do vigorous activity at least three days a week compared to 32 percent of adults 18 to 24 years of age. Seventy-three percent of ninth grade students do regular vigorous physical activity. The lack of physical education in the upper grades accounts for some of the decrease in activity among older teens. In recent years there has been a decrease in physical education in secondary schools, leading to the establishment of a national health goal for the year 2010, designed to increase physical education to promote lifetime physical activity. Another health goal for children and adolescents is to reduce the amount of time spent watching television and playing video games.

The proportion of adults meeting national health goals varies based on a variety of characteristics.

Among the major characteristics associated with different levels of physical activity are age, education level, ethnicity, geographic location, and disability status. Some statistics for various groups' characteristics are illustrated in Table 1.

Based on the data presented in Table 1, there is no doubt that a variety of characteristics affect the amount and type of physical activities adults perform. Also of importance is the influence of social class and economic status. As a recent report indicates, social and economic factors are related to differences in activity levels among ethnic groups and those from urban versus rural areas. Clearly, education level is also a factor that contributes both to inactivity and social/economic

Table 1 The Percentage of Adults Meeting Activity Goals

Characteristic	Moderate Activity	Vigorous Activity	Muscle Fitness Exercise	Flexibility Exercises	No Leisure Activity
Age					
18–24	17	32	28	36	31
25–44	15	27	21	32	34
45–64	14	21	14	28	42
65–74	16	13	10	24	51
75+	12	0	7	22	65
Education					
Grades 9–11	11	12	8	16	59
HS graduate	14	18	11	23	46
Some college	17	24	19	36	35
College graduate	17	32	26	no data	24
Ethnicity					
Native/Indian Alaskan	13	19	18	26	46
Asian or Pacific Islander	15	17	17	34	42
Black/African American	10	17	16	26	52
Hispanic/Latino	11	16	13	22	54
White/non-Hispanic	16	25	19	31	36
Geographic Location					
Urban	15	24	19	32	39
Rural	15	21	15	24	43
Disability Status					
With	12	13	14	29	56
Without	16	25	20	31	36

SOURCE: From *Healthy People 2010* (see Suggested Readings).

class. One of the two major goals of *Healthy People 2010* is to eliminate health disparities among different segments of the population. Education in general, and educating the public about the value of physical activity and other health issues in specific, would appear to be important if we are to achieve this goal.

Strategies for Action: The Facts

> A self-assessment of your current activity at each level of the pyramid can help you determine future activity goals.

Lab 4A provides you with the opportunity to assess your physical activity at each level of the pyramid. Later you will be developing a program of activity, and these assessments will provide a basis for program planning.

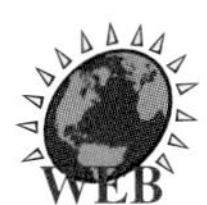

Web Review

Web review materials for Concept 4 are available at *www.mhhe.com/phys_fit/webreview01 click 06.*

American College of Sports Medicine
www.acsm.org

Healthy People 2010
www.health.gov/healthypeople

Medicine and Science in Sports and Exercise
www.acsm-msse.org

Morbidity and Mortality Weekly Reports
www.cdc.gov/mmwr

National Sports Medicine Institute of the United Kingdom
www.nsmi.org.uk

Surgeon General's Report on Physical Activity and Health
www.cdc.gov/nccdphp/sgr/sgr.htm

Suggested Readings

American College of Sports Medicine. *ACSM's Guidelines for Exercise Testing and Prescription.* 6th ed. Philadelphia: Lippincott, Williams and Wilkins, 2000.

Corbin, C. B., and Pangrazi, R. P. "Physical Activity Pyramid Rebuffs Peak Experience." *ACSM's Health and Fitness.* 2(1)(1998):12–17.

Crespo, C. J. et al. "Prevalence of Physical Inactivity and Its Relation to Social Class in U. S. Adults." *Medicine and Science in Sports and Exercise.* 31(12)(1999):1821–1826.

Howley, E. T., and Franks, B. D. *Health Fitness Instructor's Handbook.* (3rd ed.). Champaign, IL: Human Kinetics, 1997.

Medicine and Science in Sports and Exercise. "Dose-Response Issues Concerning Physical Activity and Health: An Evidence Based Symposium." *Medicine and Science in Sports and Exercise.* 33(6)(2001): entire issue.

Roitman, J. L. (ed.) *ACSM's Resource Manual for Guidelines for Exercise Testing and Prescription.* 4th ed. Philadelphia: Lippincott, Williams and Wilkins, 2001.

Spain, C. G., and Franks, B. D. "Healthy People 2010: Physical Activity and Fitness." *President's Council on Physical Fitness and Sports Research Digest.* 3(13)(2001):1–16.

U.S. Department of Health and Human Services. *Healthy People 2010.* 2nd ed. With *Understanding and Improving Health* and *Objectives for Improving Health.* 2 vols. Washington, DC: U.S. Government Printing Office, November 2000.

U.S. Department of Health and Human Services. *Physical Activity and Health: A Report of the Surgeon General.* Atlanta: U.S. Department of Health and Human Services, 1996.

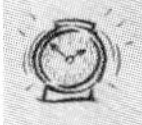

Physical Fitness News Update

The American College of Sports Medicine has published the most recent edition (6th) of its *Guidelines for Exercise Testing and Prescription,* designed to help individuals and exercise practitioners in planning activity programs for the new century. ACSM first developed guidelines in 1975 and has revised them frequently. ACSM periodically develops position statements on exercise testing and prescription. Activity recommendations presented in previous editions of this text were consistent with earlier versions of the ACSM guidelines, as well as with the 1998 position statements on "recommended quantity and quality of exercise for developing cardiorespiratory, muscular fitness, and flexibility in healthy adults," statements that have been incorporated into the new guidelines. The recommendations in this concept on "how much is enough," as well as other concepts in this text, are consistent with the new ACSM guidelines.

An important change in the new guidelines is the inclusion of more information on exercise prescription for health as opposed to fitness and performance enhancement. This shift is consistent with the Surgeon General's recommendations on physical activity and health that are featured in the new guidelines. This focus on health is emphasized in this text.

The authors of this text would like to join the American College of Sports Medicine in saluting Dr. Michael L. Pollock (1936–1998) whose research was central to the development of the guidelines of the College and the exercise recommendations in this book. Dr. Pollock was a good friend and classmate of the senior author of this text and was a model of scholarship for us all. He will be missed.

Concept 5

Learning Self-Planning Skills for Lifetime Physical Activity

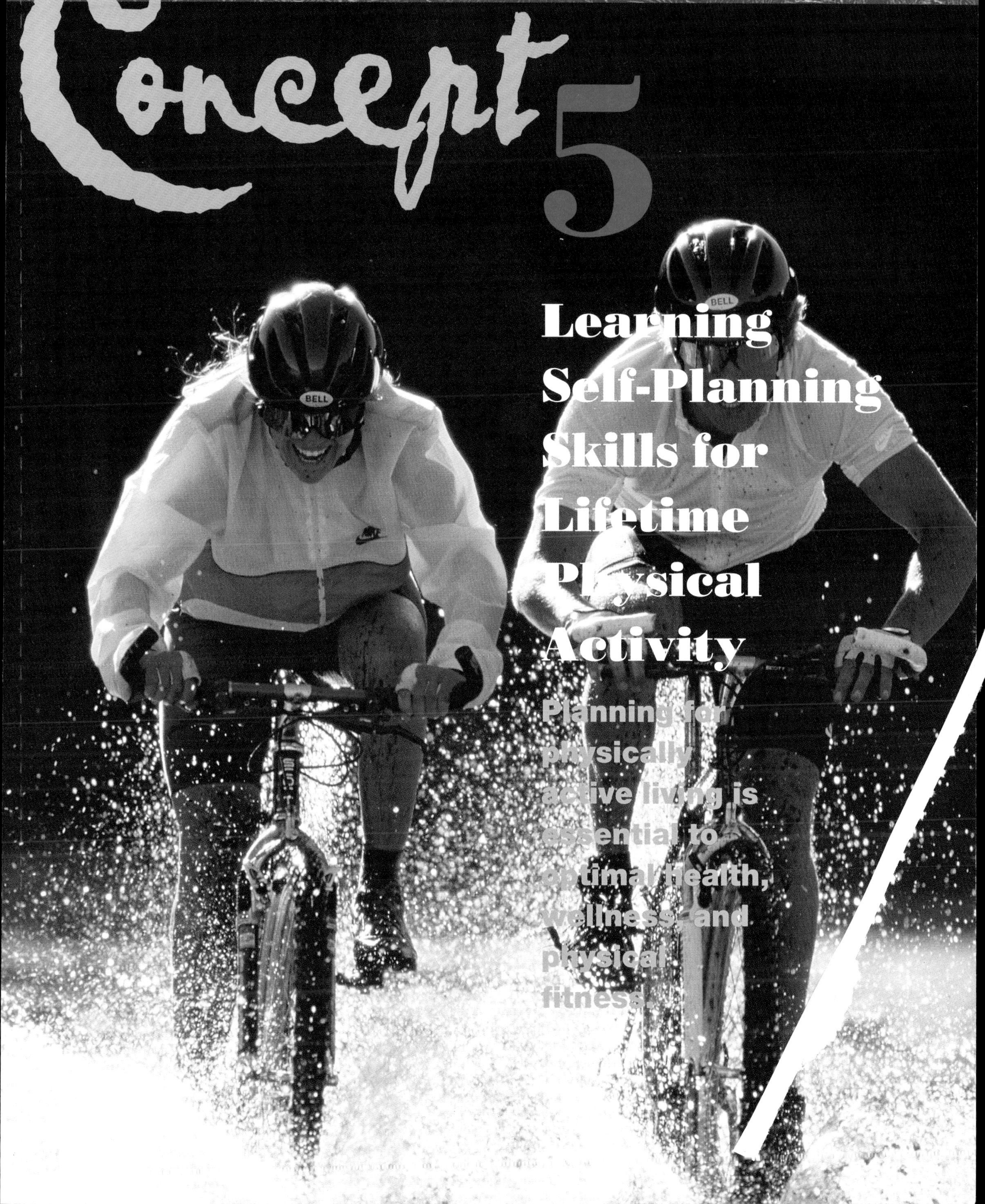

Planning for physically active living is essential to optimal health, wellness, and physical fitness.

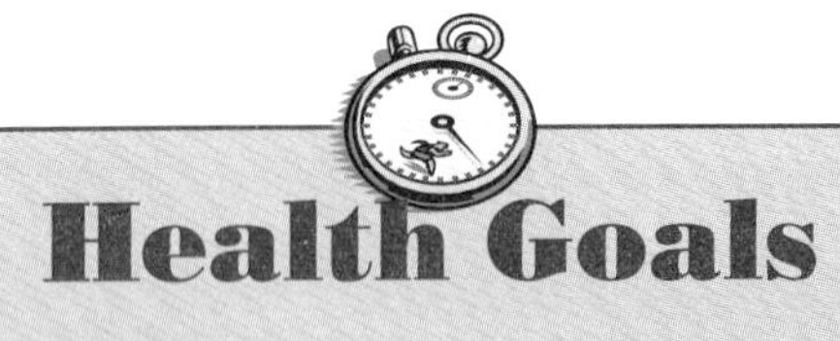

Health Goals

for year 2010

Improve the health, fitness, and quality of life of all people through the adoption and maintenance of regular, daily physical activity.

Increase leisure time physical activity.

Increase proportion of people who do moderate daily activity for 30 minutes.

Increase proportion of people who do vigorous physical activity three days a week.

Increase proportion of people who do regular muscle fitness exercise.

Increase proportion of people who do regular exercise for flexibility.

Increase prevalence of a healthy weight.

Introduction

There is no single exercise program best suited for all people, nor is there one best lifestyle for health, wellness, and fitness. When planning a program, it is important to consider your own unique needs and interests and to self-plan a program that is personal. In concept 2, you learned about self-management skills. In this concept, you will have the opportunity to practice and apply self-management skills that are especially useful in helping you plan for a lifetime of physical activity. Later you will learn self-management skills for use in developing other healthy lifestyles.

Clarifying Reasons for Participation: The Facts

Clarifying your reasons for participating, or not participating, in physical activity is an important step in self-planning.

As you continue your study in this book, you will be presented with a wide variety of physical activity choices. Your personal reasons for choosing to participate or not to participate should be clarified prior to planning your program. Over time, attitudes change, so periodic reassessment is recommended.

Knowing the most common reasons for inactivity can help you avoid sedentary living.

Some of the common reasons given by those who do not do regular physical activity are outlined in Table 1. Many of the reasons for not being active are considered by experts to be barriers that can be overcome. Overcoming barriers is a self-management skill. Using the solutions in Table 1 helps inactive people to become more active.

Knowing the reasons people give for being active can help you adopt positive attitudes.

www.mhhe.com/phys_fit/webreview05 Click 01

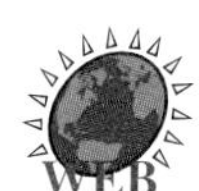

Table 2 describes some of the major reasons why people choose to be active. It also offers strategies for changing behavior if you have more than one or two negative attitudes. Active people have more positive than negative attitudes. This is referred to by experts as a positive "balance of attitudes." The questionnaire in Lab 5A gives you the opportunity to assess your balance of attitudes. If you have a negative balance score, you can analyze your attitudes and determine how you can change them to view activity more favorably.

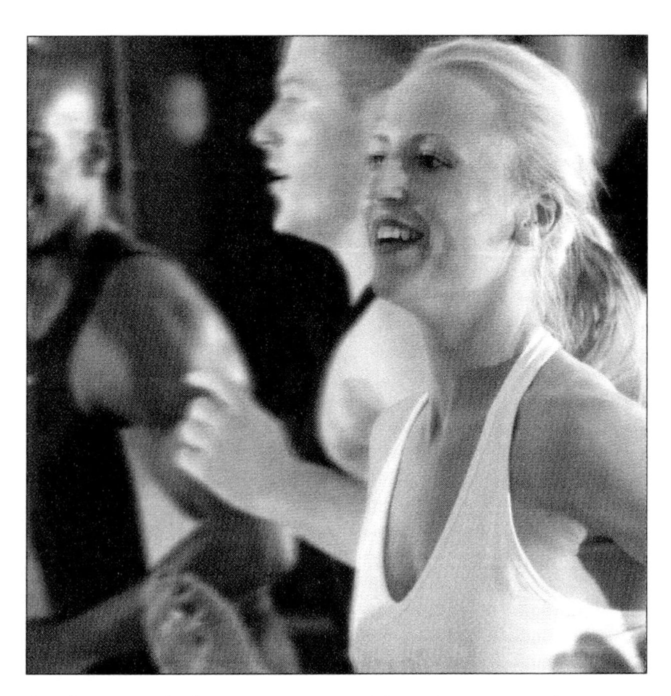

Active people have more positive than negative feelings about physical activity.

Table 1 Common Reasons People Give for Not Being Active

Reason	Description	Strategy for Change
"I don't have the time."	This is the number one reason people give for not exercising. Invariably, those who feel they don't have time indicate that they know they should do more exercise and that they plan to in the future when "things are less hectic." Young people say that they will soon be established in a career and then they will have the time to exercise. Older people say that they wish they had taken the time to be active when they were younger.	Planning a daily schedule can help you find the time for activity and avoid wasting time on things that are less important. Learning the facts in the concepts that follow will help you see the importance of activity and how you can include it in your schedule with a minimum of effort and with time efficiency.
"It's too inconvenient."	Many who avoid physical activity do so because it is inconvenient. They are procrastinators. Specific reasons for procrastinating include: "It makes me sweaty" and "It messes up my hair."	Research shows that if you have to travel more than 10 minutes to do activity or if you do not have easy access to equipment, you will avoid activity. Locating facilities and finding a time when you can shower is important.
"I just don't enjoy it."	Many do not find physical activity to be enjoyable or invigorating. These people may assume that all forms of activity have to be strenuous and fatiguing to count as exercise.	There are many activities to choose from. If you don't enjoy vigorous activity, try more moderate forms of activity such as walking.
"I'm no good at physical activity."	"People might laugh at me"; "Sports make me nervous"; and "I am not good at physical activities" are reasons some people give for not being active. These people often lack confidence in their own abilities. In some cases, this is because of their past experiences in physical education or athletics (sports).	With properly selected activities, even those who have never enjoyed exercise can get hooked. Building performance skills can help, as can changing your way of thinking. Avoiding comparisons to others can help you feel successful.
"I am not fit so I avoid activity."	Some people avoid exercise because of health reasons. Some who are unfit lack energy. Starting slowly can build fitness gradually and help you realize that you can do it.	There are good medical reasons for not doing physical activity, but many people with problems can benefit from exercise if it is properly designed. If necessary, get help adapting activity to meet your needs.
"I have no place to be active, especially in bad weather."	Regular activity is much more convenient if facilities are easy to reach and the weather is good. Still, recreational opportunities have increased considerably in recent years. Some of the most popular activities require very little equipment, can be done in or near the home, and are inexpensive.	If you cannot find a place, if it is not safe, or if it is too expensive, consider using low-cost equipment at home such as rubber bands or calisthenics. Lifestyle activity can be done by anyone at almost any time.
"I am too old."	As people grow older, many begin to feel that physical activity is something they cannot do. For most people, this is simply not true! Studies indicate that properly planned exercise for older adults is not only safe but also has many health benefits, including longer life, fewer illnesses, increased working capacity, an improved sense of well-being, and optimal functioning.	Older people who are just beginning activity should start slowly. Lifestyle activities are a good alternative. Setting realistic goals can help, as can learning new activity skills, such as resistance training and appropriate flexibility exercises.

Table 4 Self-Planning Skills

Self-Planning	Description	Self-Management Skill
Clarifying reasons	Knowing the general reasons why you might benefit helps you select activities that you will enjoy and adhere to for a lifetime.	Balancing Attitudes: Sections of this concept and Lab 5A help you determine if you have more positive than negative attitudes and help clarify your reasons for doing physical activity.
Identifying needs	If you know your strengths and weaknesses, you can plan to build on your strengths and overcome weaknesses.	Self-Assessment: In the concepts that follow, you will learn how to assess different health, wellness, and fitness characteristics. Learning these self-assessments will help you identify needs.
Establishing goals	Goals are more specific than reasons (see above). Establishing specific things that you want to accomplish can provide a basis for feedback that your program is working.	Goal Setting: Guidelines in this concept will help you set goals. In subsequent concepts, you will establish goals for different types of activity from the pyramid.
Selecting activities	A personal plan should include activities that meet your needs and goals (see steps above) and provide fun and enjoyment. Having skill improves enjoyment.	Performance Skills: In subsequent concepts, you will learn how to enhance your performance skills. Self-assessments will also help you match your abilities to specific activities.
Keeping records	Keeping records provides feedback and helps you adhere to your program.	Self-Monitoring: These skills are necessary for accurate record keeping.

Table 4 summarizes the self-planning and associated self-management skills presented in this concept.

Strategies for Action: The Facts

A self-assessment of your attitudes about physical activity is a good first step in planning for lifelong physical activity.

The physical activity attitudes questionnaire included in Lab 5A allows you the opportunity to consider your reasons for participating in physical activity. You will calculate a score for each of the nine attitudes described in Table 2. You will also calculate a balance of attitudes score that will indicate whether you have more positive than negative attitudes about physical activity. If you have low scores for certain attitudes, you should consider the strategies for action outlined in Table 2. Efforts to change attitudes are especially important for people with a negative balance of attitudes (poor or very poor ratings).

Self-planning skills can be used for each of the different types of activity in the physical activity pyramid.

In subsequent concepts, you develop self-plans for each of the types of activity in the physical activity pyramid. As you develop those plans, it will be useful to refer to the self-planning skills outlined in this concept.

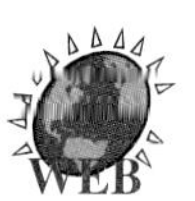

Web Review

Web review materials for Concept 5 are available at *www.mhhe.com/phys_fit/webreview05 Click 05.*

American College of Sports Medicine
www.acsm.org

The Fitness Jumpsite
www.primusweb.com/fitnesspartner

Health Canada-Physical Activity Guide
www.hc-sc.qc.ca/hppb/paguide

Planning Workouts
www.thriveonline.com

Suggested Readings

American College of Sports Medicine. *ACSM's Guidelines for Exercise Testing and Exercise Prescription.* 6th ed. Philadelphia: Lippincott, Williams and Wilkins, 2000.

Blair, S. N. et al. *Active Living Every Day.* Champaign, IL: Human Kinetics, 2001.

Brehm, B. A. "Maximizing the Psychological Benefits of Physical Activity." *ACSM's Health and Fitness Journal.* 4(6)(2000): 7–11.

Corbin, C. B., and Pangrazi, R. P. (Editors), *Towards a Better Understanding of Physical Fitness and Activity.* Scottsdale, AZ: Holcomb-Hathaway, 1999, Chapters 2 and 3.

Roitman, J. L. (ed.) *ACSM's Resource Manual for Guidelines for Exercise Testing and Prescription.* 4th ed. Philadelphia: Lippincott, Williams and Wilkins, 2001.

U.S. Department of Health and Human Services. *Physical Activity and Health: A Report of the Surgeon General.* Atlanta: U.S. Department of Health and Human Services, 1996.

Lab 5A: Physical Activity Attitude Questionnaire

Name	Section	Date

Purpose: To evaluate your feelings concerning physical activity and to determine the specific reasons why you do or do not participate in regular physical activity.

Procedures:

1. Read and answer each question in the questionnaire.
2. Make an X over the circle that best represents whether you strongly agree, agree, disagree, or strongly disagree. If you are unsure place an X on undecided.
3. Write the number in the circle of your answer in the box labeled "score" provided.
4. After you have answered all questions, add the two questions for each score and record the sum of the two items in the box provided on the questionnaire.
5. Record your scores in the chart provided in the results section.
6. Determine your rating for each score and record it in the chart in the results section.
7. Count the number of ratings that were good or excellent and record this number in the box as indicated.
8. Count the number of ratings that were fair, poor, or very poor and record this number in the box as indicated.
9. Subtract the number in the second box from the one in the first box to determine your balance of feelings score.
10. Determine your balance of feelings rating and record it in the appropriate space.

The Physical Activity Attitude Questionnaire

Directions: The term *physical activity* in the following statements refers to all kinds of activities, including sports, formal exercises, and informal activities, such as jogging and cycling. Make an X over the circle that best represents your answer to each question.

	Strongly Agree	Agree	Undecided	Disagree	Strongly Disagree	Score
1. I should do physical activity regularly for my health.	5	4	3	2	1	
2. Doing regular physical activity is good for my fitness and wellness.	5	4	3	2	1	
Health and Fitness Score (1 + 2)						
3. Regular exercise helps me look my best.	5	4	3	2	1	
4. I feel more physically attractive when I do regular physical activity.	5	4	3	2	1	
Appearance Score (3 + 4)						
5. One of the main reasons I do regular physical activity is because it is fun.	5	4	3	2	1	
6. The most enjoyable part of my day is when I am exercising or doing a sport.	5	4	3	2	1	
Enjoyment Score (5 + 6)						

	Strongly Agree	Agree	Undecided	Disagree	Strongly Disagree	Score
7. Taking part in physical activity helps me to relax.	5	4	3	2	1	
8. Physical activity helps me get away from the pressures of daily living.	5	4	3	2	1	
Relaxation Score (7 + 8)						
9. The challenge of physical training is one reason why I do physical activity.	5	4	3	2	1	
10. I like to see if I can master sports and activities that are new to me.	5	4	3	2	1	
Challenge Score (9 + 10)						
11. I like to do physical activity that involves other people.	5	4	3	2	1	
12. Exercise offers me the opportunity to meet other people.	5	4	3	2	1	
Social Score (11 + 12)						
13. Competition is a good way to make physical activity fun.	5	4	3	2	1	
14. I like to see how my physical abilities compare to others.	5	4	3	2	1	
Competition Score (13 + 14)						
15. When I do regular exercise, I feel better than when I don't.	5	4	3	2	1	
16. My ability to do physical activity is something that makes me proud.	5	4	3	2	1	
Feeling Good Score (15 + 16)						
17. I like to do outdoor activities.	5	4	3	2	1	
18. Experiencing nature is something I look forward to when exercising.	5	4	3	2	1	
Outdoor Nature Score (17 + 18)						

Results: Using the chart below record your scores as indicated in the procedures above.

Physical Activity Attitude Questionnaire Results

Attitude	Score	Rating
Health and Fitness		
Appearance		
Enjoyment		
Relaxation		
Challenge		
Social		
Competition		
Feeling Good		
Outdoor		

Rating Chart

Rating Category	Individual Scores	Balance of Feeling Score
Excellent	9–10	+5 to +9
Good	7–8	+2 to +4
Fair	5–6	0 to +1
Poor	3–4	–1 to –2
Very Poor	2	more than –2

Record the number of good and excellent ratings. ☐

Record the number of fair, poor, or very poor ratings. ☐

Subtract the number from box 2 from the number in box 1. This is your balance of feelings score. ☐

Balance of Feelings Rating ☐

Conclusions and Implications:

1. In a few sentences, discuss your results on the Physical Activity Attitude Questionnaire (ratings for the nine attitude scores). Include comments on whether you think your ratings suggest that you will be active or inactive and whether your ratings are really indicative of your feelings.

2. In a few sentences, discuss your "balance of feelings" rating. Having more positive than negative scores (positive balance of feelings) increases the probability of being active. Include comments on whether you think your ratings suggest that you will be active or inactive and whether your ratings are really indicative of your feelings. Do you think that the scores on which you were rated poor or very poor might be reasons why you would avoid physical activity? Explain.

Concept 6

The Health Benefits of Physical Activity

Physical activity and good physical fitness can reduce risk of illness and contribute to optimal health and wellness.

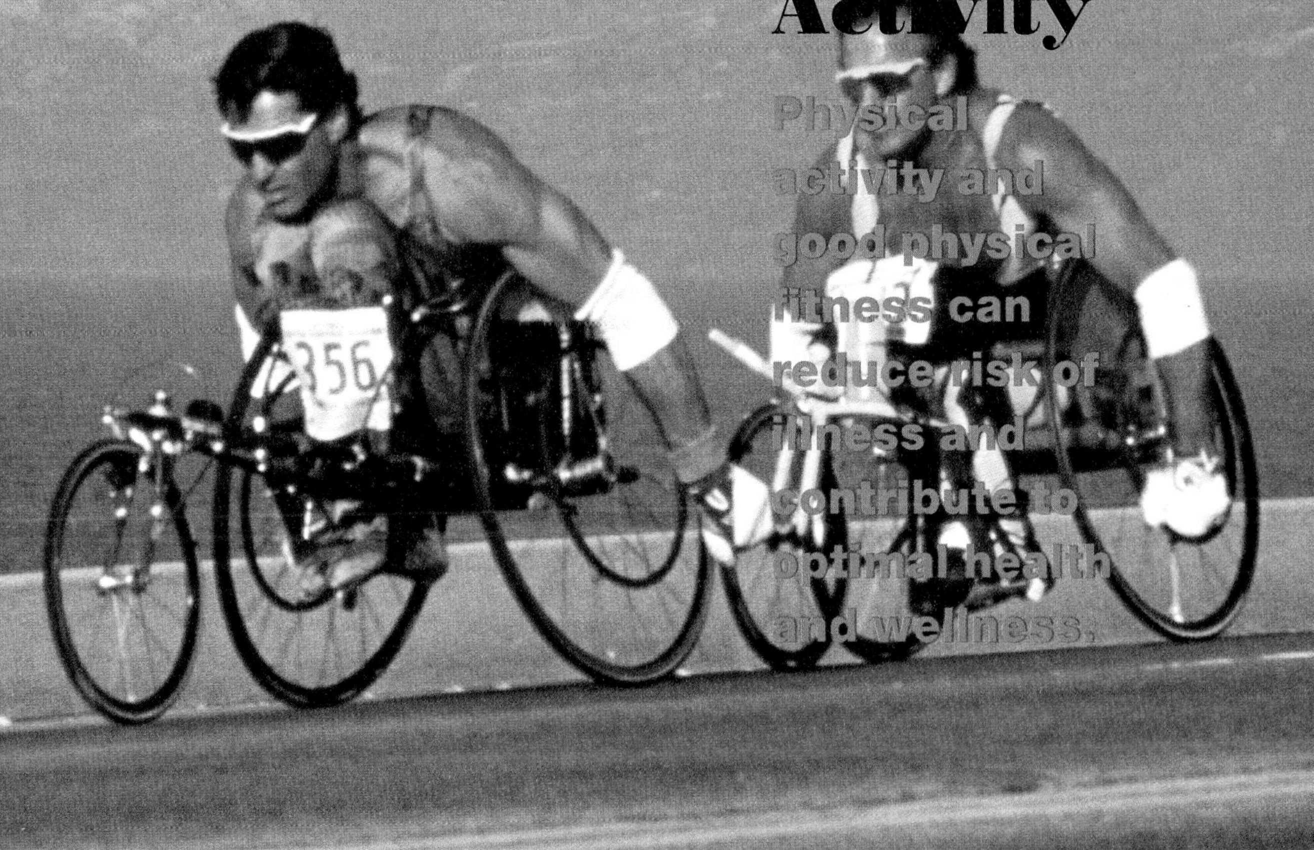

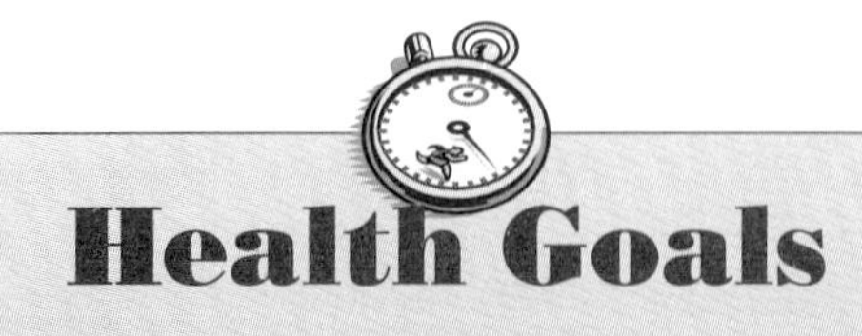

Health Goals

for year 2010

Increase quality and years of healthy life.

Increase incidence of people reporting "healthy days."

Increase incidence of people reporting "active days."

Increase the adoption and maintenance of daily physical activity.

Increase prevalence of a healthy weight and reduce prevalence of overweight.

Reduce days with pain for those with arthritis, osteoporosis, and chronic back problems.

Reduce activity limitations, especially among older adults.

Reduce incidence of and deaths from cancer.

Increase diagnosis of and reduce incidence of Type II diabetes.

Decrease incidence of depression.

Decrease incidence of heart diseases including stroke and high blood pressure.

Decrease incidence of high cholesterol levels among adults.

Introduction

At no time in our history has so much evidence been accumulated to demonstrate the health and wellness benefits of physical activity and fitness. The American Heart Association has elevated sedentary living to the status of a "primary risk factor" for heart disease, indicating that activity is of primary rather than secondary importance in preventing heart disease. The recent *Surgeon General's Report on Physical Activity and Health* is an especially powerful document summarizing the benefits of regular physical activity and good fitness. It provides definitive evidence of the value of physical activity and fitness to sound health and wellness. *Healthy People 2010*, the national health goals that take us into the twenty-first century, emphasize physical activity as one of the key healthy lifestyles contributing to optimal health, wellness, and fitness. Each of these documents is cited to support the facts in this concept.

The Facts about Physical Activity, Fitness, and Disease Prevention/Treatment

There are three major ways in which regular physical activity and good fitness contribute to optimal health and wellness.

The methods by which physical activity and fitness contribute to optimal health and wellness are illustrated in Figure 1. First, they can aid in disease/illness prevention. There is considerable evidence that the risk of **hypokinetic conditions** can be greatly reduced among people who do regular physical activity and achieve good physical fitness. Virtually all **chronic diseases** that plague society are considered to be hypokinetic, though some relate more to inactivity than others. Nearly three-quarters of all deaths among those 18 and older are a result of chronic diseases.

Leading public health officials have suggested that physical activity is related to the health of all Americans. It directly reduces the risk for several major chronic diseases. Physical activity also stimulates positive changes with respect to other risk factors for these diseases. Physical activity may produce the stimulus for the control of chronic diseases, much like immunization controlled infectious diseases.

Second, physical activity and fitness can be a significant contributor to disease/illness treatment. Even with the best disease-prevention practices, some people will become ill. Regular exercise and good fitness have been shown to be effective in alleviating symptoms and aiding rehabilitation after illness for such hypokinetic conditions as diabetes, heart attack, back pain, and others.

Finally, physical activity and fitness are methods of health and wellness promotion. They contribute to quality living associated with wellness, the positive component of good health. In the process they aid in meeting many of the nation's health goals for the year 2010.

Too many adults suffer from hypokinetic diseases.

In 1961, Kraus and Raab coined the term "hypokinetic disease." They pointed out that recent advances in medicine had been quite effective in eliminating infectious diseases but that degenerative diseases, characterized by sedentary or "take-it-easy" living, had increased in recent decades. In fact, heart disease is the leading cause of death in North America. High blood pressure, stroke, and coronary artery disease (including heart attack) afflict millions each year. The second leading medical complaint (headache is number one) is low back

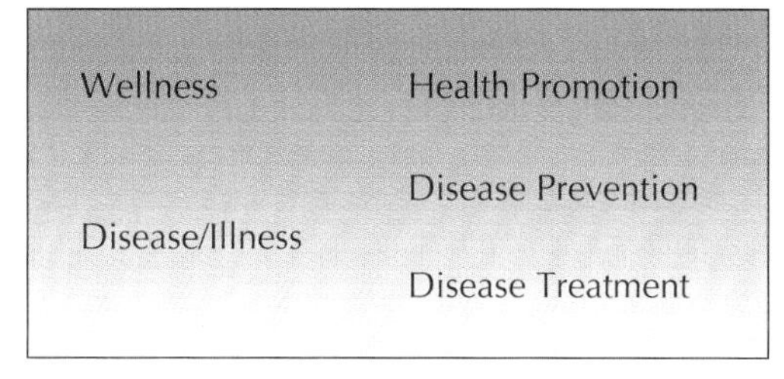

Figure 1
Contributors to optimal health and wellness.

pain, and as many as one-half of all adults are considered to be obese. Studies show that the symptoms of hypokinetic conditions begin in youth. This suggests that the incidence of hypokinetic disease in our culture will not be reduced without considerable lifestyle change in people of all ages.

The link between regular physical activity and good health is now well documented.

www.mhhe.com/phys_fit/webreview06 Click 01

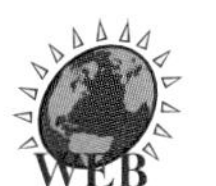

People who do regular physical activity can reduce their risk of death, regardless of the cause. Active people increase their life expectancy by two years compared to those who are inactive. Sedentary people experience a 20 percent to two-fold increase in early death compared to active people. One leading public health official indicates that increasing physical activity among the adult population would do wonders for the health of the nation because there are so many sedentary people who could benefit from active lifestyles. He notes that physical inactivity, in combination with the poor eating patterns, ranks with tobacco use among the leading preventable contributors to death for adults. If adults who lead sedentary lives would adopt a more active lifestyle, there would be enormous benefit to the public's health and to individual well-being. The major health benefits of physical activity as outlined in the *Surgeon General's Report* and other important recent reports are summarized later in this concept.

Regular physical activity over a lifetime may overcome the effects of inherited risk.

Some people with a family history of disease may conclude that there is nothing they can do because their heredity works against them. There is no doubt that heredity significantly affects risk of early death from hypokinetic diseases. New studies of twins, however, suggest that active people are less likely to die early than inactive people with similar genes. This suggests that long-term adherence to physical activity can overcome other risk factors such as heredity—at least for some people.

Hypokinetic diseases and conditions have many causes.

Regular physical activity and good physical fitness are only two of the preventative factors associated with the conditions described in this concept as hypokinetic diseases. Other healthy lifestyle factors cannot be overlooked in the prevention of these diseases.

The Facts about Physical Activity and Cardiovascular Diseases

There are many types of cardiovascular diseases.

There are many forms of **cardiovascular diseases (CVD).** Some are classified as **coronary heart disease (CHD)** because they affect the heart muscle and the blood vessels

Hypokinetic Conditions *Hypo-* means "under" or "too little," and *-kinetic* means "movement" or "activity." Thus, *hypokinetic* means "too little activity." A hypokinetic disease or condition is associated with lack of physical activity or too little regular exercise. Examples of such conditions include heart disease, low back pain, adult-onset diabetes, and obesity.

Chronic Disease A disease or illness that is associated with lifestyle or environmental factors as opposed to infectious diseases (hypokinetic diseases are considered to be chronic diseases).

Cardiovascular Disease (CVD) A broad classification of diseases of the heart and blood vessels that include CHD, as well as high blood pressure, stroke, and peripheral vascular disease.

Coronary Heart Disease (CHD) Diseases of the heart muscle and the blood vessels that supply it with oxygen, including heart attack.

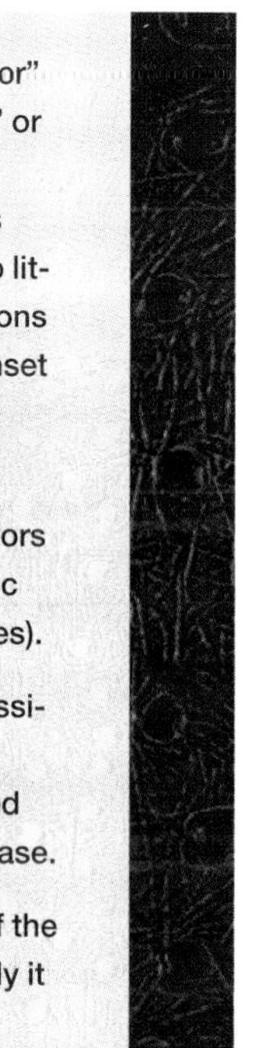

inside the heart. **Coronary occlusion** (heart attack) is a type of CHD. **Atherosclerosis** and **arteriosclerosis** are two conditions that increase risk of heart attack and are also considered to be types of CHD. **Angina pectoris** (chest or arm pain), which occurs when the oxygen supply to the heart muscle is diminished, is sometimes considered to be a type of CHD though it is really a symptom of poor circulation.

Hypertension (high blood pressure), **stroke** (brain attack), **peripheral vascular disease,** and **congestive heart failure** are other forms of CVD. Inactivity relates in some way to each of these types of disease.

> The various forms of cardiovascular disease are the leading killers in automated societies.

In the United States, coronary heart disease accounts for approximately 31 percent of all premature deaths. Stroke accounts for an additional 7 percent. Men are more likely to suffer from heart disease than women. African American, Hispanic, and Native American populations are at higher-than-normal risk. Heart disease and stroke death rates are similar in the United States, Canada, Great Britain, Australia, and other automated societies.

> There is a wealth of statistical evidence that physical inactivity is a primary risk factor for CHD.

Much of the research relating inactivity to heart disease has come from occupational studies that show a high incidence of heart disease in people involved only in sedentary work. Even with the limitations inherent in these types of studies, the findings of more and more occupational studies present convincing evidence that the inactive individual has an increased risk of coronary heart disease. A study summarizing all of the important occupational studies shows a 90 percent reduced risk of coronary heart disease for those in active versus inactive occupations.

Studies also indicate that adults who expend a significant number of calories per week in strenuous sports and other activities have reduced risk of coronary heart disease. In fact, improving activity levels is among the best ways to reduce the risk of heart disease among adults.

The American Heart Association, after carefully examining the research literature, concluded that a sedentary lifestyle is a risk factor comparable to high blood pressure, high blood cholesterol, obesity, and cigarette smoke. After reviewing hundreds of studies on exercise and heart disease, the *Surgeon General's Report on Physical Activity and Health* concluded that "physical inactivity is causally linked to atherosclerosis and coronary heart disease."

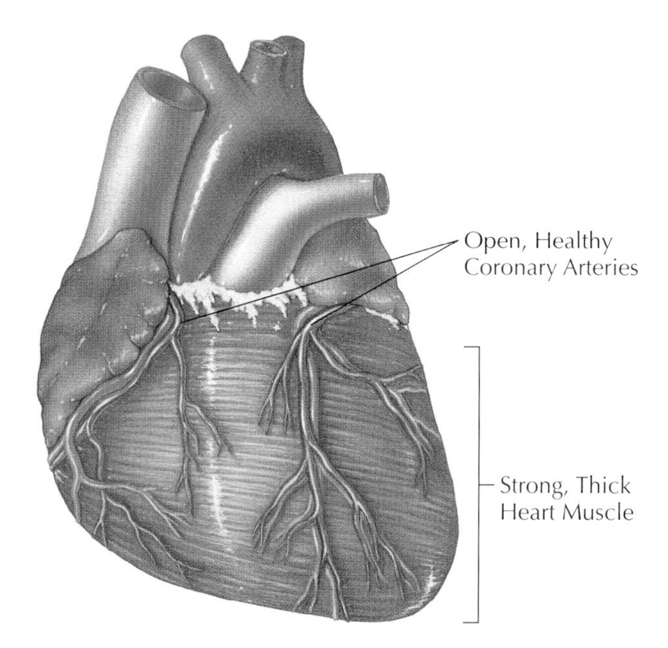

Figure 2
The fit heart muscle.

The Facts about Physical Activity and the Healthy Heart

> There is evidence that regular physical activity will increase the ability of the heart muscle to pump blood as well as oxygen.

A fit heart muscle can handle extra demands placed on it. Through regular exercise, the heart muscle gets stronger, contracts more forcefully, and therefore pumps more blood with each beat. This results in a slower heart rate (especially during physical activity), and greater heart efficiency. The heart is just like any other muscle—it must be exercised regularly to stay fit. The fit heart has open, clear arteries free of atherosclerosis. (See Figure 2.)

The hypothetical "normal" resting heart rate is said to be 72 beats per minute (bpm). However, resting rates of 50 to 85 bpm are not uncommon. People who regularly do physical activity will typically have lower resting heart rates than people who do no regular activity. Some endurance athletes have heart rates in the 30 and 40 bpm range. This is not considered unhealthy or abnormal. While resting heart rate is *not* considered to be a good measure of health or fitness, decreases in individual heart rate following training reflect positive adaptations. Low heart rates in response to a standard amount of physical activity *are* a good indicator of fitness. The bicycle and step tests presented later in this book use your heart rate response to a standard amount of exercise to estimate your cardiovascular fitness.

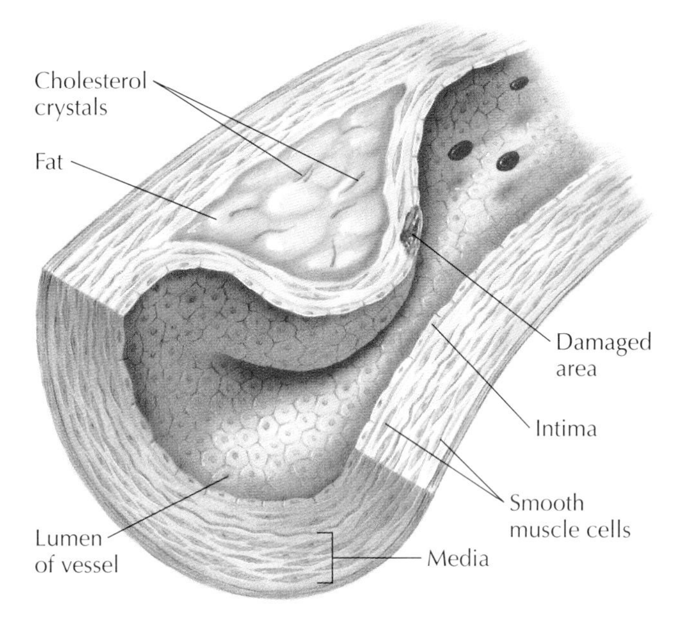

Figure 3
Atherosclerosis.

The Facts about Physical Activity and Atherosclerosis

Atherosclerosis is implicated in many cardiovascular diseases.

Atherosclerosis is a condition that contributes to heart attack, stroke, hypertension, angina pectoris, and peripheral vascular diseases. Deposits on the walls of arteries restrict blood flow and oxygen supply to the tissues. Atherosclerosis of the coronary arteries, the vessels that supply the heart muscle with oxygen, is particularly harmful. If these arteries become narrowed, the blood supply to the heart muscle is diminished, and angina pectoris may occur. Atherosclerosis increases the risk of heart attack because a fibrous clot is more likely to obstruct a narrowed artery than a healthy, open one.

Atherosclerosis, which begins early in life, is the result of a systematic buildup of deposits in an arterial wall.

Current theory suggests that atherosclerosis begins when damage occurs to the cells of the inner wall or intima of the artery (see Figure 3). Substances associated with blood clotting are attracted to the damaged area. These substances seem to cause the migration of smooth muscle cells, commonly found only in the middle wall of the artery (media), to the intima. In the later stages, fats (including cholesterol) and other substances are thought to be deposited, forming plaques or protrusions that diminish the internal diameter of the artery. Research indicates that the first signs of atherosclerosis begin in early childhood.

There is evidence that regular physical activity can help prevent atherosclerosis.

All of the ways in which regular exercise help prevent atherosclerosis are not yet known. However, three of the most plausible theories are discussed on the next page.

Coronary Occlusion The blocking of the coronary blood vessels.

Atherosclerosis The deposition of materials along the arterial walls; a type of arteriosclerosis.

Arteriosclerosis Hardening of the arteries due to conditions that cause the arterial walls to become thick, hard, and nonelastic.

Angina Pectoris Chest or arm pain resulting from reduced oxygen supply to the heart muscle.

Hypertension High blood pressure.

Stroke (Cerebrovascular Accident or CVA) A condition in which the brain, or part of the brain, receives insufficient oxygen as a result of diminished blood supply; sometimes called apoplexy.

Peripheral Vascular Disease Lack of oxygen supply to the working muscles and tissues of the arms and legs resulting from decreased blood flow.

Congestive Heart Failure The inability of the heart muscle to pump the blood at a life-sustaining rate.

Lipid Deposit Theory

www.mhhe.com/phys_fit/webreview06 Click 02

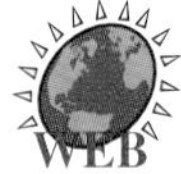

There are several kinds of **lipids** in the bloodstream, including **lipoproteins,** phospholipids, triglycerides, and cholesterol. Cholesterol is the most well-known, but it is not the only culprit. Many blood fats are manufactured by the body itself, while others are ingested in high-fat foods, particularly saturated fats. Saturated fats are fats that are solid at room temperature.

As noted earlier, blood lipids are thought to contribute to the development of atherosclerotic deposits on the inner walls of the artery. One substance, called **low-density lipoprotein (LDL),** is considered to be a major culprit in the development of atherosclerosis. LDL is basically a core of cholesterol surrounded by protein and another substance that makes it water soluble. The theory is that regular exercise can reduce blood lipid levels, including LDL-C (the cholesterol core of LDL). People with high total cholesterol and LDL-C levels have been shown to have a higher-than-normal risk of heart disease (see Table 1). New evidence indicates that there are subtypes of LDL cholesterol (characterized by their small size and high density) that pose even greater risks. These subtypes are hard to measure and not included in most current blood tests, but future research will no doubt help us better understand and measure them.

Triglycerides are another type of blood lipid. Elevated levels of triglycerides are positively related to heart disease. Triglycerides lose some of their ability to predict heart disease with the presence of other risk factors, so high levels are more difficult to interpret than other blood lipids. Normal levels are considered to be 150 mg/dL or less. Values of 151 to 199 are borderline, 200 to 499 are high, and above 500 are very high. It would be wise to include triglycerides in a blood lipid profile. Physical activity is often prescribed as part of a treatment for high triglyceride levels.

Protective Protein Theory

www.mhhe.com/phys_fit/webreview06 Click 03

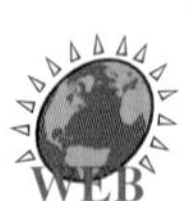

Whereas LDLs carry a core of cholesterol that is involved in the development of atherosclerosis, **high-density lipoprotein (HDL)** picks up cholesterol (HDL-C) and carries it to the liver, where it is eliminated from the body. For this reason, it is often called the "protective protein." High levels of HDL are considered to be desirable. When you have a blood test, it is wise to ask for information about total cholesterol, LDL, and HDL levels. A recent report has provided new information about healthy levels for each (see Table 1). Individuals who do regular physical activity have lower total cholesterol, lower LDL, and higher HDL levels.

Table 1 Cholesterol Classifications (mg/dL)

	Total Cholesterol	LDL-C	HDL-C
Optimal	—	<100	—
Near Optimal	—	100-129	—
Desirable	<200	—	>60
Borderline	200–240	130–160	39–59
High Risk	>240	>160	40

Source: Third Report of the National Cholesterol Education Program, 2001.

Other Theories

There are at least two other theories that relate to the build up of atherosclerosis in the arteries. The blood coagulant theory suggests that **fibrin** and platelets (types of cells involved in blood coagulation) deposit at the site of an injury on the wall of the artery contributing to the process of plaque buildup or atherosclerosis. Regular physical activity has been shown to reduce fibrin levels in the blood. The breakdown of fibrin seems to reduce platelet adhesiveness and the concentration of platelets in the blood. The immune system theory suggests that physical activity may influence the immune system in a positive way by lowering atherosclerosis promoting immune cells in the blood and by protecting the lining of the artery.

The Facts about Physical Activity and Heart Attack

Heart attack is the most prevalent and serious of all cardiovascular diseases.

A heart attack occurs when a coronary artery is blocked (see Figure 4). A clot or thrombus is the most common cause, reducing or cutting off blood flow and oxygen to the heart muscle. If the coronary artery that is blocked supplies a major portion of the heart muscle, death will occur within minutes. Occlusions of lesser arteries may result in angina pectoris or a nonfatal heart attack.

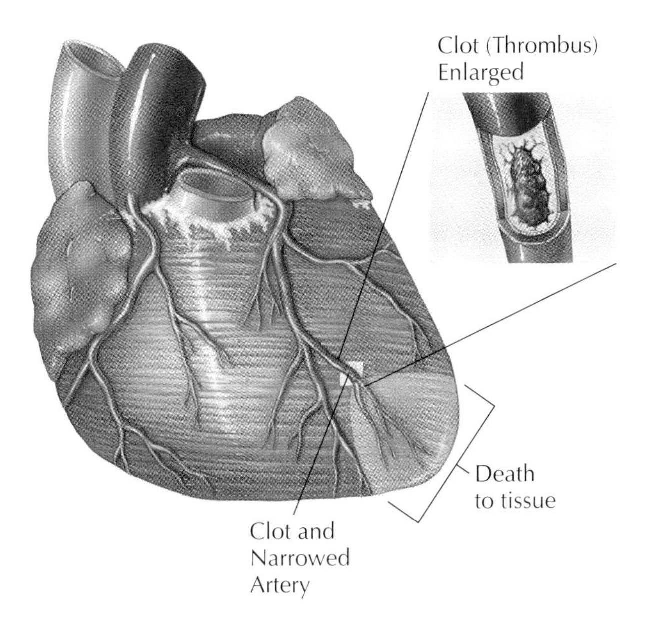

Figure 4
Heart attack.

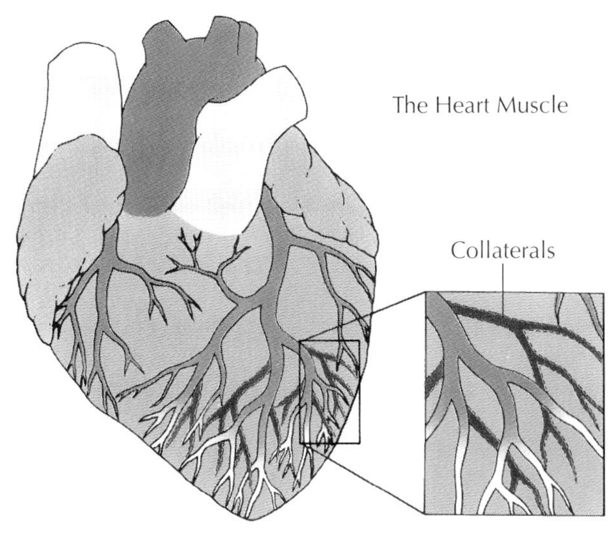

Figure 5
Coronary collateral circulation.

Regular physical activity reduces the risk of heart attack (coronary occlusion).

People who perform regular sports and physical activity have half the risk of a first heart attack compared to those who are sedentary. Possible reasons are less atherosclerosis, greater diameter of arteries, and less chance of a clot forming.

There is evidence that regular exercise can improve coronary circulation and thus reduce the chances of a heart attack or dying from one.

Within the heart, there are many tiny branches extending from the major coronary arteries. All of these vessels supply blood to the heart muscle. Healthy arteries can supply blood to any region of the heart as it is needed. Active people are likely to have greater blood-carrying capacity in these vessels, probably because the vessels are larger and more elastic. Also, the active person may have a more profuse distribution of arteries within the heart muscle (see Figure 5), which results in greater blood flow. A few studies show that physical activity may promote the growth of "extra" blood vessels, which are thought to open up to provide the heart muscle with the necessary blood and oxygen when the oxygen supply is diminished, as in a heart attack. Blood flow from extra blood vessels is referred to as **coronary collateral circulation.**

Improved coronary circulation may provide protection against a heart attack because a larger artery would require more atherosclerosis to occlude it. In addition, the development of collateral blood vessels supplying the heart may diminish the effects of a heart attack if one does occur. These extra (or collateral) blood vessels may take over the function of regular blood vessels during a heart attack.

Lipids All fats and fatty substances.

Lipoprotein Fat-carrying protein in the blood.

Low-Density Lipoprotein (LDL) A core of cholesterol surrounded by protein; the core is often called "bad cholesterol."

Triglyceride A type of blood fat associated with increased risk of heart disease.

High-Density Lipoprotein (HDL) A blood substance that picks up cholesterol and helps remove it from the body; often called "good cholesterol."

Fibrin A sticky threadlike substance that in combination with blood cells forms a blood clot.

Coronary Collateral Circulation Circulation of blood to the heart muscle associated with the blood-carrying capacity of a specific vessel or development of collateral vessels (extra blood vessels).

The heart of the inactive person is less able to resist stress and is more susceptible to an emotional storm that may precipitate a heart attack.

The heart is rendered inefficient by one or more of the following circumstances: high heart rate, high blood pressure, and excessive stimulation. All of these conditions require the heart to use more oxygen than is normal and decrease its ability to adapt to stressful situations.

The inefficient heart is one that beats rapidly because it is dominated by the **sympathetic nervous system,** which speeds up the heart rate. Thus, the heart continuously beats rapidly, even at rest, and never has a true rest period. A study of one college basketball coach who was under considerable stress indicated that his lowest resting heart rate during the day was 88 bpm. High blood pressure also makes the heart work harder and contributes to its inefficiency.

Research indicates five things concerning physical activity and the inefficient heart.

1. Regular activity leads to dominance of the **parasympathetic nervous system** rather than to sympathetic dominance; thus the heart rate is reduced and the heart works efficiently.
2. Regular activity helps the heart rate return to normal faster after emotional stress.
3. Regular activity strengthens the heart muscle, making it better able to weather an **emotional storm.**
4. Regular activity decreases sympathetic dominance and its associated hormonal effects on the heart, thus lessening the chances of altered heart contractility and the likelihood of the circulatory problems that accompany this state.
5. Regular activity reduces the risk of sudden death from ventricular fibrillation (arrhythmic heartbeat).

Regular physical activity is one effective means of rehabilitation for a person who has coronary heart disease or who has had a heart attack.

Not only does regular physical activity seem to reduce the risk of developing coronary heart disease, there is also evidence that those who already have the condition may reduce the symptoms of the disease through regular exercise. For people who have had heart attacks, regular and progressive exercise can be an effective prescription when carried out under the supervision of a physician. Remember, however, that exercise is not the treatment of preference for all heart attack victims. In some cases, it may be contraindicated.

The Facts about Physical Activity and Other Cardiovascular Diseases

Regular physical activity is associated with a reduced risk of high blood pressure (hypertension).

www.mhhe.com/phys_fit/webreview06 Click 04

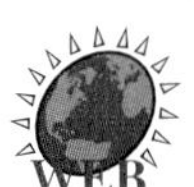

Approximately 30 percent of adults have borderline or high-risk hypertension. More men than women are likely to be hypertensive, as are more blacks than whites. Native Americans and Hispanics have a higher-than-normal incidence of hypertension, and the incidence for all groups increases as people grow older. A recent research summary indicates that the effects of physical activity on blood pressure are more dramatic than previously thought and are independent of age, body fatness, and other factors. Inactive, less-fit individuals have a 30 to 50 percent greater chance of being hypertensive than active, fit people. Regular physical activity can also be one effective method of reducing blood pressure for those with hypertension. Physical inactivity in middle age is associated with risk of high blood pressure later in life. The most plausible reason is a reduction in resistance to blood flow in the blood vessels, probably resulting from dilation of the vessels.

The hypothetical "goal" blood pressure is 120 mm Hg (**systolic blood pressure**) over 80 mm Hg (**diastolic blood pressure**). However, systolic pressures as low as 100 mm Hg and up to 130 mm Hg are considered in the normal range. Diastolic pressures of 60 to 85 mm Hg are also considered to be in the normal range. Exceptionally low blood pressures (below 100 systolic and 60 diastolic) do not pose the same risks to health as high blood pressure but can cause dizziness, fainting, and lack of tolerance to change in body positions. Classifications for blood pressure are shown in Table 2. Stage 1 hypertension is sometimes called "mild," Stage 2 "moderate," and Stage 3 "severe." Some experts do not like these terms because people with "mild" or "moderate" hypertension may not feel the need to seek medical help. All stages of hypertension should be taken seriously.

Regular physical activity can help reduce the risk of stroke.

Stroke is a major killer of adults. People with high blood pressure and atherosclerosis are susceptible to stroke. Since regular exercise and good fitness are important to the prevention of both high blood pressure and atherosclerosis, exercise and fitness are considered helpful in the prevention of stroke.

Table 2 Blood Pressure Classifications for Adults*

Category	Systolic Blood Pressure (mm Hg)	Diastolic Blood Pressure (mm Hg)
Goal	<120	<80
Normal	<130	<85
High Normal	130–139	85–89
Stage 1 Hypertension	140–159	90–99
Stage 2 Hypertension	160–179	100–109
Stage 3 Hypertension	≥180	≥110

*Not taking antihypertensive drugs and not acutely ill. When the systolic and diastolic blood pressure categories vary, the higher reading determines the blood pressure classification.

SOURCE: National Institutes for Health, 1997 (see Suggested Readings).

Regular physical activity is helpful in the prevention of peripheral vascular diseases.

www.mhhe.com/phys_fit/webreview06 Click 05

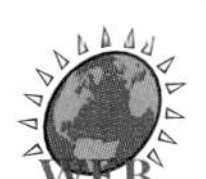

There is evidence that people who exercise regularly have better blood flow to the working muscles and other tissues than inactive, unfit people. Since peripheral vascular disease is associated with poor circulation to the extremities, regular exercise can be considered one method of preventing this condition.

The Facts about Physical Activity and Other Hypokinetic Conditions

Physical activity reduces the risk of some forms of cancer.

www.mhhe.com/phys_fit/webreview06 Click 06

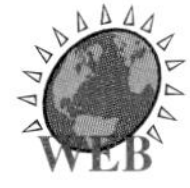

Cancer is the second leading cause of death in the United States. According to the American Cancer Society, cancer is a group of diseases characterized by uncontrollable growth and spread of abnormal cells. Several cancers are considered hypokinetic. Adequate data are now available to document the relationship of inactivity to colon cancer. Inactive people have a 50 to 250 percent greater risk of getting colon cancer than active people. Consistent findings also suggest that rectal cancer is also associated with inactivity. The relationship between fitness, exercise, and other forms of cancer is not yet fully understood. One possible reason why regular exercisers have a reduced risk of colon/rectal cancer (the second most common cause of cancer deaths among males) is the faster intestinal transit time.

Several studies have suggested that fit people who regularly perform physical activity have increased protection against reproductive system and breast cancers. One study indicates a one-third reduction in risk of breast cancer among those who do at least four hours of leisure physical activity each week as compared to those who are less active. (People who do heavy manual labor have an even greater reduction in risk.) In fact, nonathletes have been found to have a greater risk of breast cancer than athletes. On the other hand, a recent study of Harvard graduates failed to find a strong link between activity and breast cancer. Researchers who have shown a relationship between activity and breast cancer hypothesize that regular physical activity in youth may delay the onset of menstruation and reduce the lifelong exposure to estrogen. This suggests a hormonal link between physical activity and breast cancer. A causal link between activity and breast cancer has yet to be established—more research is necessary. For those who have cancer, there is evidence that physical activity can help them lead more fulfilling and productive lives.

Physical activity plays an important role in the management and treatment of Type II diabetes.

www.mhhe.com/phys_fit/webreview06 Click 07

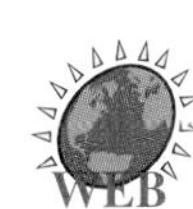

Diabetes is a group of disorders that results when there is too much sugar in the blood. It occurs when the body does not make enough

Sympathetic Nervous System Branch of the autonomic nervous system that prepares the body for activity by speeding up the heart rate.

Parasympathetic Nervous System Branch of the autonomic nervous system that slows the heart rate.

Emotional Storm A traumatic emotional experience that is likely to affect the human organism physiologically.

Systolic Blood Pressure The upper blood pressure number often called working blood pressure. It represents the pressure in the arteries at its highest level just after the heart beats.

Diastolic Blood Pressure The lower blood pressure number often called "resting pressure." It is the pressure in the arteries at its lowest level occurring just before the next beat of the heart.

insulin or when the body is not able to use insulin effectively. Diabetes is the seventh leading cause of death among people over 40. It accounts for at least 10 percent of all short-term hospital stays and has a major impact on health-care costs in Western society. By itself, exercise is not an effective treatment for Type I (insulin-dependent) diabetes. However, with medical supervision, exercise is encouraged for maintaining fitness for most diabetics.

People who perform regular physical activity are less likely to suffer from Type II (noninsulin-dependent, adult-onset) diabetes than sedentary people. For people with Type II diabetes, regular physical activity can help reduce body fatness, decrease **insulin resistance,** improve **insulin sensitivity,** and improve the body's ability to clear sugar from the blood in a reasonable time. All of these factors contribute to controlling the disease. With sound nutritional habits and proper medication, physical activity can be useful in the management of both types of diabetes.

> Regular physical activity is important to maintaining bone density and decreasing risk of osteoporosis.

www.mhhe.com/phys fit/webreview06 Click 08

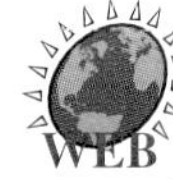

As noted in Concept 1, bone integrity is considered by some experts as a health-related component of physical fitness. Healthy bones are dense and strong. When bones lose calcium and become less dense they become porous and are at risk of fracture. The bones of young children are not especially dense, but during adolescence (see Figure 6) bone density increases to a level higher than at any other time in life (peak bone density). Though bone density often begins to decrease in young adulthood, it is not until older adulthood that bone loss becomes dramatic. As illustrated in Figure 6, many older adults have lost enough bone density to have a condition called **osteoporosis** (when bone density drops below the osteoporosis threshold). Some will have crossed the fracture threshold, putting them at risk of fractures especially to the hip, vertebrae, and other "soft" or "spongy" bones of the skeletal system. Active people have a higher peak bone mass and are more resistant to osteoporosis (see blue line in Figure 6) than sedentary people (see red line in Figure 6).

Women, especially post-menopausal women, have a higher risk of osteoporosis than men. Males typically have a higher peak bone mass than females and for this reason can lose more bone density over time without reaching the osteoporosis or fracture thresholds. More women reach the osteoporosis and fracture thresholds at earlier ages than men. Other risk factors for osteoporosis are northern European ancestry, smoking, alcohol use, current or previous eating disorders, early menstruation, and low dietary calcium intake. People who are confined to bed rest are especially at risk of osteoporosis because regular exercise is necessary for good bone health.

Guidelines for building bone integrity and preventing osteoporosis include the following:

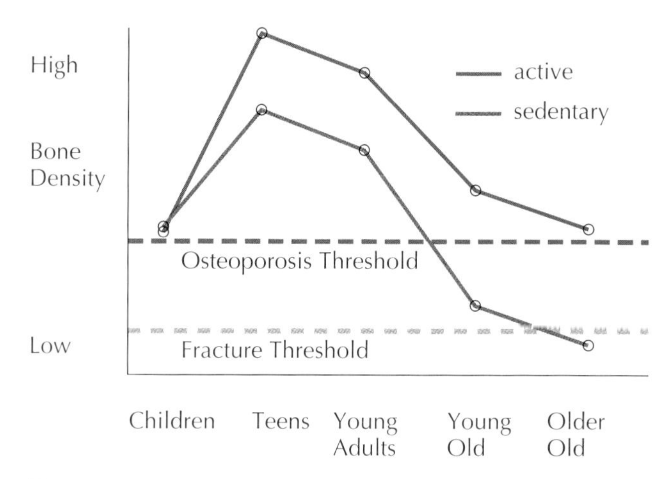

Figure 6
Changes in Bone Density with Age.

- Do regular weight bearing exercise and resistance training that stresses the bones of the body. The load bearing and pull of the muscles in these types of exercises builds bone density.
- Eat a diet rich in calcium. Calcium is necessary to build strong bones. At risk groups should consider a calcium supplement.
- Post-menopausal women should consider a calcium supplement, special medication to prevent bone loss, and/or an estrogen supplement.
- Start early in life to build strong bones because peak bone mass is developed in the teen years.
- It is never too late to start. Following these guidelines has been shown to help people of all ages, including those 80 and over.
- Older people with osteoporosis should consider protective pads shown to prevent fractures from falls.

> Active people who possess good muscle fitness are less likely to have back and other musculoskeletal problems than inactive, unfit people.

Because few people die from it, back pain does not receive the attention given to such medical problems as heart disease and cancer. But back pain is considered to be the second leading medical complaint in the United States, second only to headaches. Only common colds and flu cause more days lost from work. At some point in our lives, approximately 80 percent of all adults will experience back pain that limits their ability to function normally. Recent National Safety Council data indicated that the back was the most frequently injured of all body parts, and the injury rate was double that of any other part of the body.

Many years ago, medical doctors began to associate back problems with the lack of physical fitness. It is now known that the great majority of back ailments are the result of poor muscle strength and endurance, and poor flexibility. Tests on patients with back problems show weakness and lack of flexibility in key muscle groups.

Though lack of fitness is probably the leading reason for back pain in Western society, there are many other factors that increase the risk of back ailments, including poor posture, improper lifting and work habits, heredity, and disease states, such as scoliosis and arthritis.

Physical activity is important in maintaining a healthy body weight and avoiding the numerous health conditions associated with obesity.

Obesity, as well as lesser degrees of fatness, is not a disease state in itself but is a hypokinetic condition associated with a multitude of far-reaching complications. Obesity is associated with a variety of organic impairments, psychosocial problems, and shortened life span. Recent studies show that fat people who are fit are not especially at high risk of early death. However, "metabolic syndrome"—sometimes called syndrome X—that includes high body fatness, especially high abdominal fatness, combined with high blood fat levels, high blood sugar levels, insulin resistance, and high blood pressure is associated with risk for heart disease, diabetes, and other chronic diseases. Because physical activity, together with sound nutritional management, is an effective means of lowering body fat and other symptoms of metabolic syndrome, it can be helpful in reducing the risk of a variety of chronic diseases.

Physical activity reduces the risk and severity of a variety of common mental (emotional) health disorders. Such disorders can be considered hypokinetic conditions.

Some mental (emotional) health conditions are prevalent in modern society. According to the *Surgeon General's Report on Physical Activity and Health,* nearly one of every two adult Americans will report having a mental health disorder at some point in life. A recent summary of studies revealed that there are several mental/emotional disorders that are associated with inactive lifestyles.

Depression is a stress-related condition experienced by many adults. Thirty-three percent of inactive adults report that they often feel depressed. For some, depression is a serious disorder that physical activity alone will not cure; however, recent research does indicate that activity, combined with other forms of therapy, can be effective.

Anxiety is an emotional condition characterized by worry, self-doubt, and apprehension. More than a few studies have shown that symptoms of anxiety can be reduced by regular activity. Low-fit people who do regular aerobic activity seem to benefit the most. In one study, one-third of very active people felt that regular activity helped them to better cope with life's pressures.

Physical activity is also associated with better and more restful sleep. People with insomnia (the inability to sleep) seem to benefit from regular activity if it is not done too vigorously right before going to bed. A recent study indicates that 52 percent of the population feel that physical activity helps them sleep better. Regular aerobic activity is associated with reduced brain activation that can result in greater ability to relax or fall asleep.

Even more common than depression and insomnia is the condition called Type A behavior. Type A personalities are stress-prone individuals with a greater than normal incidence of diseases. A Type A person is tense, overcompetitive, and worried about meeting time schedules. Apparently all Type A personalities are not equally stressed. It has been suggested that aggressive Type A personalities are most likely to be prone to negative consequences of stress. Regular physical activity can benefit the Type A person—especially the aggressive Type A. Noncompetitive activities would probably be best for this stress-prone personality type.

A final benefit of regular physical activity is increased self-esteem. Improvements in fitness and appearance can improve self-confidence and self-esteem. The ability to regulate behavior and perform new tasks can also promote higher self-esteem.

Regular physical activity can have positive effects on some non-hypokinetic conditions.

Some non-hypokinetic conditions that can benefit from physical activity are:

- Arthritis. Many, if not most, arthritics are in a deconditioned state resulting from a lack of activity. The traditional advice that arthritics should avoid physical activity is now being modified in view of the findings that carefully prescribed exercise can improve general fitness and, in some cases, reduce the symptoms of the disease.

Insulin A hormone secreted by the pancreas that regulates levels of sugar in the blood.

Insulin Resistance A condition that occurs when insulin becomes ineffective or less effective than is necessary to regulate sugar levels in the blood.

Insulin Sensitivity A person with insulin resistance (see above) is said to have decreased insulin sensitivity. The body's cells are not sensitive to insulin so they resist it and sugar levels are not regulated effectively.

Osteoporosis A condition associated with low bone density and subsequent bone fragility leading to high risk of fracture.

- Asthma. Asthmatics often have physical activity limitations. New evidence suggests that, with proper management, activity can be part of their daily life. In fact, when done properly, activity can reduce airway reactivity and medication use. Because exercise can trigger bronchial constriction, it is important to choose appropriate types of activity and to use inhaled medications to prevent bronchial constriction caused by exercise or other triggers such as cold weather. Cold weather exercise should typically be avoided.
- Immune system disorders. Recent evidence suggests that regular moderate physical activity can enhance immune system function and help people resist infections. However, vigorous training can temporarily reduce immune function, so people with systemic infections such as colds or flu should avoid heavy training. There is evidence that regular activity for immune system disorders such as HIV can enhance quality of life.
- Premenstrual syndrome (PMS). PMS, a mixture of physical and emotional symptoms that occurs prior to menstruation, has many causes. However, current evidence suggests that changes in lifestyle, including regular exercise, may be effective in relieving PMS symptoms.
- Other conditions. Aerobic activity and resistance training are currently being prescribed for some people who have chronic pain (persistent pain without relief) and evidence suggests that active people have a 30 percent lesser chance of having gallstones than inactive people.

The Facts about Physical Activity and Aging

> Regular physical activity can improve fitness and improve functioning among older adults.

www.mhhe.com/phys_fit/webreview06 Click 09

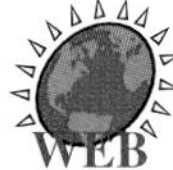

Approximately 30 percent of adults age 70 and over have difficulty with one or more activities of daily living. Women have more limitations than men, and low-income groups have more limitations than higher-income groups. Nearly half get no assistance with the activity in which they are limited.

The inability to function effectively as you grow older is associated with lack of fitness and inactive lifestyles. This loss of function is sometimes referred to as "acquired aging" as opposed to "time-dependent" aging. Because so many people experience limitations in daily activities and often find it difficult to get assistance, it is especially important for older people to stay active and fit. In Africa, Asia, and South America, where older adults maintain an active lifestyle, individuals do not acquire many of the characteristics commonly associated with aging in North America.

The *Surgeon General's Report* indicates that, in general, older adults become much less active than younger adults. Losses in muscle fitness are associated with loss of balance, greater risk of falling, and less ability to function independently. Though the amount of activity performed must be adapted as people grow older, fitness benefits discussed in the next section and throughout this book apply to people of all ages.

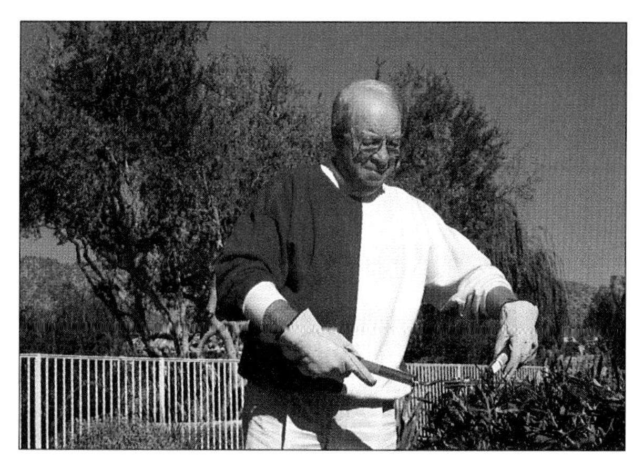

Fitness improves work efficiency.

> Regular physical activity can compress illness into a shorter period of our life.

www.mhhe.com/phys_fit/webreview06 Click 10

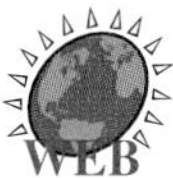

An important national health goal is to increase the years of healthy life. Living longer is important, but being able to function effectively during all years of life is equally—if not more—important. "Compression" refers to shortening the total number of years that illnesses and disabilities occur. The average person lives to the national average of 77 years and has nearly 12 years of illness. Compressing the illness means dramatically decreasing the years of illness. Healthy lifestyles, including regular physical activity, have been shown to compress illness and increase years of effective functioning.

Facts about Health, Fitness, and Wellness Promotion

> Physical activity enhances metabolic fitness that can reduce risk of a variety of health problems.

Metabolism refers to the chemical and physiological processes of the body that lead to the production of energy. When the metabolic systems of the body do not work effectively, it can lead to risk of chronic diseases such as diabetes and heart disease. Metabolic fitness is the positive

Table 3 Health and Wellness Benefits of Physical Activity and Fitness

Major Benefit	Related Benefits
Improved cardiovascular fitness and health	• Stronger heart muscle • Lower heart rate • Better electric stability of heart • Decreased sympathetic control of heart • Increased O_2 to brain • Reduced blood fat, including low-density lipids (LDLs) • Increased protective high-density lipids (HDLs) • Delayed development of atherosclerosis • Increased work capacity • Improved peripheral circulation • Improved coronary circulation • Resistance to "emotional storm" • Reduced risk of heart attack • Reduced risk of stroke • Reduced risk of hypertension • Greater chance of surviving a heart attack • Increased oxygen-carrying capacity of the blood
Greater lean body mass and less body fat	• Greater work efficiency • Less susceptibility to disease • Improved appearance • Less incidence of self-concept problems related to obesity
Improved strength and muscular endurance	• Greater work efficiency • Less chance of muscle injury • Reduced risk of low back problems • Improved performance in sports • Quicker recovery after hard work • Improved ability to meet emergencies
Bone development	• Greater peak bone density • Less chance of osteoporosis
Reduced cancer risk	• Reduced risk of colon cancer • Possible reduced risk of rectal, reproductive, and breast cancers
Improved metabolic fitness	• Decreased diabetes risk • Quality of life for diabetics • Less risk of Syndrome X
Enhanced mental health and function	• Relief of depression • Improved sleep habits • Fewer stress symptoms • Ability to enjoy leisure and work • Improved brain function
Opportunity for social interactions	• Improved quality of life
Resistance to fatigue	• Ability to enjoy leisure • Improved quality of life • Improved ability to meet some stressors
Opportunity for successful experience	• Improved self-concept • Opportunity to recognize and accept personal limitations • Improved sense of well-being • Enjoy life—fun
Improved appearance	• Better figure/physique • Better posture • Fat control
Reduced effect of acquired aging	• Improved ability to function in daily life • Better short-term memory • Fewer illnesses • Greater mobility • Greater independence • Greater ability to operate an automobile
Improved flexibility	• Greater work efficiency • Less chance of muscle injury • Less chance of joint injury • Decreased chance of low back problems • Improved sports performance
Other health benefits	• Extended life • Decrease in dysfunctional years • Aids some people who have arthritis, PMS, asthma, and chronic pain

states of these systems, evidenced by healthy blood fat (lipid) profiles, healthy blood pressure, healthy blood sugar and insulin levels, and other nonperformance measures including a healthy body fatness level. It is apparent that many of the factors that constitute metabolic fitness are common to more than a few of the hypokinetic conditions described in this concept. For this reason, good metabolic fitness is important to an overall reduced risk of disease. Good metabolic fitness is, for all practical purposes, the opposite of metabolic syndrome or Syndrome X described previously.

Good health-related physical fitness and regular physical activity are important to health promotion and feeling well.

Optimal health is more than freedom from disease. Regular physical activity and good fitness not only help prevent illness and disease but also promote quality of life and feeling well. Good health-related fitness can help you feel good, look good, and enjoy life. Table 3 presents a summary of some of the more specific benefits associated with physical activity.

Good physical fitness can help an individual enjoy his or her leisure time.

A person who is lean, has no back problems, does not have high blood pressure, and has reasonable skills in a lifetime of sports is more likely to get involved and stay regularly involved in leisure-time activities than one who does not have these characteristics. It is said that enjoying your leisure time may not add years to your life, but can add life to your years.

Good physical fitness can help an individual work effectively and efficiently.

A person who can resist fatigue, muscle soreness, back problems, and other symptoms associated with poor health-related fitness is capable of working productively and having energy left over at the end of the day. Surveys of employees who are involved with employee fitness programs indicate that 75 percent have an improved sense of well-being. Employers indicate that absenteeism decreased by up to 50 percent among program participants. People with good skill-related fitness may be more effective and efficient in performing specific motor skills required for certain jobs.

Good physical fitness is essential to effective living.

Although the need for each component of physical fitness is specific to each individual, every person requires enough fitness to perform normal daily activities without undue fatigue. Whether it be walking, performing household chores, or merely feeling good and enjoying the simple things in life without pain or fear of injury, good fitness is important to all people.

Good physical fitness may help you function safely and assist you in meeting unexpected emergencies.

Emergencies are never expected, but when they do arise, they often demand performance that requires good fitness. For example, flood victims may need to fill sandbags for hours without rest, and accident victims may be required to walk or run long distances for help. Also, good fitness is required for such simple tasks as safely changing a spare tire or loading a moving van without injury.

Physical fitness is the basis for dynamic and creative activity.

Though the following quotation by former President John F. Kennedy is more than 30 years old, it clearly points out the importance of physical fitness.

> The relationship between the soundness of the body and the activity of the mind is subtle and complex. Much is not yet understood, but we know what the Greeks knew: that intelligence and skill can only function at the peak of their capacity when the body is healthy and strong, and that hardy spirits and tough minds usually inhabit sound bodies. Physical fitness is the basis of all activities in our society; if our bodies grow soft and inactive, if we fail to encourage physical development and prowess, we will undermine our capacity for thought, for work, and for the use of those skills vital to an expanding and complex America.

President Kennedy's belief that activity and fitness are associated with intellectual functioning has now been backed up with research. A recent research summary suggests that, though modest, the effect of activity and fitness on intellectual functioning is positive. One study shows activity to foster new brain cell growth. Time taken to be active during the day has been shown to help children learn more, even though less time is spent in intellectual pursuits.

There are many economic benefits associated with employee physical activity.

A comprehensive review of the literature indicates that worksite physical activity programs can improve health, wellness, and fitness; reduce health care costs; and decrease absenteeism. The costs associated with providing physical activity for employees more than offsets the cost of medical care and lost days of work associated with inactivity. Nearly half of worksites offer some type of program. A national goal is to increase this to 75 percent.

The Facts about Risk Factors

There are many different positive lifestyles that can reduce the risk of disease.

Many of the factors that contribute to optimal health and quality of life are also considered risk factors. Changing these risk factors can dramatically reduce the risk of hypokinetic diseases such as heart disease, back pain, diabetes, and cancer. Lack of physical activity, poor nutrition, smoking, and inability to cope with stress are all risk factors associated with various diseases (see Table 4).

Not all risk factors are under your personal control.

Some factors that can contribute to the increased risk of disease are not under your personal control. Three uncontrollable

Table 4 Hypokinetic Disease Risk Factors

Factors That Cannot Be Altered

1. **Age**—As you grow older, your risk of contracting hypokinetic diseases increases. For example, the risk of heart disease is approximately three times as great after 60 as before. The risk of back pain is considerably greater after 40.
2. **Heredity**—People who have a family history of hypokinetic disease are more likely to develop a hypokinetic condition, such as heart disease, hypertension, back problems, obesity, high blood lipid levels, and other problems. African Americans are 45 percent more likely to have high blood pressure than Caucasians; therefore, they suffer strokes at an earlier age with more severe consequences.
3. **Gender**—Men have a higher incidence of many hypokinetic conditions than women. However, differences between men and women have decreased recently. This is especially true for heart disease, the leading cause of death for both men and women. Postmenopausal women have a higher heart disease risk than pre-menopausal women.

Factors That Can Be Altered

4. **Body fatness**—Having too much body fat is now a primary risk factor for heart disease and is a risk factor for other hypokinetic conditions as well. For example, loss of fat can result in relief from symptoms of adult-onset diabetes, can reduce problems associated with certain types of back pain, and can reduce the risks of surgery.
5. **Diet**—There is a clear association between hypokinetic disease and certain types of diets. The excessive intake of saturated fats, such as animal fats, is linked to atherosclerosis and other forms of heart disease. Excessive salt in the diet is associated with high blood pressure.
6. **Diseases**—People who have one hypokinetic disease are more likely to develop a second or even a third condition. For example, if you have diabetes,* atherosclerosis, or high blood pressure, your risk of having a heart attack or stroke increases dramatically. People with poor posture have a high risk of experiencing back pain, and those with too much body fat have a greater-than-normal risk of diabetes. Although you may not be entirely able to alter the extent to which you develop certain diseases and conditions, reducing your risk and following your doctor's advice can improve your odds significantly.
7. **Regular physical activity**—As noted throughout this book, regular exercise can help reduce the risk of hypokinetic disease.
8. **Tobacco use**—Smokers have a much higher risk of developing and dying from heart disease than nonsmokers. The risk of heart attack is twice as great among young smokers as among young nonsmokers. (Most striking is the difference in risk between older women smokers and nonsmokers.) Smokers have five times the risk of heart attack as nonsmokers. Tobacco use is also associated with the increased risk of high blood pressure, cancer, and several other medical conditions. Apparently, the more you use, the greater the risk. Stopping tobacco use even after many years can significantly reduce the hypokinetic disease risk.
9. **Stress**—There is evidence that people who are subject to excessive stress are predisposed to various hypokinetic diseases including heart disease and back pain. Statistics indicate that hypokinetic conditions are common among those in certain high-stress jobs and those having type A personality profiles.

*Some types of diabetes cannot be altered.

risk factors are age, heredity, and gender. These factors that cannot be altered by lifestyle changes are presented in Table 4.

Altering risk factors can help reduce the risk of more than one adverse condition at the same time.

By altering the risk factors that are controllable, you can reduce the risk of several hypokinetic conditions. For example, controlling body fatness reduces the risk of diabetes, hypertension, and back problems. Altering your diet can reduce the chances of developing high levels of blood lipids, and thus reduce the risk of atherosclerosis.

Risk reduction does not guarantee freedom from disease.

Reducing risk alters the probability of disease, but does not assure disease immunity.

Too much physical activity can lead to hyperkinetic diseases or conditions.

www.mhhe.com/phys_fit/webreview06 Click 11

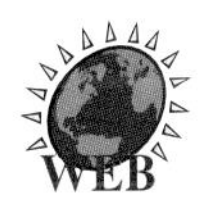

The information presented in this concept points out the health benefits of physical activity performed in appropriate amounts. When done in excess or incorrectly, physical activity can result in **hyperkinetic conditions.** The most common hyperkinetic condition is overuse injury to muscles, connective tissue, and bones. Recently, anorexia nervosa and body neurosis have been identified as conditions associated with inappropriate amounts of physical activity. These conditions will be discussed in the concept on performance.

Hyperkinetic Condition A disease/illness or health condition caused by or contributed to by too much physical activity.

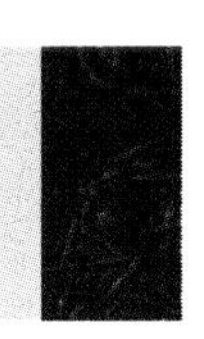

Strategies for Action: The Facts

> A self-assessment of risk factors can help you modify your lifestyle to reduce risk of heart disease.

The Heart Disease Risk Factor Questionnaire in Lab 6A will help you assess your personal risk for heart disease. While this questionnaire considers the major risk factors, there are two recently identified factors that are not included: C-reactive protein (CRP) and homocysteine. Women with high CRP have four times the risk of having heart disease as those with low CRP. Used along with other blood tests, the CRP may prove to be useful in the future. Screening for CRP is currently available with regular blood lipid tests, though data are lacking for men.

High levels of the amino acid homocysteine have also been associated with increased risk of heart disease, though the American Heart Association says it is too soon to do general screening for it. Adequate folic acid, vitamin B6, and Vitamin B12 help prevent high homocysteine in the blood, so eating foods that insure adequate daily intake of these vitamins is recommended. Because evidence is only preliminary at this point, these two risk factors are not included in this questionnaire.

You can use your self-assessments on the questionnaire to determine your alterable, unalterable, and total risk scores. These scores should be useful in preparing a plan for lifestyle change to reduce risk.

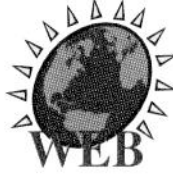

Web Review

Web review materials for Concept 6 are available at *www.mhhe.com/phys_fit/webreview06 Click 12.*

American Cancer Society
www.cancer.org

American Diabetes Association
www.diabetes.org

American Heart Association
www.americanheart.org

Centers for Disease Control and Prevention
www.cdc.gov

Healthy People 2010
www.health.gov/healthypeople

National Stroke Association
www.stroke.org

National Osteoporosis Foundation
www.nof.org

Suggested Readings

Booth, F. W. et al. "Waging War on Modern Chronic Diseases: Primary Prevention through Exercise Biology." *Journal of Applied Physiology.* 88(2)(2000): 774–787.

Brehm, B. A. "Maximizing the Psychological Benefits of Physical Activity." *ACSM's Health and Fitness Journal.* 4(6)(2000): 7–11.

Brill, P. A. et al. "Muscular Strength and Physical Function." *Medicine and Science in Sports and Exercise.* 32(2)(2000): 412–416.

Colberg, S. R. "Exercise: A Diabetes "Cure" for Many." *ACSM's Health and Fitness Journal.* 5(2)(2001): 20–26.

Dembo, L., and McCormick, K. M. "Exercise Prescription to Prevent Osteoporosis." *ACSM's Health and Fitness Journal.* 4(1)(2000): 32–38.

Durak, E. "The Use of Exercise in the Cancer Recovery Process." *ACSM's Health and Fitness Journal.* 5(1)(2001): 6–10.

Etnier, J. L. et al. "The Influences of Physical Fitness and Exercise Upon Cognitive Functioning: A Meta Analysis." *The Journal of Sport and Exercise Psychology.* 19(3)(1997):249.

Lee, I., and Paffenbarger, R.S. "Preventing Coronary Heart Disease: The Role of Physical Activity." *The Physician and Sports Medicine.* 29(2)(2001):37–52.

Leutholtz, B. C. "Exercise Can Reduce Incidence and Severity of Hypertension." *ACSM's Health and Fitness.* 2(5)(1998):36.

Manilow, M. R., Bostom, A. G., and Krauss, R. M. "Homocysteine, Diet and Cardiovascular Disease: A Statement for Health Care Professionals from the Nutrition Committee of the American Heart Association." *Circulation.* 99(1)(1999): 178–182.

McGill, S. M. "Low Back Stability." *Exercise and Sports Science Reviews.* 29(1)(2001): 26–31.

Metcalf, L. et al. "Postmenopausal Women and Exercise for Prevention of Osteoporosis." *ACSM's Health and Fitness Journal.* 5(3)(2001): 6–11.

Moseley, P. L. "Exercise, Stress, and the Immune Conversation." *Exercise and Sport Sciences Reviews.* 28(3)(2000): 128–132.

National Cholesterol Education Program. "Executive Summary of the Third Report of the National Cholesterol Education Program Expert Panel on Detection, Evaluation, and Treatment of High Blood Cholesterol in Adults." *Journal of the American Medical Association.* 285(2001): 2486–2497.

National Institutes of Health. The Sixth Report of the Joint National Committee on Detection, Evaluation, and Treatment of High Blood Pressure, NIH Publication Number 98-4080, 1997.

Nieman, D. C. "Does Exercise Alter Immune Function and Respiratory Infections?" *President's Council on Physical Fitness and Sports Research Digest.* 3(13)(2001): 1–8.

Nieman, D. C. "Exercise Soothes Arthritis: Joint Effects." *ACSM's Health and Fitness Journal.* 4(3)(2000):20–28.

Ortal, M., and Sherman, C. "Exercise Against Depression." *The Physician and Sports Medicine.* 26(10)(1998):55–60.

Physician and Sports Medicine. "Homocysteine and Heart Disease: A Culprit or Just a Suspect?" *Physician and Sports Medicine.* 27(7)(1999): 13–16.

Rosenfeld, I. "What Women Can Do About PMS." *Parade Magazine.* February 13, 2000, pp. 14–16.

Smith, J. K. "Exercise and Atherogenesis." *Exercise and Sports Science Reviews.* 29(2)(2001): 49–53.

Spain, C. G., and Franks, B. D. "Healthy People 2010: Physical Activity and Fitness." *President's Council on Physical Fitness and Sports Research Digest.* 3(13)(2001): 1–16.

U.S. Department of Health and Human Services. *Healthy People 2010.* (2nd ed.) With *Understanding and Improving Health* and *Objectives for Improving Health.* 2 vols. Washington, DC: U.S. Government Printing Office, November 2000.

U.S. Department of Health and Human Services. (1996). *Physical Activity and Health: A Report of the Surgeon General.* Atlanta: U.S. Department of Health and Human Services, Chapter 6.

Wells, C. L. "Physical Activity and Cancer Prevention: Focus on Breast Cancer." *ACSM's Health and Fitness Journal.* 3(1)(1999): 13–18.

Whaley, M. H. et al. "Physical Fitness and Clustering of Risk Factors Associated with Metabolic Syndrome." *Medicine and Science in Sports and Exercise.* 31(2)(1999): 287–293.

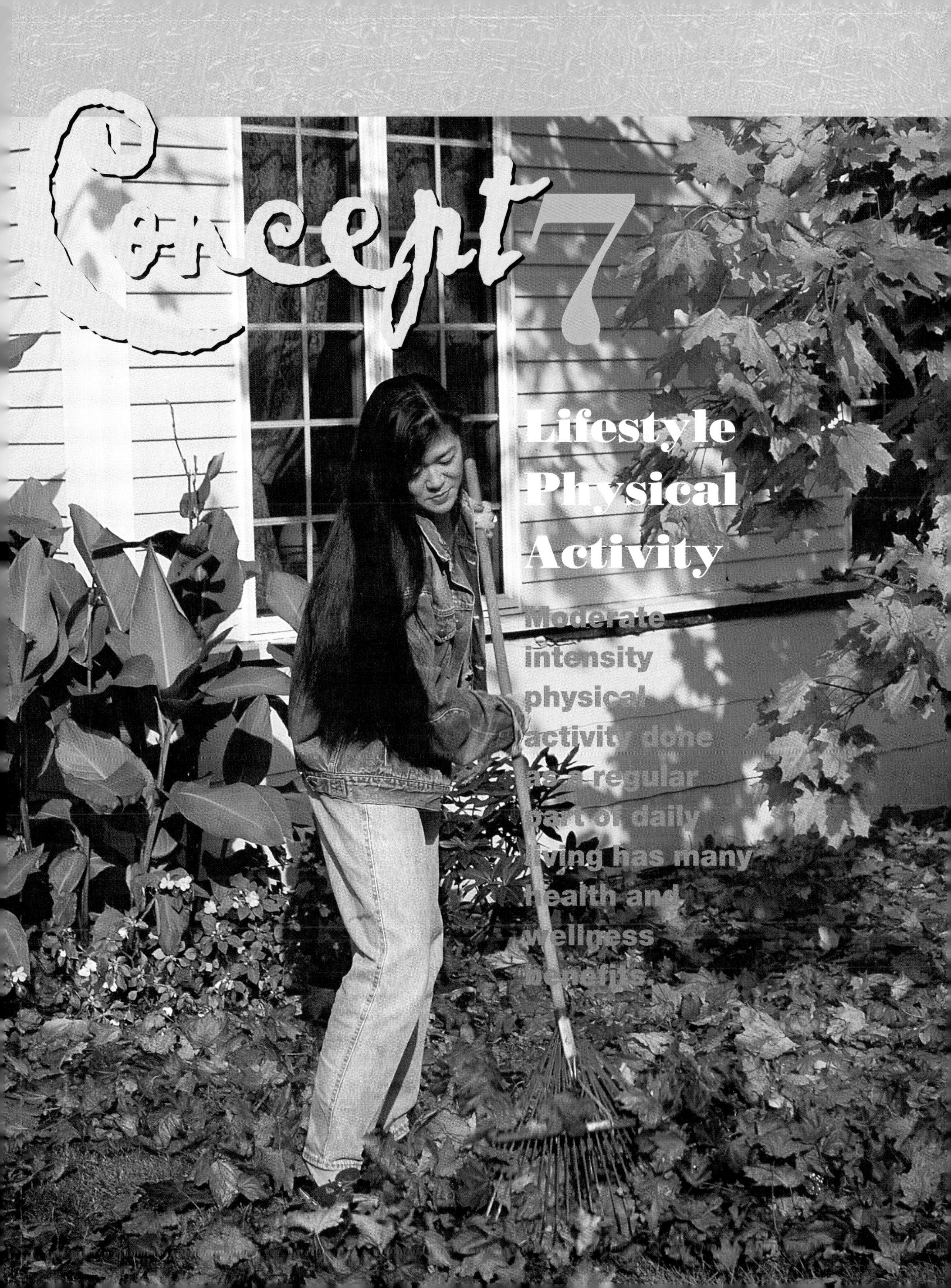

Concept 7

Lifestyle Physical Activity

Moderate intensity physical activity done as a regular part of daily living has many health and wellness benefits.

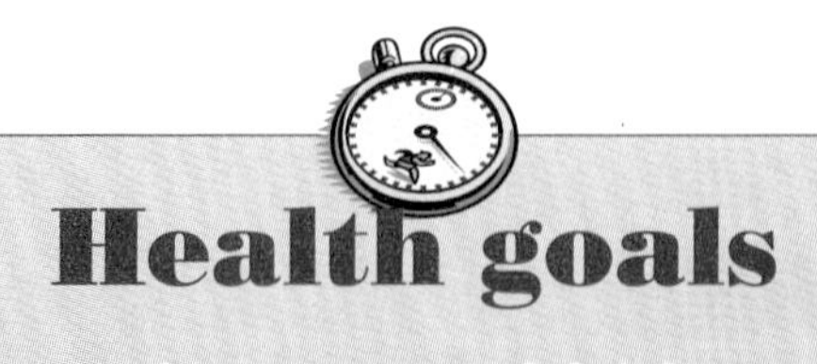

Increase the adoption and maintenance of daily physical activity.

Increase incidence of people reporting "active days."

Increase leisure time physical activity.

Increase proportion of people who do daily activity for 30 minutes.

Increase travel by walking and by bicycle.

Introduction

The *Surgeon General's Report on Physical Activity and Health* and a recommendation on *Physical Activity and Public Health* from the Centers for Disease Control and Prevention and the most recent prescription guidelines of the American College of Sports Medicine emphasize the value of **moderate physical activity** to good health. These reports refer to moderate intensity physical activity as lifestyle physical activity, which is located at the base of the physical activity pyramid. In this concept, lifestyle physical activity will be explained in detail.

The Facts about Lifestyle Activity

Lifestyle physical activities can easily be integrated into daily living.

During rest, the body is able to meet all of its energy needs. This is done by the aerobic system that allows the body to produce energy by breaking down a food in the presence of oxygen. Thus, sedentary activities like sitting, playing a musical instrument, or even watching television can technically be considered "aerobic" in nature. To improve our health and fitness, activities must challenge the body to work above this resting level on a regular basis. One of the best ways to do this is to perform physical activity as part of your daily routine. Moderate intensity lifestyle physical activities that involve the larger muscle groups of the body are **aerobic physical activities** that are often referred to as lifestyle activities. Lifestyle activities include daily living activities such as walking to work or to the store, housework, gardening or yard work, and climbing the stairs.

Lifestyle physical activities should expend much more energy than normally expended at rest.

www.mhhe.com/phys_fit/webreview07 Click 01

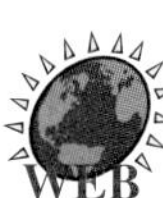

Scientists have devised a method to classify levels of activity by intensity. With this system, all activities are compared against the amount of activity needed at rest. The amount of energy expended at rest is referred to as one metabolic equivalent (1 **MET**). Activities listed as 2 METs require twice the energy of rest, and activities listed as 4 METs require four times the energy required for rest. Table 1 defines different intensity levels so that the reader can distinguish among the various terms used later in this book. You can see that moderate-intensity activities typically require 4.7–7.0 METs. The table also indicates that nearly all people can perform moderate activity aerobically. This means that the aerobic system can meet the energy demands for this activity, and the activity can be performed for relatively long periods of time without stopping.

www.mhhe.com/phys_fit/webreview07 Click 02

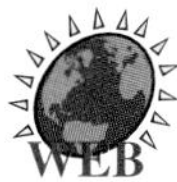

Anaerobic physical activities are those that are so vigorous that your body cannot supply adequate oxygen to meet the energy demand using the aerobic system. In these instances, the body must rely on short-term energy provided by the anaerobic metabolic system. As indicated in Table 1, those activities classified as hard, very hard, or maximum may be anaerobic in nature (or at least partially anaerobic). Because these activities cannot be sustained, they are not considered lifestyle physical activities.

Activities considered to be "light" when you are young may be considered moderate at older ages.

As noted in Table 1, brisk walking for a young person (20s and 30s) typically requires a 4.7 to 7 MET energy expenditure. The activity is 4.7 to 7 times more intense than lying down doing nothing. As a person grows older, the MET equivalent of the activity can decrease and still result in benefits. This is because fitness levels tend to decrease and less activity is needed to challenge the body. From the 40s to age

Table 1 Classification of Different Intensities of Aerobic and Anaerobic Physical Activity*

Classification	Description	Type	Examples
Very light	Activity that is about 2 to 2 1/2 times as intense as lying or sitting at rest (2 to 2.5 METs).	Aerobic	Washing your face, dressing yourself, typing, driving a car
Light	Activity that is 2 1/2 to 4 2/3 times as intense as rest (2.5 to 4.7 METs).	Aerobic	Normal walking, walking downstairs, bowling, mopping
Moderate	Activity about 4 2/3 to 7 times as intense as rest (4.7 to 7 METs).	Aerobic	Brisk walking, lawn mowing, shoveling, social dancing
Hard	Activities more than 7 and up to 10 times as intense as rest (7 to 10 METs).	Anaerobic for some, aerobic for others	Digging, level jogging (5 mph, 12 min. mile), cycling (13 mph), skiing, fencing
Very hard	Activities more than 10 and up to 12 times as intense as rest (10 to 12 METs).	Anaerobic for most, partly aerobic for some	Running (8.5 mph, 7 min. mile), handball, full-court competitive basketball
Maximum	Activities more than 12 times as intense as rest (12+ METs).	Anaerobic for virtually all	Running (10 mph, 6 min. mile)

*This table is based on values for healthy adults 20–39 years of age. As you grow older, it takes less intensity to achieve higher level classifications.

65, expending 4–6 METs provides benefits similar to those of 5–7 METs for people in their 20s and 30s. From 65 to 80, an expenditure of 3–5 METs is considered moderate activity. For the older old adults (80+), moderate activity is equal to 2–3 METs. Because the multiples of resting expenditure need not be as great as you grow older, it is easy to see that the speed of walking need not be the same among older people as among the young. The intensity of all activities should be adjusted as you grow older.

Because they are relatively easy to perform, lifestyle activities are very popular among adults.

www.mhhe.com/phys_fit/webreview07 Click 03

WEB According to the *Surgeon General's* report, walking is the most popular of all leisure-time activities among adults 18 years of age and over. Approximately 39 percent of all men and 48 percent of all women walked for exercise in the past two weeks. Also, among the 10 most popular activities among adults is gardening (including yard work), which is done by 34 percent of all male and 25 percent of all female adults. Approximately 10 percent of men and 12 percent of women report that they regularly use the stairs to increase their activity levels.

One very interesting fact about lifestyle physical activities is that the number of people participating in them increases with age. For example, only 33 percent of men 18 to 29 walk regularly, but 50 percent of men over 65 walk for exercise. Among young women, 47 percent walk, while 50 percent over 65 are walkers. Nearly twice as many older men than young men do gardening, and the difference

Moderate Activity Physical activity of moderate intensity; referred to as moderate activity in this concept.

Aerobic Physical Activity or Exercise Aerobic means "in the presence of oxygen." Aerobic activity is activity or exercise for which the body is able to supply adequate oxygen to sustain performance for long periods of time.

MET One MET equals the amount of energy a person expends at rest. METs are multiples of resting activity (two METS equals twice the resting energy expenditure).

Anaerobic Physical Activity or Exercise Anaerobic means "in the absence of oxygen." Anaerobic exercise is performed at an intensity so great that the body's demand for oxygen exceeds its ability to supply it.

among women is almost as dramatic. As lifetime physical activity participation increases with age, involvement in sports dramatically decreases.

> Some sports and recreational activities may be considered to be lifestyle physical activities if classified as light or moderate in intensity.

Some sports that are of light or moderate intensity can be classified as lifestyle physical activities. Golf, shuffleboard, bocci ball, table tennis, and bowling are examples. Recreational activities of light and moderate intensity can also be classified as lifestyle physical activities. Examples are fishing, canoeing, horseback riding, and gardening.

For children, play is considered to be a lifestyle physical activity because play is a normal activity for this age group. For retired adults, light- to moderate-intensity sports and recreational activities are truly lifestyle activities because they are a part of normal daily living.

Light- to moderate-intensity sports and recreational activities are very popular among adults, especially older adults. A recent Gallup poll indicated that fishing was the second most popular lifetime activity, bowling the fourth, and camping fifth. Though golf is not one of the top 10 participation activities, it is a very popular activity among older adults. More people over 65 play golf than those in the 18–30 group, perhaps because older people have more time for activities that take several hours and because its intensity is more appropriate for older adults.

> Lifestyle physical activities can easily be performed by most people regardless of fitness level.

www.mhhe.com/phys_fit/webreview07 Click 04

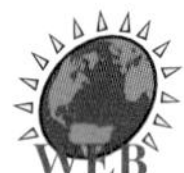

Prior to the last two decades, the conventional wisdom concerning physical activity was that it had to be vigorous to provide health and fitness benefits. Long-term studies of large populations were conducted with a variety of groups showing that moderate activity produced many benefits. For example, postal carriers who delivered mail showed benefits not present in the postal workers who sorted the mail, and bus drivers in England did not get the benefits found for conductors who climbed the stairs in double-deck busses many times during the day. More recently, a study in Finland showed that people who do gardening are much less likely to have health problems than sedentary people, and people who hunt and hike in the forest have even more dramatic reductions in health conditions. A recent study found that people who commuted to work by bicycle had fewer health problems and less early death than those who drove. These are only a few of the studies now available to show the benefits of lifestyle physical activity.

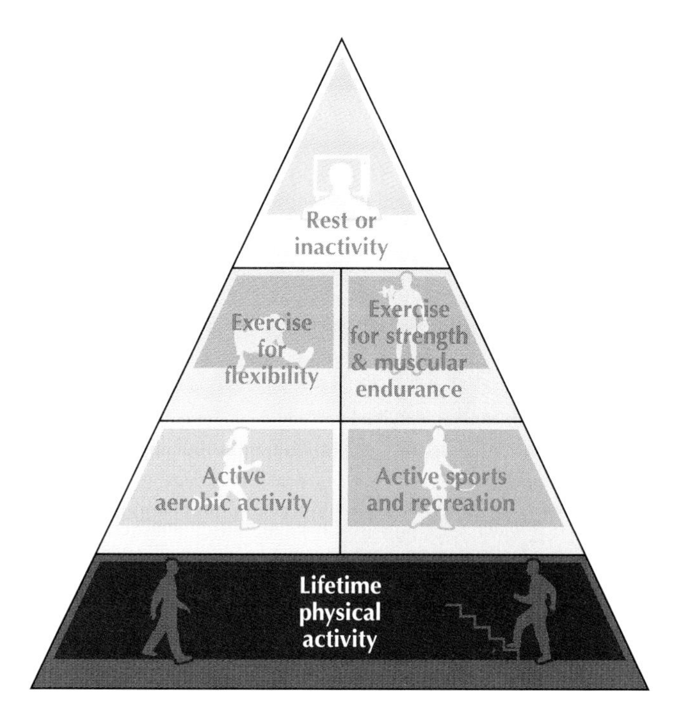

Figure 1
The physical activity pyramid: Level 1.

Because lifestyle activities are moderate, most people can easily perform them. This is one reason lifestyle physical activities are placed at the bottom of the pyramid (see Figure 1). They are basic and provide a foundation for other activities.

> Moderate activity is more attractive than vigorous activity to many people.

As the intensity of physical activity increases, it becomes less enjoyable to many people. Studies show that vigorous physical activity is a deterrent for more than a few people. This is another reason why lifestyle physical activities are placed at the base of the physical activity pyramid. Not only does this type of activity provide many health benefits, its intensity level makes it especially attractive to the people who most need to be active.

About 40 percent of all adult Americans do no leisure-time physical activity at all. They are totally sedentary. Statistics indicate that hundreds of thousands of premature deaths could be prevented if sedentary people would become active. Moderate physical activity is an alternative to vigorous activity that may be especially attractive to sedentary and/or less-fit adults.

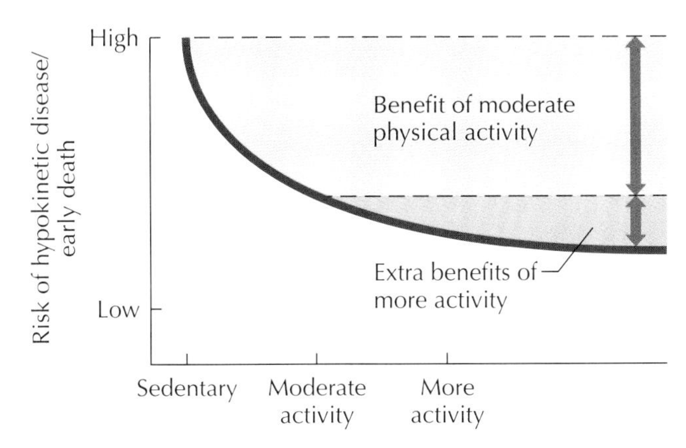

Figure 2
The benefits of moderate lifestyle physical activity.

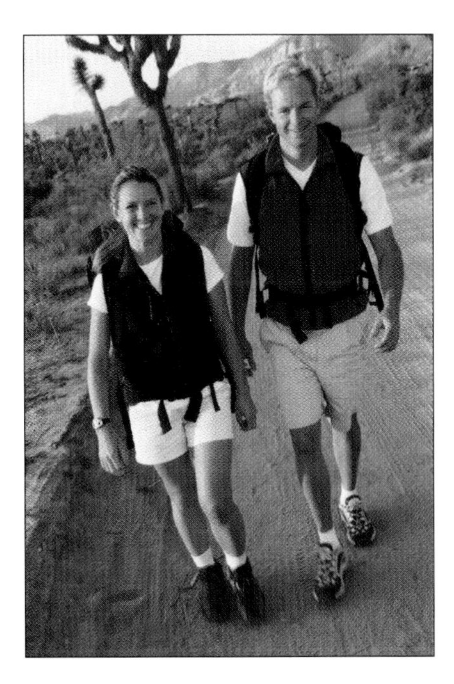

Moderate lifestyle activity has many health benefits.

The Health Benefits of Lifestyle Physical Activity

> Many health benefits can be achieved as a result of participation in lifestyle physical activities.

Figure 2 illustrates the fact that disease risk and early death are greatly reduced by moderate lifestyle physical activity. This figure, based on several large studies done worldwide, shows that a great proportion of the **health benefits** of physical activity described in this book result from participation in moderate lifestyle physical activities. Though additional benefits occur with more vigorous activity, they do not produce the proportional gain resulting from moderate activity.

The benefits of moderate or lifestyle physical activities are illustrated by the long arrow in Figure 2. The shorter arrow shows the additional benefits that result from more vigorous activity. The principle of diminishing returns applies. Even modest increases in physical activity are better than doing no activity at all. Clearly, the adage that "something is better than nothing" applies to physical activity.

> Lifestyle physical activity promotes metabolic fitness.

www.mhhe.com/phys_fit/webreview07 Click 05

WEB Metabolic fitness has been previously defined as fitness of the systems that provide the energy for effective daily living. Indicators of good metabolic fitness include normal blood lipid levels, normal blood pressure, normal blood sugar levels, and healthy body fat levels.

While lifestyle physical activity does not promote high-level cardiovascular fitness, commonly referred to as a **performance benefit,** it is effective in promoting metabolic fitness associated with health and wellness benefits. This type of activity can produce enough cardiovascular fitness to help unfit people escape from the low-fit category.

> Lifestyle physical activity has wellness benefits.

Reduction in disease risk and early death are important. But equally important is quality of life. Many of the wellness benefits previously described result from moderate lifestyle physical activity. For example, people who do very moderate exercise have been shown to take less time to go to sleep and sleep nearly an hour longer. A very recent study shows that functional limitations are much lower in moderately active people than those who are sedentary. Lifestyle activity and its accompanying metabolic fitness benefits are also associated with enhanced self-esteem and less incidence of depression and anxiety.

Health Benefits Health benefits refer to reduction in hypokinetic disease risk, decreased risk of early death, and improved quality of life.

Performance Benefits Performance benefits refer to improved ability to score well on physical fitness tests or to perform well in athletic or work activities requiring high-level performance.

How Much Lifestyle Physical Activity Is Enough? The Facts

> The Surgeon General and the American College of Sports Medicine have outlined a basic recommendation for lifestyle physical activity.

The recommendation for lifestyle physical activity is that adults accumulate 30 minutes or more of moderate-intensity physical activity on most, preferably all, days of the week. Brisk walking is an example of activity that typifies moderate activity. Table 2 provides some other examples of activities that meet the activity recommendation.

Near-daily activity is recommended because each activity session actually has short-term benefits that do not occur if activity is not relatively frequent. This is sometimes referred to as the **last bout effect.** Activity is beneficial only if you do the next bout before the effect of the last bout wears off.

> There are a variety of ways to determine if a person is doing enough to receive the health benefits of physical activity

The threshold of training (minimum amount of activity) for producing many of the health benefits can be determined in several ways. Much of the early research was done based on calories expended per day or per week. As illustrated in Figure 3, people who expend as few as 500 to 1,000 calories per week can greatly reduce the risk of early death compared to those who do no regular physical activity. Expending 1,000 to 2,000 calories per week decreases risk even more and people who expend this number of calories meet the national health goal of performing 30 minutes of moderate activity per day (see Table 3).

The easiest method for beginners is to keep track of lifestyle activities performed with a goal of accumulating at least 30 minutes each day of the week (equal in intensity to brisk walking). More sophisticated methods for determining if activity is likely to produce health benefits include counting heart rate and using ratings of perceived exertion. You will learn more about these methods in the concept on cardiovascular fitness that follows. As you begin monitoring your lifestyle physical activity it is best to keep track of all of the activities that you perform, and try to accumulate at least 30 minutes in lifestyle activities per day (Lab 7A). Using METs (see Table 1) or calories expended per week (Table 4) are alternative methods that may be useful. Later you can use heart rate or RPE methods as you gain more experience.

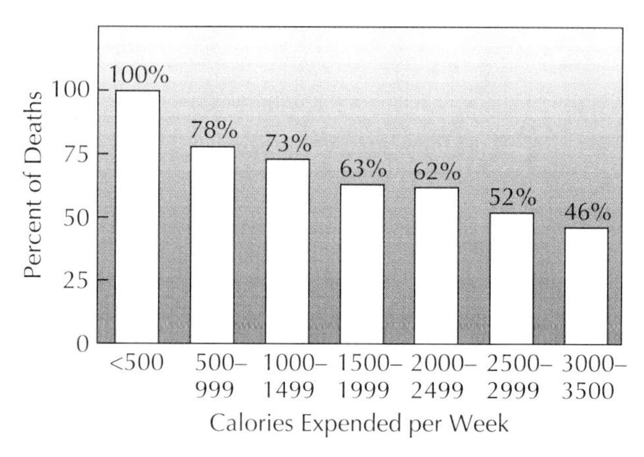

Figure 3
Deaths decrease as caloric expenditure increases.

> You can "accumulate" lifestyle physical activity to meet the recommendation.

Previous recommendations suggested that physical activity had to be continuous to be effective. The evidence now indicates that all of the activity need not be done in one session to be effective. To achieve the health benefits you can "accumulate activity" throughout the day. While the bulk of the energy or calories expended should be in moderate activities, some light activity can also be beneficial. When some

Table 2 Examples of Lifestyle Physical Activities

Activity	Length of time	
Washing and waxing a car	45–60 minutes	Less vigorous, more time
Washing windows or floors	45–60 minutes	↑
Gardening	30–45 minutes	
Wheeling self in wheelchair	30–40 minutes	
Social dancing	30 minutes	
Pushing a stroller (1 1/2 miles)	30 minutes	
Raking leaves	30 minutes	↓
Walking (2 miles)	30 minutes	More vigorous, less time

Adapted from the *Surgeon General's Report on Physical Activity and Health.*

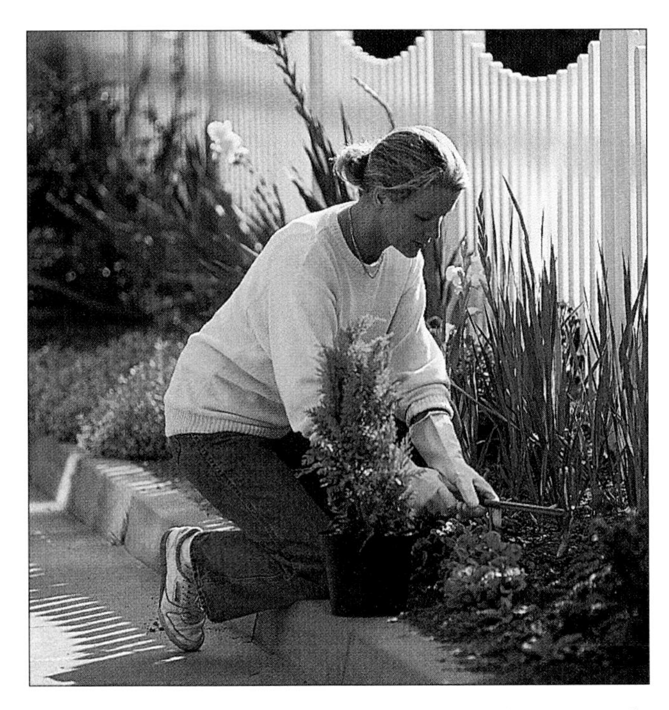

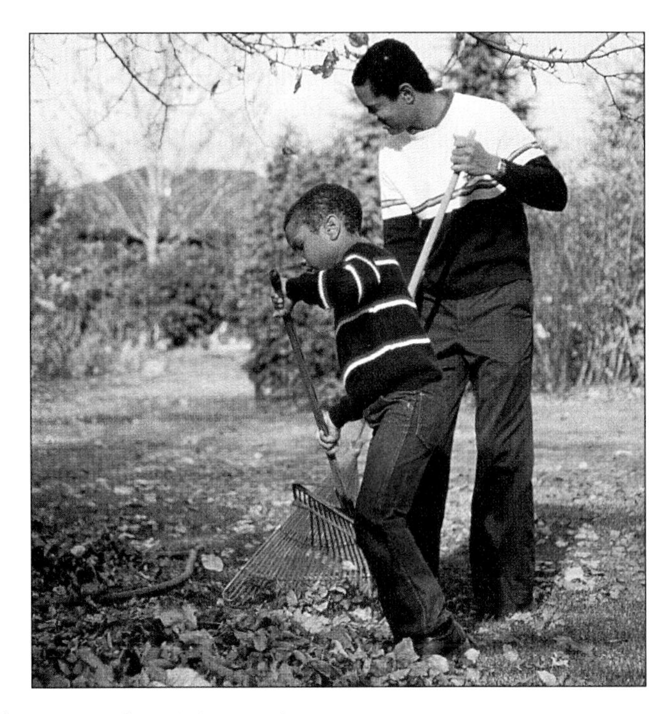

Moderate lifestyle physical activity can be accumulated in several activity sessions.

of the accumulated activity is in light activity, the duration of the activity must be increased (e.g., washing windows and floors as seen in Table 2). Some lifestyle physical activities, such as shoveling snow and climbing the stairs, are actually considered to be vigorous in nature. These activities can be counted in the accumulation of daily activities. Performing some of these activities can offset the performance of light activity and make it possible to expend adequate calories in a 30-minute period.

If the goal is to build cardiovascular fitness activity, sessions need to be at least moderate in nature, and activity sessions should probably be at least 10 minutes in length. You will learn more about this in the concept on cardiovascular fitness.

There is a FIT formula for lifestyle physical activity.

Table 3 summarizes the FIT formula for lifestyle physical activity. Both threshold of training (minimum amounts to get a benefit) and target zones (optimal activity levels) are presented.

Last Bout Effect Some of the benefits of physical activity are short-term in nature. If the benefit of a bout of exercise lasts 24 hours, it is beneficial only if the last bout of activity was done before 24 hours elapsed.

Table 3 The FIT Formula for Lifestyle Physical Activity

	Threshold of Training	Target Zone
Frequency	Most days of the week	All, or most, days of the week
Intensity	• Equal to brisk walking • Approximately 150 calories accumulated per day • 4.0 METs	• Equal to brisk to fast walking • Approximately 150–300 calories accumulated per day • 4.0 to 7 METs
Time (duration)	30 minutes or three 10 minute sessions per day.	30–60 minutes accumulated in sessions of at least 10 minutes.

*Heart rate and relative perceived exertion can also be used to determine intensity (see Concept 8).

log of the lifestyle activities you perform during a one-week time period. This is a short-term record sheet. However, charts such as this can be copied to make a log book to allow long-term activity self-monitoring.

> Because lifestyle physical activity is moderate in nature, a specific warm-up may not be necessary.

Lifestyle activities are very similar to the cardiovascular portion of the warm-up described in the concept on preparing for physical activity. For this reason, it may not be necessary to perform a special warm-up prior to doing activities such as walking. It would be wise to perform the stretching activities after the walk as a cool-down.

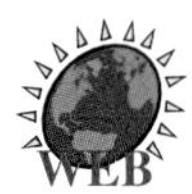

Web Review

Web review materials for Concept 7 are available at *www.mhhe.com/phys_fit/webreview07 Click 07.*

American College of Sports Medicine
www.acsm.org

ACSM's Health and Fitness Journal
www.acsm-healthfitness.org

Centers for Disease Control and Prevention
www.cdc.gov

Ordering Information for Pedometers
www.digiwalkerinfo.com

Surgeon General's Report on Physical Activity and Health
www.cdc.gov/nccdphp/sgr/sgr.htm

The Fitness Jumpsite
www.primusweb.com/fitnesspartner

Suggested Readings

Ainsworth, B. E., Haskell, W. L., Leon, A. S., Jacobs, D. R., Montoye, H. J., Sallis, J. F., and Paffenberger, R. S. "Compendium of Physical Activities: Classification of Energy Costs of Human Activities." *Medicine and Science in Sports and Exercise.* 25(1993): 71–80.

American College of Sports Medicine. *ACSM's Guidelines for Exercise Testing and Prescription.* 6th ed. Philadelphia: Lippincott, Williams and Wilkins, 2000.

American College of Sports Medicine. "Exercise and Physical Activity for Older Adults." *Medicine and Science in Sports and Exercise.* 30(6)(1998):992.

Bassett, D. R., Cureton, A. L., and Ainsworth, B. E. "Measurement of Daily Walking Distance-Questionnaire versus Pedometer." *Medicine and Science in Sports and Exercise.* 32(5)(2000): 1018–1023.

Blair, S. N. et al. *Active Living Every Day.* Champaign, IL: Human Kinetics, 2001.

Corbin, C. B., and Pangrazi, R. P. "Physical Activity Pyramid Rebuffs Peak Experience." *ACSM's Health and Fitness Journal.* 2(1)(1998): 12–17.

Manson, W. C. et al. "A Prospective Study of Walking as Compared with Vigorous Exercise in the Prevention of Coronary Heart Disease in Women." *New England Journal of Medicine.* 341(9)(1999): 650–658.

Public Health Service. *Surgeon General's Report on Physical Activity and Health.* Washington, D.C.: U.S. Government Printing Office, 1996.

Quittner, J. "High-tech Walking." *Time.* 24 July 2000, 77.

Schniffing, L. "Can Exercise Gadgets Motivate Patients?" *The Physician and Sports Medicine.* 29(1)(2001): 15–18.

Talbot, L. A., Metter, E. J., and Fleg, J. L. "Leisure-time Physical Activities and their Relationship to Cardiovascular Fitness in Healthy Men and Women 18–95 Years." *Medicine and Science in Sports and Exercise.* 32(2)(2000): 417–423.

Thompson, P. D. "Cardiovascular Risks of Exercise." *The Physician and Sports Medicine.* 29(4)(2001): 33–47.

U.S. Department of Health and Human Services. *Healthy People 2010.* 2nd ed. With *Understanding and Improving Health* and *Objectives for Improving Health.* 2 vols. Washington, DC: U. S. Government Printing Office. November 2000.

Welk, G. J. et al. "The Utility of the Digi-Walker Step Counter to Assess Daily Physical Activity Patterns." *Medicine and Science in Sports and Exercise.* 32(9)(2000): 5481–5488.

Wilde, B. E., Sidman, C. L., and Corbin, C. B. "A 10,000 Step Count as a Physical Activity Standard for Sedentary Women." *Research Quarterly for Exercise and Sport.* 72(1)(2001): 411–414.

Physical Fitness News Update

In recent years researchers have searched for new and different ways to monitor physical activity. Several types of electronic or computerized monitors now exist, including heart rate monitors, accelerometers, and pedometers. Heart rate monitors count heart rate to determine exercise intensity and are now relatively inexpensive. They are popular with runners and bikers. Accelerometers are mini-computers that are worn on the belt and count movement in several dimensions. They are considered to be a good way of objectively monitoring activity. Unfortunately, even the least expensive monitors cost several hundred dollars and for this reason accelerometers are not practical for use by most people.

One of the most popular devices currently in use is the electronic pedometer. These devices are worn on the waist and count the number of steps taken each day. As noted earlier in this concept, 10,000 steps per day is considered a goal target for lifestyle physical activity. A limitation of pedometers is that they will record fewer steps for running than for walking. However, if used for tracking lifestyle activities such as walking, they can be highly effective. Most units sell for approximately $20. Some versions convert steps per day to miles per day and calories per day. (See the Web Review for more information on pedometers.)

Lab 7A: Planning and Logging Your Lifestyle Physical Activity

Name **Section** **Date**

Purpose: To establish goals for one week of lifestyle physical activity, to prepare a lifestyle physical activity plan, to self-monitor progress in your one-week plan.

Procedures:

1. On chart 1, check the lifestyle activities you plan to perform during the week. Try to plan for at least 30 minutes each day.
2. Keep a one-week log of your actual participation using chart 2. If possible, keep the log with you during the day. List all lifestyle activities you perform for each day, including ones that you didn't originally plan to do. For each activity, record the number of minutes you were active using combinations of 5- or 10-minute blocks. For example, if you perform 15 minutes, you would select one 10-minute block and one 5-minute block. If you perform an activity for a total of 20 minutes, you could check two 10-minute blocks. If you cannot keep the log with you, fill in the log at the end of the day. If you choose to keep a log for more than one week, make extra copies of the log before you begin.
3. Sum the total number of minutes for each day by tallying the number of activity blocks.
4. Answer the questions in the Results section.

Chart 1 Lifestyle Physical Activity Plan

Write the number of minutes you plan to do each activity each day. You may mix activities each day.	Day 1	Day 2	Day 3	Day 4	Day 5	Day 6	Day 7
Brisk walking							
Yard work							
Active house work							
Gardening							
Social dancing							
Occupational activity							
Wheeling self in wheelchair							
Bicycling							
Walking							
Walking up and down stairs							
Other							
Daily Totals							

Results:

Did you do 30 minutes of activity each day? 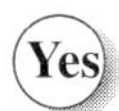 Yes 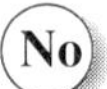 No Did you do 30 minutes of activity on most days? 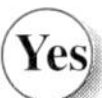 Yes  No

Conclusions and Interpretations:

1. Do you feel that you will use lifestyle physical activity as a regular part of your lifetime physical activity plan, either now or in the future? Use several sentences to explain your answer.
2. Did the logging of your activity make you more aware of your daily activity patterns? Explain why or why not.

Directions: Record the number of 5- or 10-minute blocks of lifestyle activity you did each day.

Chart 2 Lifestyle Activity Log

		5-Minute Blocks										10-Minute Blocks						Total Minutes
Day 1	**Date:**	1	2	3	4	5	6	7	8	9	10	1	2	3	4	5	6	
Activity:																		
Activity:																		
Activity:																		
Activity:																		
Activity:																		
																	Daily Total:	
Day 2	**Date:**	1	2	3	4	5	6	7	8	9	10	1	2	3	4	5	6	
Activity:																		
Activity:																		
Activity:																		
Activity:																		
Activity:																		
																	Daily Total:	
Day 3	**Date:**	1	2	3	4	5	6	7	8	9	10	1	2	3	4	5	6	
Activity:																		
Activity:																		
Activity:																		
Activity:																		
Activity:																		
																	Daily Total:	
Day 4	**Date:**	1	2	3	4	5	6	7	8	9	10	1	2	3	4	5	6	
Activity:																		
Activity:																		
Activity:																		
Activity:																		
Activity:																		
																	Daily Total:	
Day 5	**Date:**	1	2	3	4	5	6	7	8	9	10	1	2	3	4	5	6	
Activity:																		
Activity:																		
Activity:																		
Activity:																		
Activity:																		
																	Daily Total:	
Day 6	**Date:**	1	2	3	4	5	6	7	8	9	10	1	2	3	4	5	6	
Activity:																		
Activity:																		
Activity:																		
Activity:																		
Activity:																		
																	Daily Total:	
Day 7	**Date:**	1	2	3	4	5	6	7	8	9	10	1	2	3	4	5	6	
Activity:																		
Activity:																		
Activity:																		
Activity:																		
Activity:																		
																	Daily Total:	

Weekly Total ☐

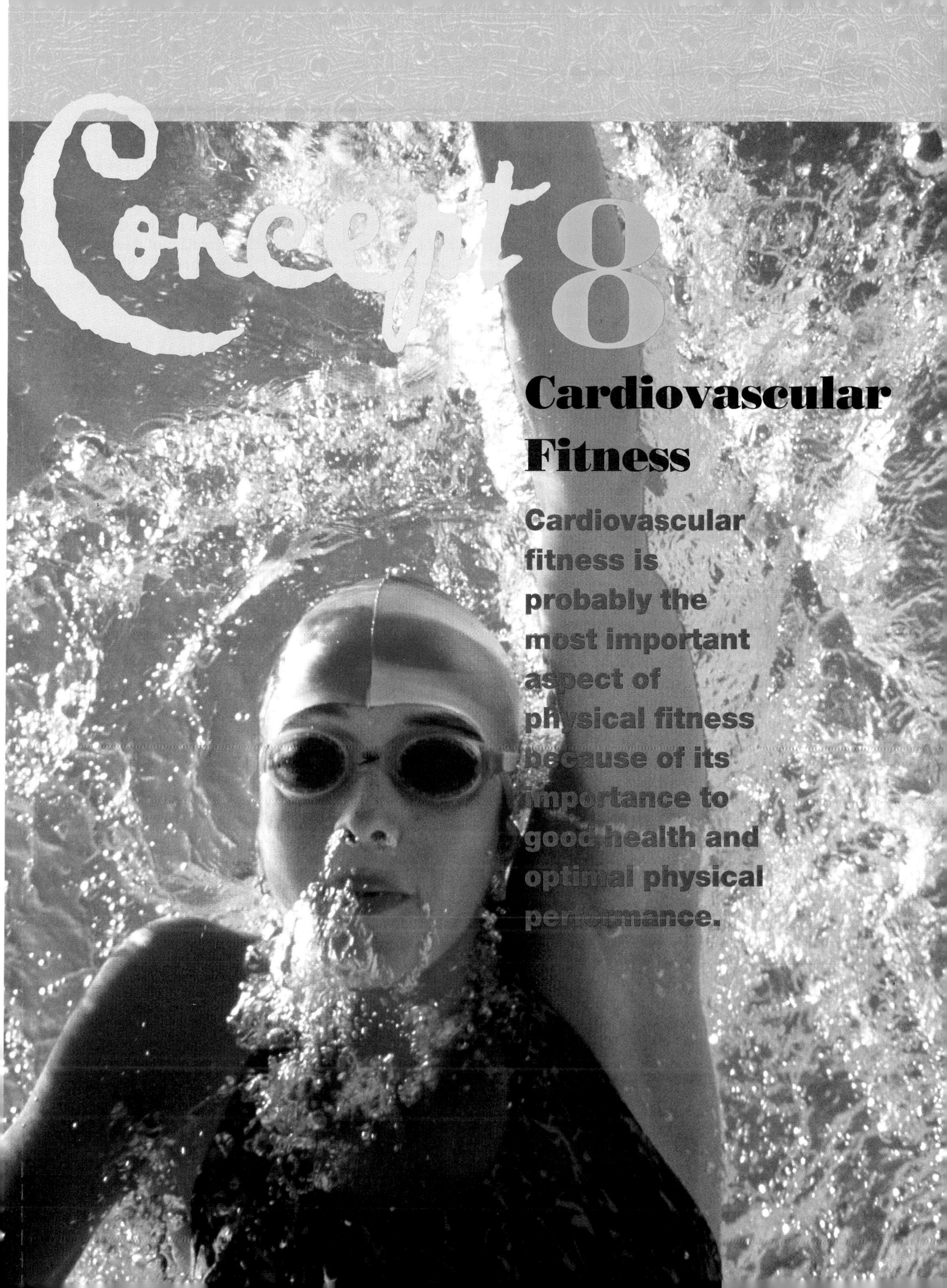

Concept 8

Cardiovascular Fitness

Cardiovascular fitness is probably the most important aspect of physical fitness because of its importance to good health and optimal physical performance.

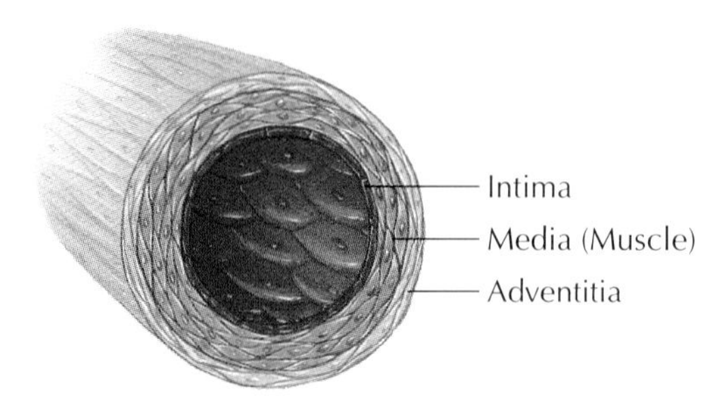

Figure 2
Healthy, elastic artery.

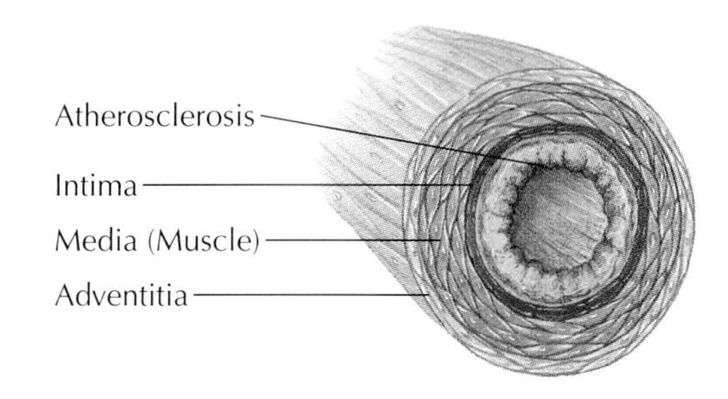

Figure 3
Unhealthy artery.

Veins have thinner, less-elastic walls than arteries, as shown in Figure 4. Also, veins contain small valves to prevent the backward flow of blood. Skeletal muscles assist the return of blood to the heart. The veins are intertwined in the muscle; therefore, when the muscle is contracted, the vein is squeezed, pushing the blood back to the heart. A malfunction of the valves results in a failure to remove used blood at the proper rate. As a result, venous blood pools, especially in the legs, causing a condition known as varicose veins. Regular physical activity helps reduce pooling of blood in the veins and helps keep the valves of the veins healthy.

Capillaries are the transfer stations where oxygen and fuel are released, and waste products, such as carbon dioxide, are removed from the tissues. The veins receive the blood from the capillaries for the return trip to the heart.

Good cardiovascular fitness requires a fit respiratory system and fit blood.

The process of taking in oxygen (through the mouth and nose) and delivering it to the lungs, where it is picked up by the blood, is called external respiration. External respiration requires fit lungs as well as blood with adequate **hemoglobin** in the red blood cells (erythrocytes). Insufficient oxygen-carrying capacity of the blood is called anemia, a condition caused by lack of hemoglobin.

Delivering oxygen to the tissues from the blood is called internal respiration. Internal respiration requires an

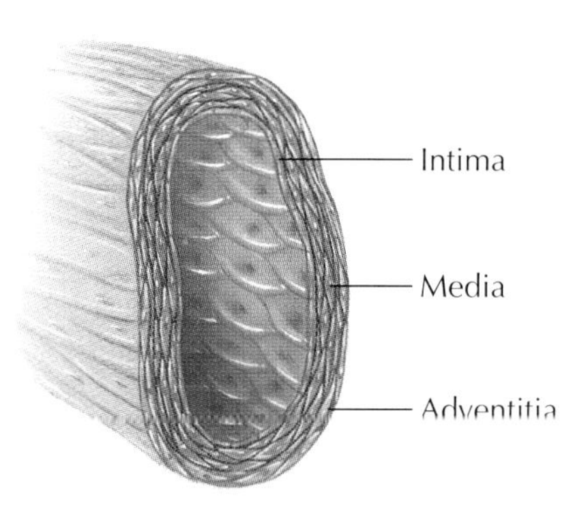

Figure 4
Healthy, nonelastic vein.

adequate number of healthy capillaries. In addition to delivering oxygen to the tissues, these systems remove carbon dioxide. Good cardiovascular fitness requires fitness of both the external and internal respiratory systems.

Cardiovascular fitness requires fit muscle tissue capable of using oxygen.

Once the oxygen is delivered, the muscle tissues must be able to use oxygen to sustain physical performance. Physical activity that promotes cardiovascular fitness stimulates changes in muscle fibers that make them more effective in using oxygen. Outstanding distance runners have high numbers of well-conditioned muscle fibers that can readily use oxygen to produce energy for sustained running. Training in other activities would elicit similar adaptations in the specific muscles used in those activities.

The Facts about Cardiovascular Fitness and Health Benefits

Good cardiovascular fitness reduces risk of heart disease, other hypokinetic conditions, and early death.

The best evidence indicates that cardiovascular fitness is associated with reduced risk for heart disease. A classic research study at The Cooper Institute for Aerobics Research showed that low-fit people are especially at risk. In addition, it has now been demonstrated that improving your fitness (moving from low-fitness to the good-fitness zone) can reduce risk of early death and produce the other health benefits described earlier in this text. Among those who are not low in fitness, further fitness increases bring additional health benefits. However, it is generally acknowledged that the principle of diminished returns applies. Figure 5 illustrates that additional fitness

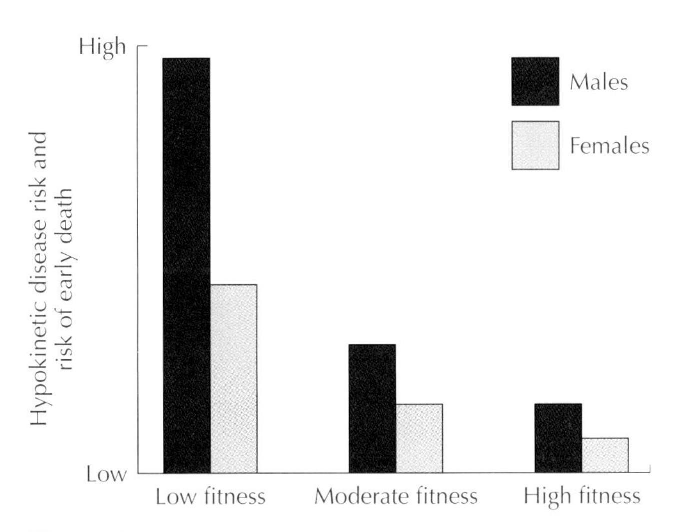

Figure 5
Risk reduction associated with cardiovascular fitness.
Adapted from Blair et al., 1996 (see Suggested Readings).

Table 1 Relative Risk of Major Risk Factors on Heart Disease and Early Death*

Risk Factor	Relative Risk of Heart Disease	Relative Risk of Early Death (All Causes)
Low Cardiovascular Fitness	2.69	2.03
Smoking	2.01	1.89
High Systolic Blood Pressure	2.07	1.67
High Cholesterol	1.86	1.45
Obesity (BMI)	1.70	1.33

*Statistically adjusted to assure independence of risk factors.
Based on Blair, S. N. et al. 1996 (see Suggested Readings).

yields additional benefits but not equal in magnitude to the benefits received from getting out of the low-fitness category.

Low cardiovascular fitness is associated with greater disease risk, and is independent of other risk factors.

Good cardiovascular fitness has been shown to be independent of other risk factors in reducing heart disease risk and of reduction in early death from all causes. Table 1 shows the relative risk of cardiovascular disease in the first column and the relative risk of early death from all causes in the second column. People with virtually no risk factors have a relative risk of 1.0. A person with a relative risk of 2.0 would have two times the risk of a risk-free person. The highest relative risk for heart disease is among people low in cardiovascular fitness (2.69). Those with low cardiovascular fitness also have the highest relative risk of early death (2.03). All of the values in the table were adjusted statistically to exclude the influence of other risk factors. This illustrates that the benefits of good cardiovascular fitness are independent of other primary risk factors for heart disease and early death from all causes.

Good cardiovascular fitness can reduce risk for most people, including those who are overweight.

www.mhhe.com/phys_fit/webreview08 Click 02

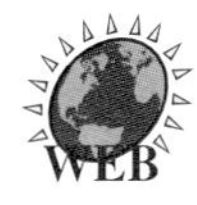

Some people think that they cannot be fit if they are overweight or overfat. It is now known that appropriate physical activity can build cardiovascular fitness in all types of people, including those with excess body fatness. In fact, having good cardiovascular fitness greatly reduces risk for those who are overweight. Poor cardiovascular fitness on the other hand, increases risk for both lean and overfat people. The greatest risk is among people who are both unfit and overfat.

Good cardiovascular fitness enhances the ability to perform various tasks, improves the ability to function, and is associated with a feeling of well-being.

Moving out of the low-fitness zone is of obvious importance to disease risk reduction. Achieving the good zone on tests further reduces disease and early death risk and promotes optimal wellness benefits and a recent position statement by the American College of Sports Medicine also shows an improved ability to function among older adults. Other wellness benefits include the ability to enjoy leisure activities and meet emergency situations, as well as the health and wellness benefits described earlier in this book. Cardiovascular fitness in the high-performance zone enhances the ability to perform in certain athletic events

Hemoglobin Oxygen-carrying pigment of the red blood cells.

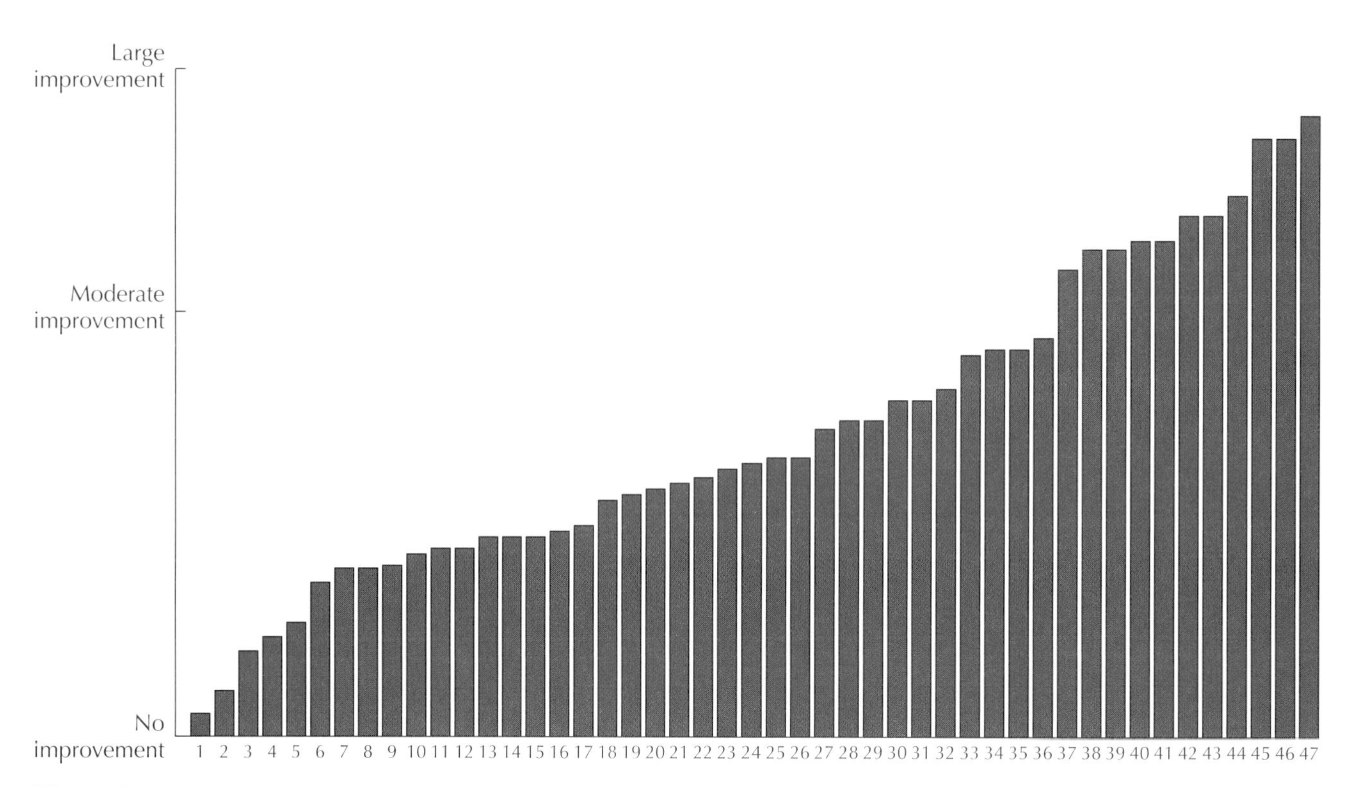

Figure 6

Difference in cardiovascular fitness improvement in 47 different people doing the same activity program for 15 to 20 weeks.

SOURCE: Adapted from Bouchard, 1999 (see Suggested Readings).

and in occupations that require high-level performance (e.g., firefighters). These benefits are commonly referred to as **performance benefits.**

Heredity influences your cardiovascular fitness.

It would be nice if all people who did appropriate physical activity achieved high levels of cardiovascular fitness. Genetic researchers have shown that the type of cardiovascular system you inherit has a good deal to do with your cardiovascular fitness. Further, we do not all respond similarly to physical activity because of our heredity. Figure 6 shows that after 15 to 20 weeks of training, different people who performed the exact same amount of physical activity varied greatly in their cardiovascular fitness improvement. This research led the researchers to draw the following conclusion: "Not only is it important to recognize that there are individual differences in the response to regular physical activity, but research indicates that there are non-responders in the population. Heredity may account for fitness differences as large as 3 to 10 fold when comparing low and high responders who have performed the same physical activity program" (Bouchard 1999).

As illustrated in Figure 6 one person showed virtually no gain, while one showed dramatic improvements in cardiovascular fitness even though the activity levels were the same. Those with low fitness in the beginning made more improvements than those who were already fit, but the researchers indicated that heredity was more of a factor than beginning fitness level.

You should not conclude from this information that achieving good cardiovascular fitness is impossible for some people. Rather, you should understand that it is harder for some people to get fit than others. No matter who you are, you can improve your cardiovascular fitness, but it takes longer for some than others. This study also points out the futility of comparing your own performance to others. Comparing yourself to fitness standards associated with good health is more reasonable. The research cited above suggests that achieving high-performance levels of cardiovascular fitness will be very difficult for some people.

Threshold and Target Zones for Improving Cardiovascular Fitness

> Aerobic physical activity that is more vigorous than lifestyle physical activities is necessary to produce optimal gains in cardiovascular fitness.

Lifestyle physical activity at the base of the pyramid promotes many health benefits and has positive effects on metabolic fitness. Activities at the second level of the physical activity pyramid—including active aerobics and active sports and recreation—are recommended for promoting good cardiovascular fitness (Figure 7). The word *active* implies that these activities must be relatively vigorous in nature.

> Cardiovascular fitness can be developed in three to six days per week.

Unlike less-intense lifestyle physical activities, the types of activities that promote cardiovascular fitness may be done as few as three days a week. Additional benefits occur with added days of activity. However, because more vigorous physical activity has been shown to increase risk of orthopedic injury if done too frequently, most experts recommend at least one day a week off.

> There are several methods for assessing the intensity of physical activity for building cardiovascular fitness.

www.mhhe.com/phys_fit/webreview08 Click 03

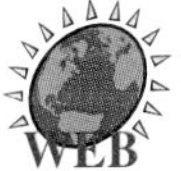

The best measure of cardiovascular fitness is **maximum oxygen uptake** ($\dot{V}O_2$ max). This test is usually done on a treadmill. Oxygen use is monitored minute by minute as exercise becomes harder and harder. When the exercise becomes very hard, oxygen use reaches its maximum. The highest amount of oxygen used in one minute of maximum intensity physical activity is your maximum oxygen uptake. Your **resting oxygen uptake** subtracted from your maximum oxygen uptake is your **oxygen uptake reserve** ($\dot{V}O_2R$). Calculating a percentage of your $\dot{V}O_2R$ is the most accurate way to determine if your exercise is intense enough to promote improvements in cardiovascular fitness.

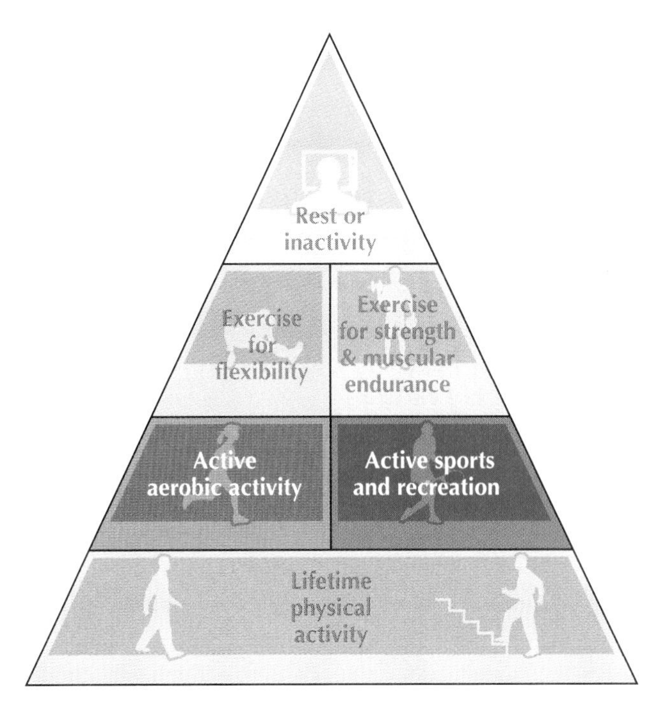

Figure 7
Select activities from level 2 of the pyramid for optimal cardiovascular fitness.

Maximum Oxygen Uptake ($\dot{V}O_2$ max) A laboratory measure held to be the best measure of cardiovascular fitness. Commonly referred to as $\dot{V}O_2$ max or the volume ($\dot{V}$) of oxygen used when a person reaches his or her maximum (max) ability to supply it during exercise.

Resting Oxygen Uptake This is the amount (volume) of oxygen used at rest; also called resting metabolism. One MET is another unit of measure representing resting oxygen uptake.

Oxygen Uptake Reserve ($\dot{V}O_2R$) This is the difference between your maximum oxygen uptake and your resting oxygen uptake. A percentage of this value is often used to determine appropriate intensities for physical activities.

Performance Benefit In this concept, performance benefit refers to an improved score on a cardiovascular fitness test or in performance of activities requiring cardiovascular fitness.

Unfortunately, $\dot{V}O_2R$ is hard to assess in normal day-to-day activities. For this reason, two different heart rate measures have been developed to help you estimate your $\dot{V}O_2R$. The first method is called percentage of **heart rate reserve (HRR),** which is the preferred method because it correlates very well with $\dot{V}O_2R$. A second method is called percentage of maximum heart rate (max HR). Both of these methods will be described in detail later (see Tables 4 and 5).

Ratings of perceived exertion (RPE) have also been shown to be useful in assessing the intensity of aerobic physical activity. This method will also be described in more detail in a later section (see Table 6).

As noted in a previous concept, calorie counting is useful for assessing the intensity of moderate lifestyle physical activities. The American College of Sports Medicine (ACSM) has cautioned against using this technique for determining intensity of aerobic activity for promoting cardiovascular fitness development; instead, they recommend heart rate monitoring and measures of relative perceived exertion.

Table 2 Threshold of Training and Target Zones for Activities Designed to Promote Cardiovascular Fitness*

	Threshold of Training	Target Zone
Frequency	3 days a week	At least 3 days and no more than 6 days a week
Intensity		
Heart rate reserve (HRR)	40%*	40–85%
Maximum heart rate (max HR)	55%*	55–90%
Relative perceived exertion (RPE)	12*	12–16
Time	20 minutes	20 to 60 minutes

*These values are for beginners—the threshold for fit individuals reaches higher into the target zone.

The duration of physical activity for building cardiovascular fitness is 20 to 60 minutes.

In the past, it was thought that the 20 to 60 minutes of active aerobic activity necessary to promote cardiovascular fitness should be done continuously in one session. Recent ACSM guidelines indicate that activity can be either intermittent or continuous if the total amount of exercise is the same and if the shorter sessions last at least 10 minutes. In other words, three 10-minute exercise sessions appear to give you the same benefit as one 30-minute session if the exercise is at the same intensity level.

There is a FIT formula for building cardiovascular fitness.

Table 2 illustrates the threshold of training and target zones for performing physical activity designed to promote cardiovascular fitness and cardiovascular health.

Your current fitness status and activity patterns should influence the type and amount of activity you do to promote cardiovascular fitness.

Making proper decisions about how much physical activity you should do is an art that is based on science. It is important that you listen to your body and not try to do too much too soon. Part of the art of making good decisions about activity is using the principle of progression. The amount of activity performed by a beginner differs from that performed by a person who is more advanced.

Beginners with low fitness may choose to start with lifestyle physical activity of relatively moderate intensity. Performing this type of activity at about 40 percent of HRR or 12 RPE for several weeks will allow the beginner to adapt gradually. Initial bouts of activity may be less than the recommended 20 minutes, but as fitness increases, at least 20 minutes a day should be accumulated. As fitness improves from the low to marginal range, the frequency, intensity, and time of activity can be increased (see Table 3). Cardiovascular fitness improvements for fit and active people are best when activity is at least 50 percent HRR, 65 percent max HR, and 13 RPE. Your current fitness and activity status will affect how quickly you progress. The type of activity you choose should be appropriate for the intensity of activity at each stage of the progression.

Learning to count heart rate at rest and after activity can help you monitor the intensity of your activity to determine if it is adequate to promote cardiovascular fitness.

To determine the intensity of physical activity for building cardiovascular fitness, it is important to know how to count your pulse. Each time the heart beats, it pumps blood into the arteries. The surge of blood causes a pulse that can be felt by holding a finger against an artery. Major arteries

Table 3 Progression of Activity Frequency, Intensity, and Time Based on Fitness Level

	Low Fitness	Marginal Fitness	Good Fitness
Frequency	3 days a week	3 to 5 days a week	3 to 6 days a week
Intensity			
Heart rate reserve (HRR)	40–50%	50–60%	60–85%
Maximum heart rate (max HR)	55–65%	65–75%	75–90%
Relative perceived exertion (RPE)	12–13	13–14	14–16
Time	10–30	20–40	30–60

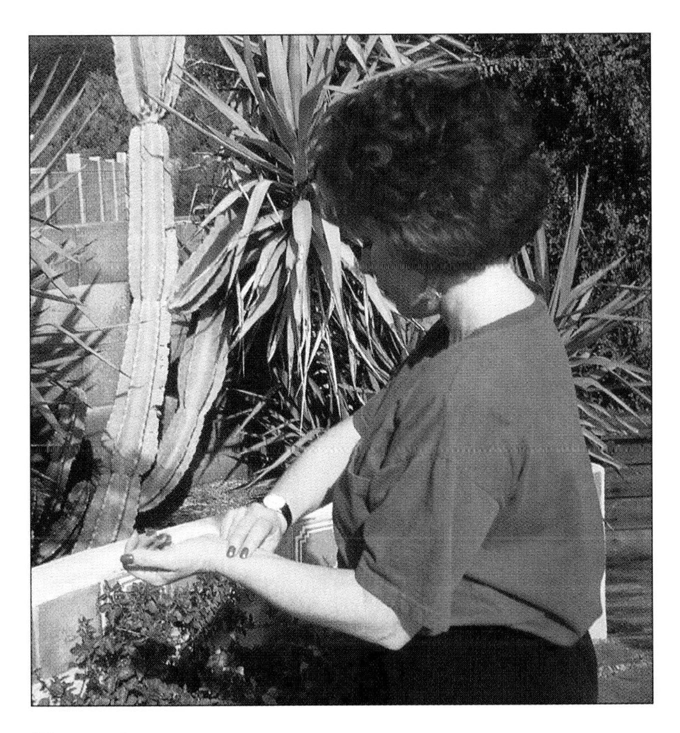

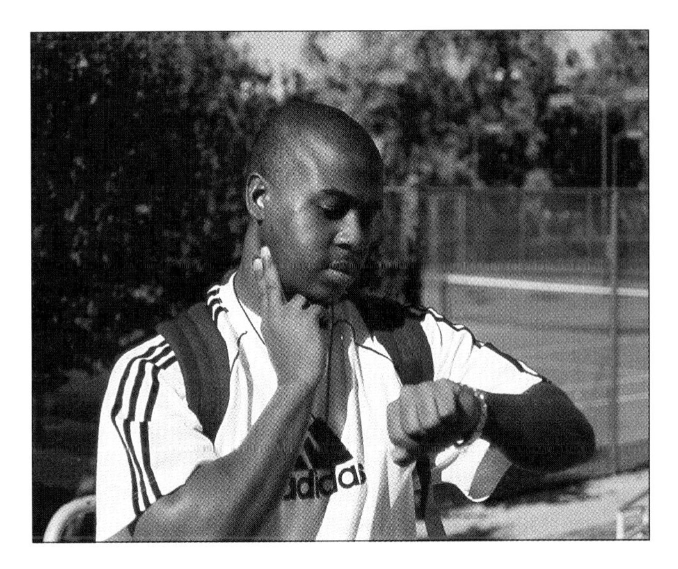

Figure 8

Counting your own pulse: (*A*) wrist (radial) and (*B*) neck (carotid).

that are easy to locate and are frequently used for pulse counts include the carotid on either side of the Adam's Apple, and the radial just below the base of the thumb on the wrist (see Figure 8). In lab 8A you will have the opportunity to practice counting your resting and postexercise heart rates.

To count the pulse rate, simply place the fingertips (index and middle finger) over the artery at one of the previously mentioned locations. Move the fingers around until a strong pulse can be felt. Press gently so as not to cut off the

Heart Rate Reserve (HRR) The difference between your maximum heart rate (highest heart rate in vigorous activity) and your resting heart rate (lowest heart rate at rest).

Ratings of Perceived Exertion (RPE) The assessment of the intensity of exercise based on how the participant feels; a subjective assessment of effort.

Physical Fitness News Update

In this book you use this formula (220 – your age in years) to calculate your predicted maximum heart rate (MaxHR). Recent evidence suggests that this formula may overestimate Max HR in young people and underestimate it among older adults. Researchers have proposed a new formula [208 – (.7 x age)]. For a thirty-year-old, the new formula would predict a MaxHR of 187 while the old formula would predict 190. For a sixty-year-old, the new formula would predict 166 as compared to 160 for the old formula.

Experts generally agree that determining your "true" rather than predicted MaxHR would be desirable. The problem is that a maximum effort or test in necessary to determine true MaxHR, and such an effort would not be wise for unfit people without supervision. You may choose to use a true MaxHR when calculating target heart rate zones if you know that your heart rate at its highest point exceeds predicted values, or you can use either the new or old MaxHR calculation technique. The old formula is considered acceptable because target zones were developed using this technique. You may also want to try the new formula as an alternative.

Bouchard, C. "Heredity and Health-Related Fitness." In Corbin, C. B., and Pangrazi, R.P. *Toward a Better Understanding of Physical Fitness and Activity.* Scottsdale, AZ: Holcomb-Hathaway, 1999.

Lee, I., and Phaffenbarger, R. S. "Preventing Coronary Heart Disease: The Role of Physical Activity." *The Physician and Sports Medicine.* 29(2)(2001): 37–52.

Schnirring, L. "New Formula Estimates Maximal Heart Rate." *The Physician and Sports Medicine.* 29(7)(2001): 13–14.

Spain, C. G., and Franks, B. D. "Healthy People 2010: Physical Activity and Fitness." *President's Council on Physical Fitness and Sports Research Digest.* 3(13)(2001): 1–16.

U.S. Department of Health and Human Services. *Healthy People 2010.* (2nd ed.) With *Understanding and Improving Health* and *Objectives for Improving Health.* 2 vols. Washington, DC: U.S. Government Printing Office, November 2000, Chapter 22.

U.S. Department of Health and Human Services. *Physical Activity and Health: A Report of the Surgeon General.* Atlanta: U.S. Department of Health and Human Services, 1996.

Williams, P. T. "Physical Fitness and Activity as Separate Heart Disease Risk Factors: A Meta-analysis." *Medicine and Science in Sports and Exercise.* 33(5)(2001): 754–761.

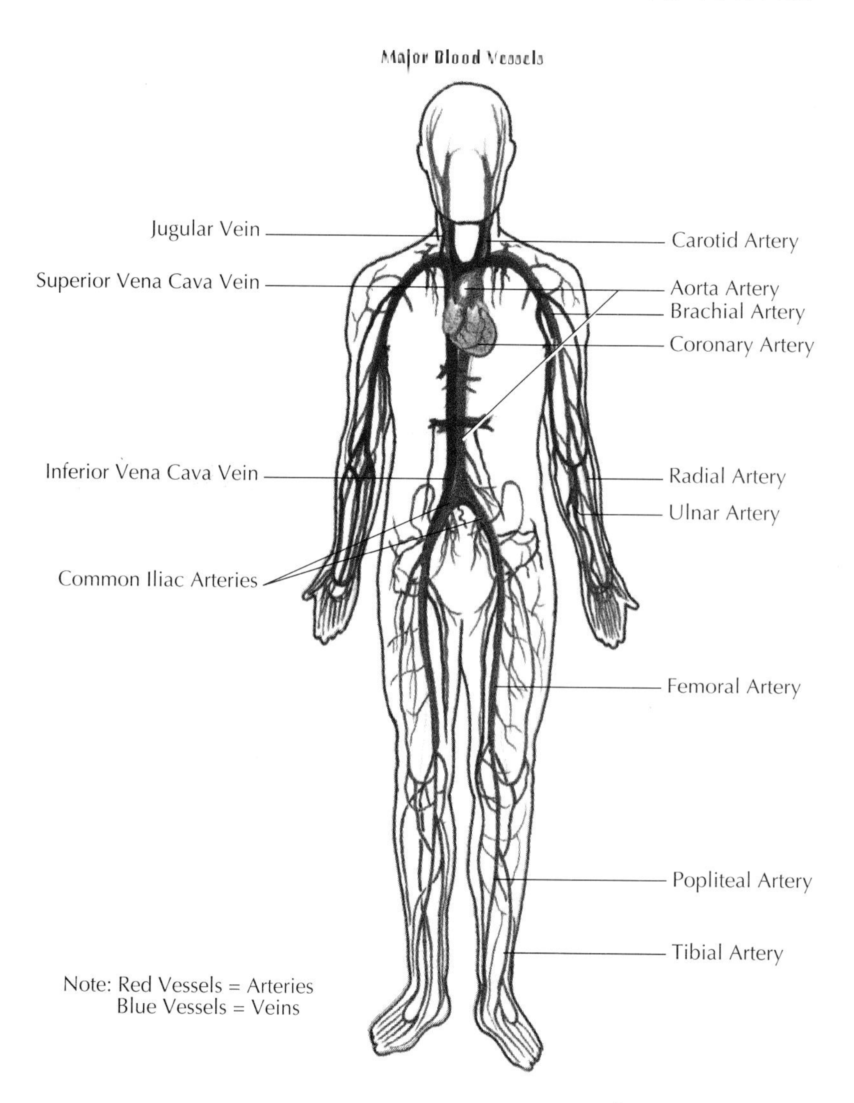

Lab Resource Materials: Evaluating Cardiovascular Fitness

The Walking Test

- Warm-up, then walk 1 mile as fast as you can without straining. Record your time to the nearest second.
- Immediately after the walk, count your heart rate for 15 seconds, then multiply by 4 to get a 1-minute heart rate. Record your heart rate.
- Use your walking time and your post-exercise heart rate to determine your rating using chart 1.

Chart 1 Walking Ratings for Males and Females

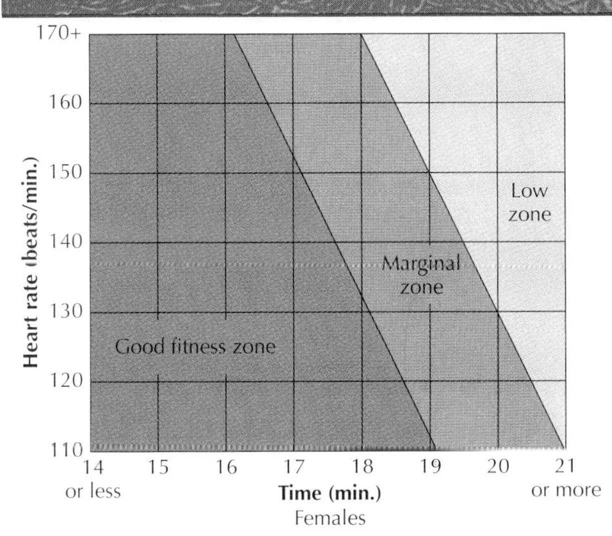

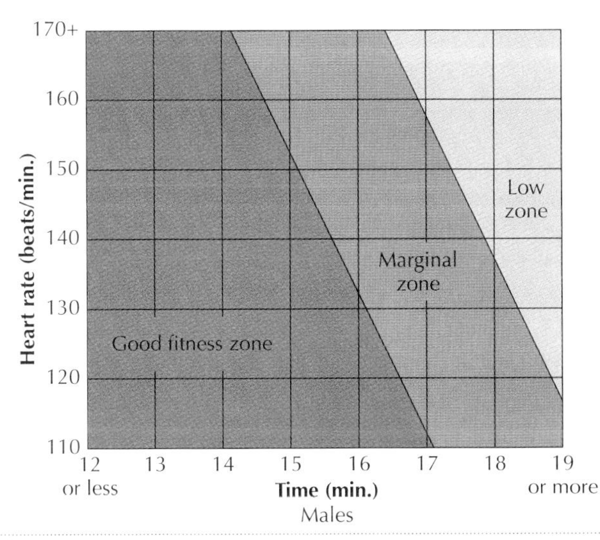

The ratings in chart 1 are for ages 20–29. They provide reasonable ratings for people of all ages.

Note: The walking test is not a good indicator of high performance, the running or bicycle tests are recommended.

Source: Test adapted from the *One Mile Walk Test,* with permission of the author, James M. Rippe, M.D.

The Step Test

- Warm-up prior to exercise, and after finishing be sure to cool-down.
- Step up and down on a 12-inch bench for 3 minutes at a rate of 24 steps per minute. One step consists of four beats; that is, "up with the left foot, up with the right foot, down with the left foot, down with the right foot."
- Immediately after the exercise, sit down on the bench and relax. Don't talk.
- Locate your pulse or have another person locate it for you.
- Five seconds after the exercise ends, begin counting your pulse. Count the pulse for 60 seconds.
- Your score is your 60-second heart rate. Locate your score and your rating on chart 2.

Chart 2 Step Test Rating Chart

Classification	60-Second Heart Rate
High-performance zone	84 or less
Good fitness zone	85–95
Marginal zone	96–119
Low zone	120 and above

As you grow older, you will want to continue to score well on this rating chart. Because your maximal heart rate decreases as you age, you should be able to score well if you exercise regularly.

Source: Data from F. W. Kasch and J. L. Boyer, *Adult Fitness: Principles and Practices,* 1968, Mayfield Publishing Company, Palo Alto, CA.

The 12-Minute Run Test

- Locate an area where a specific distance is already marked, such as a school track or football field, or measure a specific distance using a bicycle or automobile odometer.
- Use a stopwatch or wristwatch to accurately time a 12-minute period.
- For best results, warm-up prior to the test, then run at a steady pace for the entire 12 minutes (cool-down after the tests).
- Determine the distance you can run in 12 minutes in fractions of a mile. Depending upon your age, locate your score and rating in chart 3.

Chart 3 Twelve-Minute Run Test Rating Chart (Scores in Miles)

	Men (Age)			
Classification	17–26	27–39	40–49	50+
High-performance zone	1.80+	1.60+	1.50+	1.40+
Good fitness zone	1.55–1.79	1.45–1.59	1.40–1.49	1.25–1.39
Marginal zone	1.35–1.54	1.30–1.44	1.25–1.39	1.10–1.24
Low zone	<1.35	<1.30	<1.25	<1.10
	Women (Age)			
Classification	17–26	27–39	40–49	50+
High-performance zone	1.45+	1.35+	1.25+	1.15+
Good fitness zone	1.25–1.44	1.20–1.34	1.15–1.24	1.05–1.14
Marginal zone	1.15–1.24	1.05–1.19	1.00–1.14	.95–1.04
Low zone	<1.15	<1.05	<1.00	<.94

For a metric version of this chart, see Appendix B. Based on data from Cooper, see suggested readings.

The Astrand-Ryhming Bicycle Test

- Ride a stationary bicycle ergometer for 6 minutes at a rate of 50 pedal cycles per minute (one push with each foot per cycle). Cool down after the test.
- Set the bicycle at a workload between 300 to 1,200 kpm. For less fit or smaller people, a setting in the range of 300 to 600 is appropriate. Larger or fitter people will need to use a setting of 750 to 1,200. The workload should be enough to elevate the heart rate to at least 125 bpm but no more than 170 bpm during the ride.
- During the sixth minute of the ride (if the heart rate is in the correct range—see previous step), count the heart rate for the entire sixth minute. The carotid or radial pulse may be used.
- Use Chart 4 (males) or 5 (females) to determine your predicted oxygen uptake score in liters per minute. Locate your heart rate for the sixth minute of the ride in the left column and the workload (in KPM/min) across the top. The number in the chart where the heart rate and workload intersect represents your predicted O_2 uptake in liters per minute. The bicycle you use must allow you to easily and accurately determine the workload in KPM/min.
- Ratings are typically assigned based on milliliters per kilogram of body weight per minute. To convert your score to milliliters per kilogram (ml/kg/min) the first step is to multiply your score from Chart 4 or 5 by 1,000. This converts your score from liters to milliliters. Then divide your weight in pounds by 2.2. This converts your weight to kilograms. Then divide your score in milliliters by your weight in kilograms. This gives you your score in ml/kg/min.
- Example: An oxygen uptake score of 3.5 liters is equal to a 3,500 milliliter score (3.5 × 1,000). If the person with this score weighed 150 pounds, his or her weight in kilograms would be 68.18 kilograms (150 divided by 2.2). The person's oxygen uptake would be 51.3 ml/kg/min (3,500 divided by 68.18).
- Use your score in ml/kg/min to determine your rating (Chart 6).

Chart 4 Determining Oxygen Uptake Using the Bicycle Test—Men (liters O_2)

Heart Rate	Workload KPM/min 450	600	900	1,200
123	3.3	3.4	4.6	6.0
124	3.3	3.3	4.5	6.0
125	3.2	3.2	4.4	5.9
126	3.1	3.2	4.4	5.8
127	3.0	3.1	4.3	5.7
128	3.0	3.1	4.2	5.6
129	2.9	3.0	4.2	5.6
130	2.9	3.0	4.1	5.5
131	2.8	2.9	4.0	5.4
132	2.8	2.9	4.0	5.3
133	2.7	2.8	3.9	5.3
134	2.7	2.8	3.9	5.2
135	2.7	2.8	3.8	5.1
136	2.6	2.7	3.8	5.0
137	2.6	2.7	3.7	5.0
138	2.5	2.7	3.7	4.9

Heart Rate	Workload KPM/min 450	600	900	1,200	1,500
139	2.5	2.6	3.6	4.8	6.0
140	2.5	2.6	3.6	4.8	6.0
141	2.4	2.6	3.5	4.7	5.9
142	2.4	2.5	3.5	4.6	5.8
143	2.4	2.5	3.4	4.6	5.7
144	2.3	2.5	3.4	4.5	5.7
145	2.3	2.4	3.4	4.5	5.6
146	2.3	2.4	3.3	4.4	5.6
147	2.3	2.4	3.3	4.4	5.5
148	2.2	2.4	3.2	4.3	5.4
149	2.2	2.3	3.2	4.3	5.4
150	2.2	2.3	3.2	4.2	5.3
151	2.2	2.3	3.1	4.2	5.2
152	2.1	2.3	3.1	4.1	5.2
153	2.1	2.2	3.0	4.1	5.1
154	2.0	2.2	3.0	4.0	5.1

Heart Rate	Workload KPM/min 450	600	900	1,200	1,500
155	2.0	2.2	3.0	4.0	5.0
156	1.9	2.2	2.9	4.0	5.0
157	1.9	2.1	2.9	3.9	4.9
158	1.8	2.1	2.9	3.9	4.9
159	1.8	2.1	2.8	3.8	4.8
160	1.8	2.1	2.8	3.8	4.8
161	1.7	2.0	2.8	3.7	4.7
162	1.7	2.0	2.8	3.7	4.6
163	1.7	2.0	2.8	3.7	4.6
164	1.6	2.0	2.7	3.6	4.5
165	1.6	1.9	2.7	3.6	4.5
166	1.6	1.9	2.7	3.6	4.5
167	1.5	1.9	2.6	3.5	4.4
168	1.5	1.9	2.6	3.5	4.4
169	1.5	1.9	2.6	3.5	4.3
170	1.4	1.8	2.6	3.4	4.3

Chart 5 Determining Oxygen Uptake Using the Bicycle Test—Women (ml/O_2/kg)

Heart Rate	Workload KPM/min 300	450	600	750	900
123	2.4	3.1	3.9	4.6	5.1
124	2.4	3.1	3.8	4.5	5.1
125	2.3	3.0	3.7	4.4	5.0
126	2.3	3.0	3.6	4.3	5.0
127	2.2	2.9	3.5	4.2	4.8
128	2.2	2.8	3.5	4.2	4.8
129	2.2	2.8	3.4	4.1	4.8
130	2.1	2.7	3.4	4.0	4.7
131	2.1	2.7	3.4	4.0	4.6
132	2.0	2.7	3.3	3.9	4.6
133	2.0	2.6	3.2	3.8	4.5
134	2.0	2.6	3.2	3.8	4.4
135	2.0	2.6	3.1	3.7	4.4
136	1.9	2.5	3.1	3.6	4.3
137	1.9	2.5	3.0	3.6	4.2
138	1.8	2.4	3.0	3.5	4.2

Heart Rate	Workload KPM/min 300	450	600	750	900
139	1.8	2.4	2.9	3.5	4.0
140	1.8	2.4	2.8	3.4	4.0
141	1.8	2.3	2.8	3.4	3.9
142	1.7	2.3	2.8	3.3	3.9
143	1.7	2.2	2.7	3.3	3.8
144	1.7	2.2	2.7	3.2	3.8
145	1.6	2.2	2.7	3.2	3.7
146	1.6	2.2	2.6	3.2	3.7
147	1.6	2.1	2.6	3.1	3.6
148	1.6	2.1	2.6	3.1	3.6
149	1.5	2.1	2.6	3.0	3.5
150	1.5	2.0	2.5	3.0	3.5
151	1.5	2.0	2.5	3.0	3.4
152	1.4	2.0	2.5	2.9	3.4
153	1.4	2.0	2.4	2.9	3.3
154	1.4	2.0	2.4	2.8	3.3

Heart Rate	Workload KPM/min 450	600	750	900
155	1.9	2.4	2.8	3.2
156	1.9	2.4	2.8	3.2
157	1.8	2.3	2.7	3.2
158	1.8	2.3	2.7	3.1
159	1.8	2.3	2.7	3.1
160	1.8	2.2	2.6	3.0
161	1.8	2.2	2.6	3.0
162	1.8	2.2	2.6	3.0
163	1.7	2.2	2.5	2.9
164	1.7	2.1	2.5	2.9
165	1.7	2.1	2.5	2.9
166	1.7	2.1	2.5	2.8
167	1.6	2.0	2.4	2.8
168	1.6	2.0	2.4	2.8
169	1.6	2.0	2.4	2.8
170	1.6	2.0	2.4	2.7

Chart 6 Bicycle Test Rating Scale (ml/O_2/kg)

Women

Age	17–26	27–39	40–49	50–59	60–69
High-performance zone	46+	40+	38+	35+	32+
Good fitness zone	36–45	33–39	30–37	28–34	24–31
Marginal zone	30–35	28–32	24–29	21–27	18–23
Low zone	<30	<28	<24	<21	<18

Men

Age	17–26	27–39	40–49	50–59	60–69
High-performance zone	50+	46+	42+	39+	35+
Good fitness zone	43–49	35–45	32–41	29–38	26–34
Marginal zone	35–42	30–34	27–31	25–28	22–25
Low zone	<35	<30	<27	<25	<22

Charts 4, 5, and 6 based on data from P. O. Astrand and K. Rodahl, *Textbook of Work Physiology*, 1986.

Chart 7 Threshold of Training and Target Zone Heart Rates

Resting Heart Rate		Age: Less than 25	25–29	30–34	35–39	40–44	45–49	50–54	55–59	60–64	Over 65
below 50	Threshold Target Zone	108 108–173	106 106–172	104 104–167	102 102–163	100 100–159	98 98–155	96 96–150	94 94–146	92 92–142	90 90–139
50–54	Threshold Target zone	111 111–174	109 109–172	107 107–168	105 105–163	103 103–160	101 101–155	99 99–151	97 97–146	95 95–143	93 93–140
55–59	Threshold Target Zone	114 114–174	112 112–173	110 110–168	108 108–164	106 106–160	104 104–156	102 102–151	100 100–147	96 98–143	96 96–140
60–64	Threshold Target Zone	117 117–175	115 115–174	113 113–169	111 111–165	109 109–161	107 107–156	105 105–152	103 103–148	101 101–144	99 99–141
65–69	Threshold Target Zone	120 120–176	118 118–173	116 116–170	114 114–165	112 112–161	110 110–157	108 108–153	106 106–149	104 104–144	102 102–142
70–74	Threshold Target Zone	123 123–177	121 121–173	119 119–171	117 117–166	115 115–162	113 113–158	111 111–154	109 109–150	107 107–145	105 105–143
75–79	Threshold Target Zone	126 126–177	124 124–174	122 122–171	120 120–167	118 118–163	126 116–159	124 114–154	112 112–150	110 110–146	108 108–143
80–85	Threshold Target Zone	129 129–178	127 127–175	125 125–172	123 123–168	121 121–164	129 119–159	127 117–155	115 115–151	113 113–147	111 111–144
86 and over	Threshold Target Zone	132 132–179	130 130–176	128 128–173	126 126–169	124 124–164	122 122–160	130 120–156	118 118–152	116 116–147	114 114–145

*Threshold for beginners. Mid target or above recommended after becoming a regular exerciser.

Concept 9

Active Aerobics, Sports, and Recreational Activities

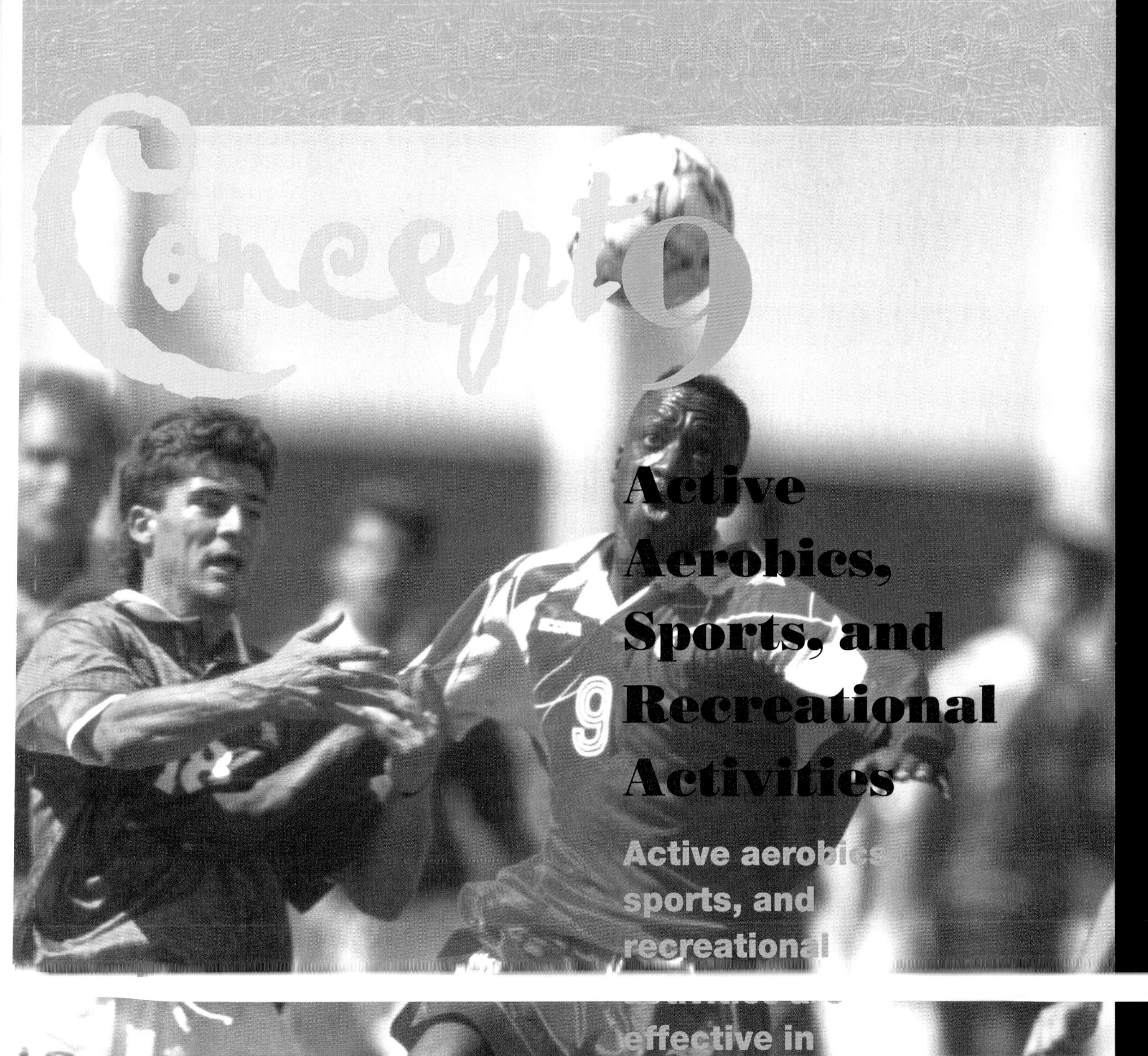

Active aerobics, sports, and recreational activities are effective in promoting health benefits, as well as developing fitness and enhancing performance.

Conclusions and Implications:

1. In several sentences, give an overall evaluation of your jogging technique.

2. In several sentences, indicate whether jogging is an appropriate activity for you. Indicate your reasons for your answer.

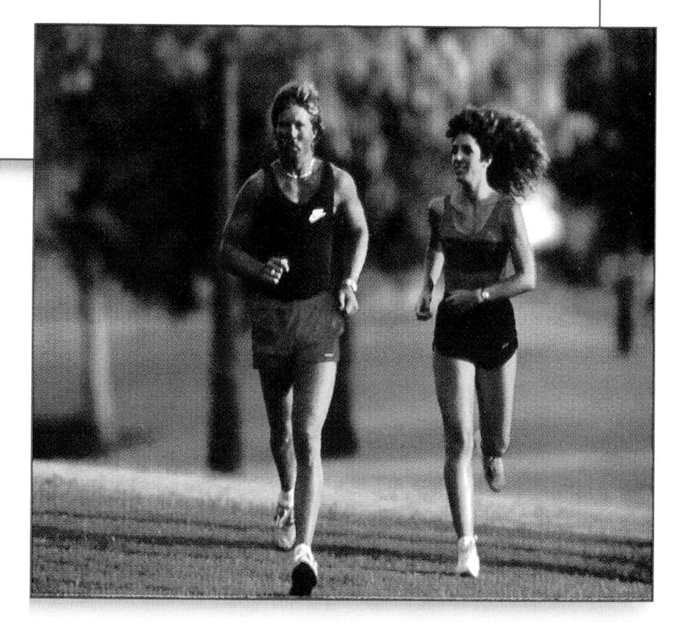

Lab 9B: Planning and Logging Participation in Active Aerobics, Sports, and Recreation

Name	Section	Date

Purpose:

To set one-week lifestyle physical activity goals, to prepare a plan, and to self-monitor progress in your one-week act aerobics, active sports, and active recreation plan.

Procedures:

1. Use the planning calendar (Chart 1) to schedule several aerobic exercise sessions for the week. Tr an at least three sessions but be realistic in your plan. Schedule activities that you enjoy and that you can conve ntly perform. You may mix different activities each day for variety. Indicate the days you expect to do them and the gth of time you expect to do the activity.
2. Keep a one-week log of your actual participation using Chart 2. If possible, keep the lo ith you during the day. Any time you perform an activity for 10 minutes, check one of the boxes. If you perform re than 10 minutes of activity in one session, check additional 10-minute blocks. If you cannot keep the log with , fill in the log at the end of the day. If you choose to keep a log for more than one week, use the extra log sheet o ake copies of the extra log sheet.
3. Log only those activities for which you meet the target zone for cardio ar fitness. Remember that 5 to 6, rather than 7 days a week of more vigorous activity, is recommended. You c ate a log book using several log sheets.
4. Sum the total number of minutes for each day by tallyir mber of activity blocks.
5. Answer the questions in the Results section.

Chart 1 Planning Calendar

Write the number of minutes you plan to do each activity each day: You may mix activities each day.	Mo ay	Tuesday	Wednesday	Thursday	Friday	Saturday	Sunday
Aerobic exercise machines							
Cycling (including stationary)							
Circuit training or calisthenics							
Dance or step aerobics							
Hiking or backpacking							
Jogging or running (or walking)							
Skating/cross-country skiing							
Swimming							
Water activity							
Sport							
Other							
Other							
Daily Totals							

Results:

	Yes	No
Did you do 20 or more minutes at each session?	○	○
Did you do 20 or more minutes of activity on at least 3 days?	○	○

Chart 3 Extra Aerobic Activity Log

Record the type and length of each activity you performed.	10-Minute Blocks						Total Minutes	Comments*
Day 1 Date:	1	2	3	4	5	6		
Activity:								
Activity:								
Activity:								
	Daily Total							
Day 2 Date:	1	2	3	4	5	6		
Activity:								
Activity:								
Activity:								
	Daily Total							
Day 3 Date:	1	2	3	4	5	6		
Activity:								
Activity:								
Activity:								
	Daily Total							
Day 4 Date:	1	2	3	4	5	6		
Activity:								
Activity:								
Activity:								
	Daily Total							
Day 5 Date:	1	2	3	4	5	6		
Activity:								
Activity:								
Activity:								
	Daily Total							
Day 6 Date:	1	2	3	4	5	6		
Activity:								
Activity:								
Activity:								
	Daily Total							

*Optional: Record heart rate, pace, calories, or other details of your session.

Concept 10

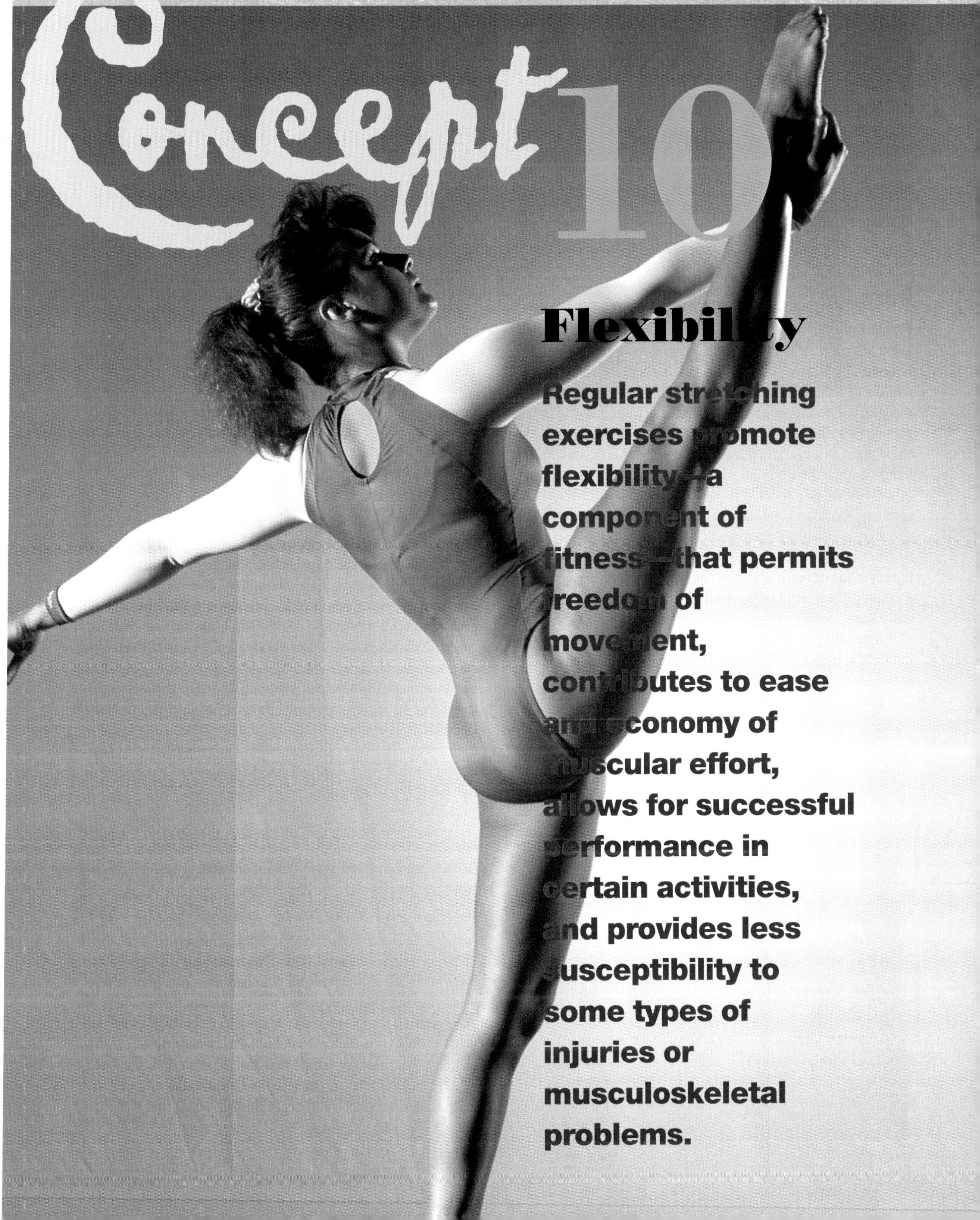

Flexibility

Regular stretching exercises promote flexibility—a component of fitness—that permits freedom of movement, contributes to ease and economy of muscular effort, allows for successful performance in certain activities, and provides less susceptibility to some types of injuries or musculoskeletal problems.

Table 4
The Basic 8 for Stretching Exercises

1. Calf Stretcher

This exercise stretches the calf muscles and Achilles tendon. Face a wall with your feet 2 or 3 feet away. Step forward on your left foot to allow both hands to touch the wall. Keep the heel of your right foot on the ground, toe turned in slightly, knee straight, and buttocks tucked in. Lean forward by bending your front knee and arms and allowing your head to move nearer the wall. Hold. Bend right knee, keeping heel on floor. Stretch and hold. Repeat with other leg.

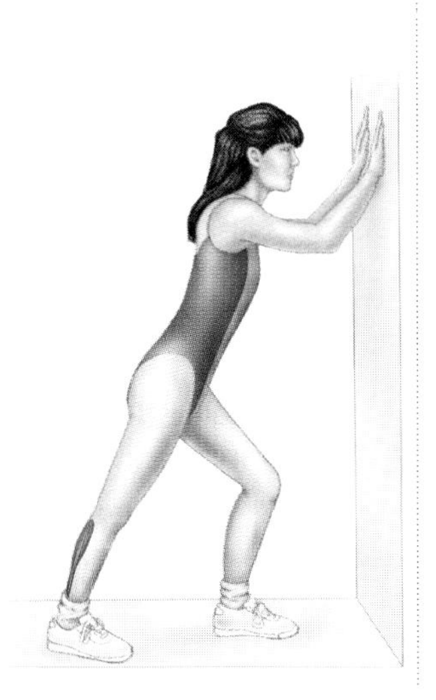

2. Hip and Thigh Stretcher

This exercise stretches the hip (iliopsoas) and thigh muscles (quadriceps) and is useful for people with lordosis and back problems. Place right knee directly above right ankle and stretch left leg backward so knee touches floor. If necessary, place hands on floor for balance.

1. Tilt the pelvis forward by tucking in the abdomen and flattening the back.
2. Then shift the weight forward until a stretch is felt on the front of the thigh; hold. Repeat on opposite side. Caution: Do not bend front knee more than 90 degrees.

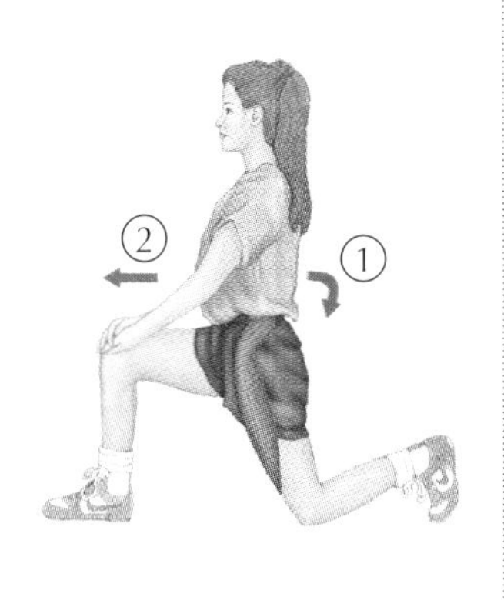

3. Sitting Stretcher

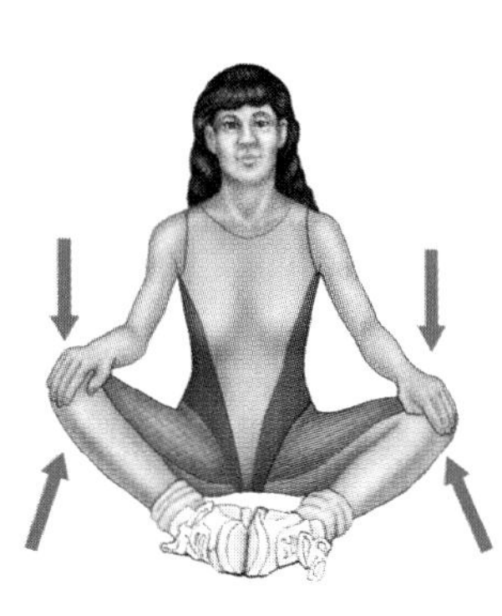

This exercise stretches the muscles on the inside of the thighs. Sit with soles of feet together; place hands on knees or ankles and lean forearms against knees; resist (contract) by attempting to raise knees. Hold; then relax and press the knees toward the floor as far as possible; hold. This exercise is useful for pregnant women and anyone whose thighs tend to rotate inward causing backache, knock-knees, and flat feet.

4. Hamstring Stretcher

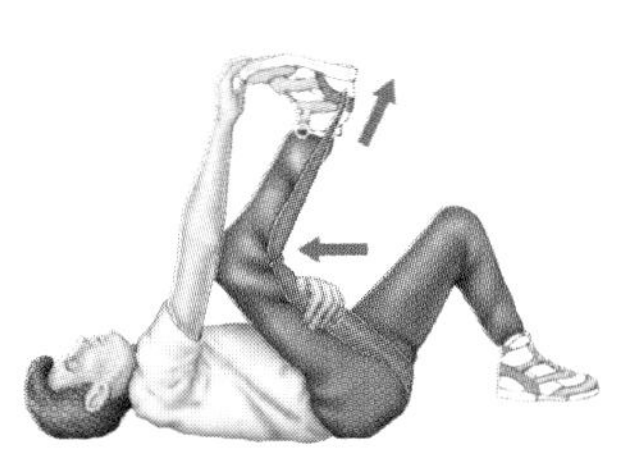

This exercise stretches the muscles on the back of the hip, thigh, knee, and ankle. Lie on your back with your knees bent. Bring right knee to chest and grasp toes with right hand. Place left hand on back of right thigh. Pull knee toward chest and push heel toward ceiling and pull toes toward shin. Attempt to straighten knee. Stretch and hold. Repeat on left side.

Table 4
The Basic 8 for Stretching Exercises (*continued*)

5. Leg Hug

This exercise stretches the lower back and gluteals. Lie on your back with your knees bent in a hook-lying position. Contract gluteals and lumbar muscles. Lift hips. Hold for 3 seconds. Relax and pull knees to chest with arms as hard as possible; hold. Useful for people with backache and lordosis. Do not place the hands over the knees to apply stretch.

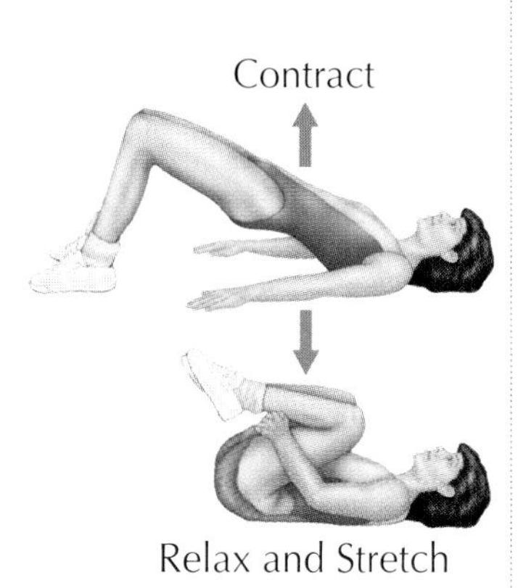

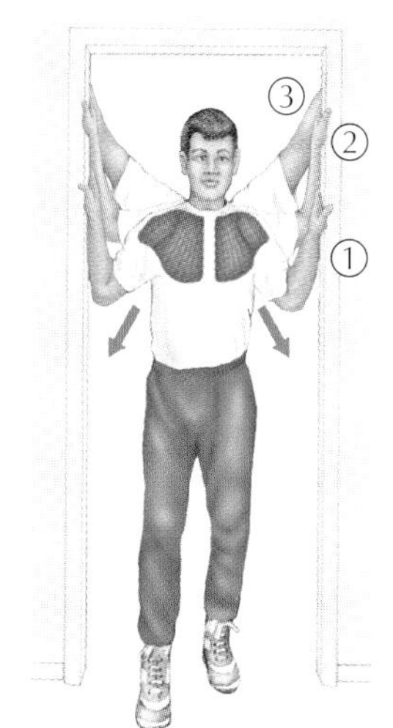

7. Pectoral Stretch

This exercise stretches the chest muscle (pectorals).

1. Stand erect in doorway with arms raised 45 degrees, elbows bent, and hands grasping doorjamb; feet in front-stride position. Press out on door frame, contracting the arms maximally for 3 seconds. Relax and shift weight forward on legs; lean into doorway so muscles on front of shoulder joint and chest are stretched; hold.
2. Repeat with arms raised 90 degrees.
3. Repeat with arms raised 135 degrees. Useful to prevent or correct round shoulders and sunken chest.

6. Trunk Twister

This exercise stretches the trunk muscles and muscles on the outside of hip. Sit with right leg extended, left leg bent and crossed over the right knee. Place right arm on the left side of the left leg and push against that leg while turning the trunk as far as possible to the left. Place left hand on floor behind buttocks. Stretch and hold. Reverse position and repeat on opposite side.

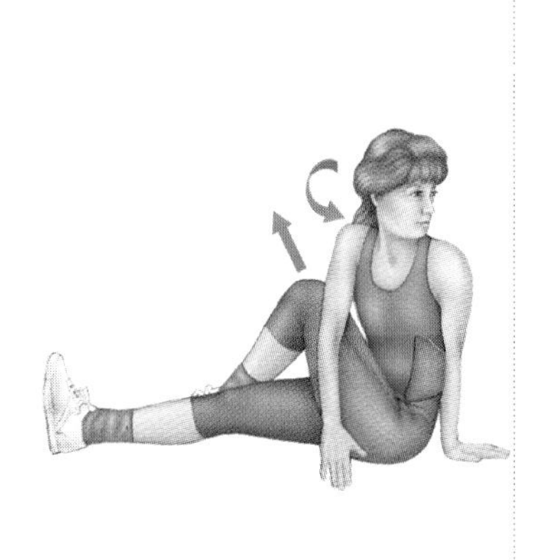

8. Arm Stretcher

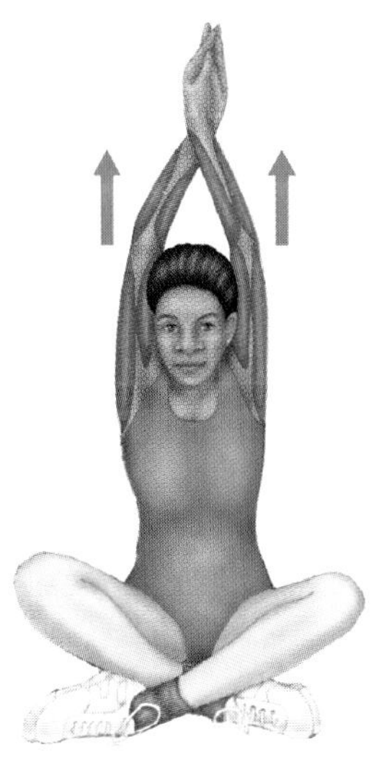

This exercise stretches the arm and chest muscles. Cross arms and turn palms of hands together. Raise arms overhead behind ears. Extend elbows. Stretch as high as possible. Hold.

Table 5
Supplemental Stretching Exercises for Flexibility

1. Lower Leg Stretcher

This exercise stretches the calf muscles and Achilles tendon. Stand with the toes on a stair step or thick book. Use hands to balance by holding a rail or wall. Keep toes pointed straight ahead or slightly inward. Rise up on toes (contract) as far as possible and hold for 3 seconds. Relax and lower heels to floor as far as possible; hold. Static stretch may alleviate spasms or cramps in calf muscles.

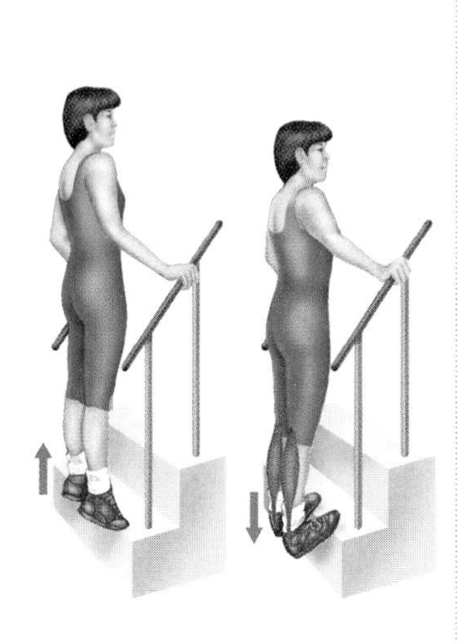

2. Standing Thigh Stretcher

This exercise stretches the hip flexor (iliopsoas) and thigh muscles (quadriceps). Stand near a wall so you can use one hand for balance. Place the top of one foot on a flat surface slightly higher than knee height (use a chair or table). Keep the knee of the elevated foot bent. Slide the leg backward until a stretch is felt on the front of the thigh. Keep the top of the pelvis tilted backward so the back does not arch. Repeat with the opposite leg.

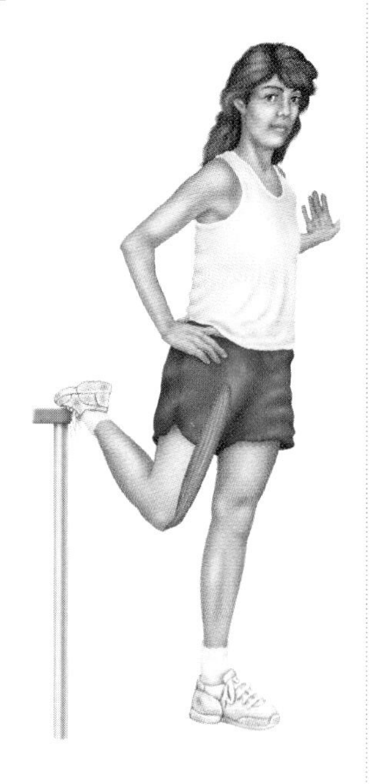

3. Lateral Thigh and Hip Stretch

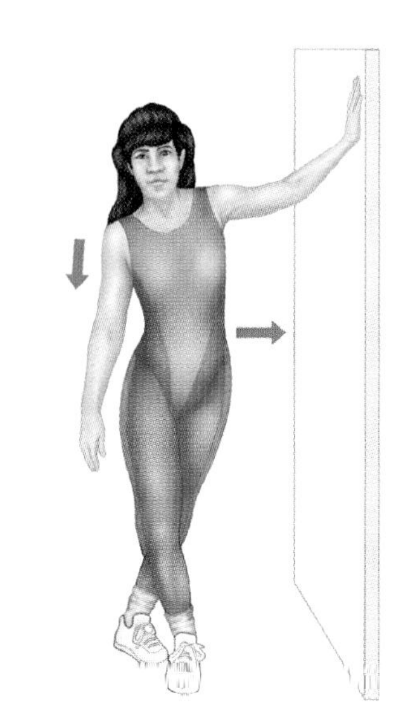

This exercise stretches the muscles and connective tissue on the outside of the legs (iliotibial band and tensor fascia lata). Stand with left side to wall, left arm extended and palm of hand flat on wall for support. Cross the left leg behind right and turn toes of both feet out slightly. Bend left knee slightly and shift pelvis toward wall (left) as trunk bends toward right. Adjust until tension is felt down outside of left hip and thigh. Stretch and hold. Repeat on other side.

4. Back-Saver Hamstring Stretch

This exercise stretches the hamstrings and calf muscles and helps prevent or correct backache caused in part by short hamstrings. Sit on the floor with the feet against the wall or an immovable object. Bend left knee and bring foot close to buttocks. Clasp hands behind back. Contract the muscles of the back of the upper leg (hamstrings) by pressing the heel downward toward the floor; hold; relax. Bend forward from hips, keeping lower back as straight as possible. Let bent knee rotate outward so trunk can move forward. Lean forward keeping back flat; hold and repeat on each leg.

Table 5
Supplemental Stretching Exercises for Flexibility *(continued)*

5. One-Leg Stretcher

This exercise stretches the lower back and hamstring muscles. Stand with one foot on a bench, keeping both legs straight. Contract the hamstrings and gluteals by pressing down on bench with the heel for 3 seconds, then relax and bend the trunk forward, toward the knee. Hold for 10–15 seconds. Return to starting position and repeat with opposite leg. As flexibility improves, the arms can be used to pull the chest toward the legs. Do not allow either knee to lock. This exercise is useful in relief of backache and correction of lordosis (swayback).

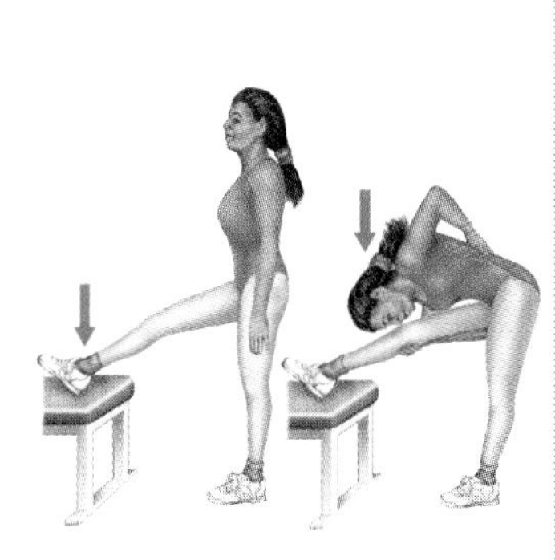

6. Lateral Trunk Stretcher

This exercise stretches the trunk muscles. Sit on the floor. Stretch the left arm over head to right. Bend to the right at waist, reaching as far to right as possible with left arm and as far as possible to the left with right arm; hold. Do not let trunk rotate. Repeat on opposite side. For less stretch, overhead arm may be bent at elbow. This exercise can be done in the standing position but is less effective.

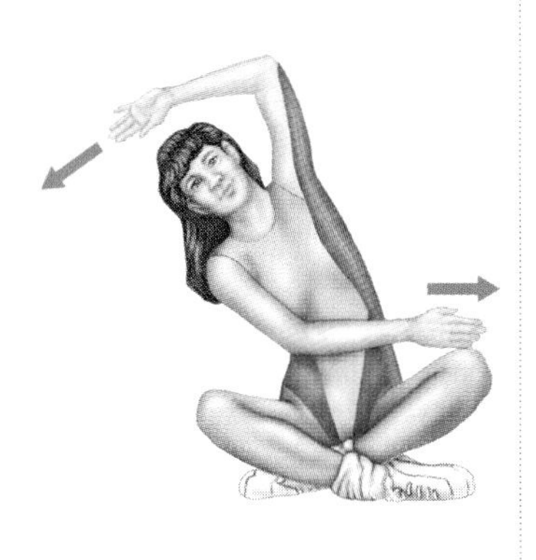

7. Wand Exercise

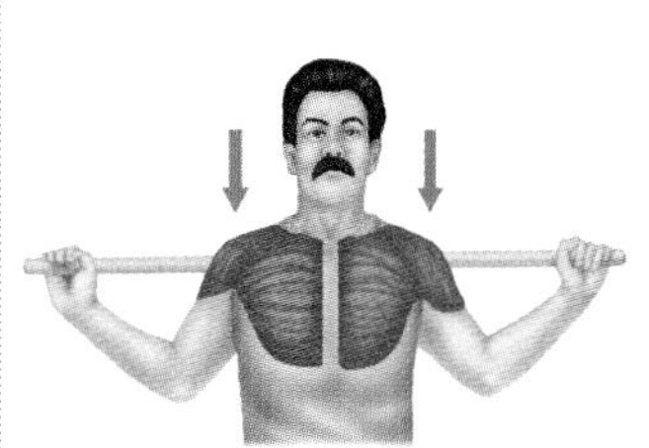

This exercise stretches the front of the shoulders and chest. Sit with wand grasped at ends. Raise wand overhead. Be certain that the head does not slide forward. Keep the chin tucked and neck straight. Bring wand down behind shoulder blades. Keep spine erect. Hold. Press forward on the wand simultaneously by pushing with the hands. Relax, then try to move the hands lower, sliding the wand down the back. Hold again. Hands may be moved closer together to increase stretch on chest muscles. If this is an easy exercise for you, try straightening the elbows and bringing the wand to waist level in back of you.

8. Arm Pretzel

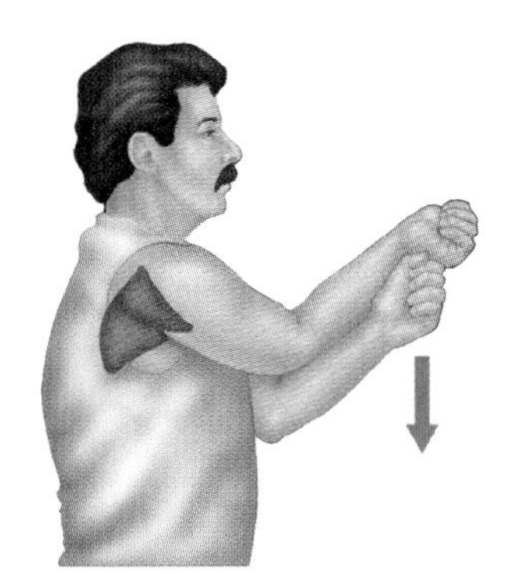

This exercise stretches the shoulder muscles (lateral rotators). Stand or sit with elbows flexed at right angles, palms up. Cross right arm over left; grasp right thumb with left hand and pull gently downward, causing right arm to rotate laterally. Stretch and hold. Reverse arm position and repeat on left arm.

Table 5
Supplemental Stretching Exercises for Flexibility *(continued)*

9. Shin Stretcher

This exercise relieves shin muscle soreness by stretching muscles on front of shin. Kneel on both knees, turn to right, and press down and stretch right ankle with right hand. Move pelvis forward. Hold. Repeat on opposite side. Except when they are sore, most people need to strengthen rather than stretch these muscles.

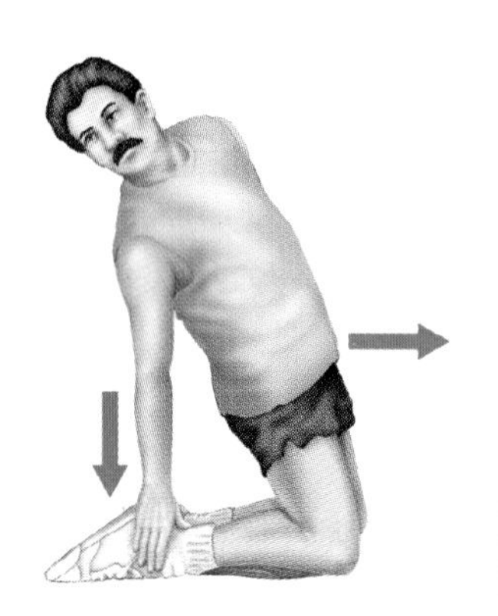

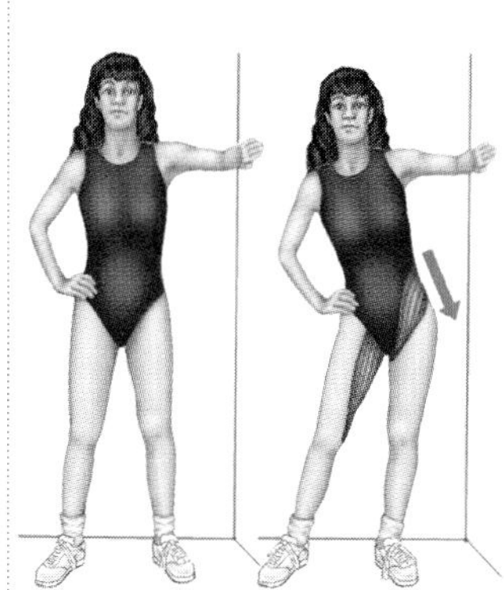

11. Billig's Exercise

This exercise stretches the pelvic fascia, hip flexors, and muscles of the inside thigh. Stand with side to a wall and place the elbow and forearm against the wall at shoulder height. Tilt the pelvis backward, tightening the gluteal and abdominal muscles. Place opposite hand on hip and push the hips toward the wall. Push forward and sideward (45 degrees) with the hips. Do not twist the hips. Hold. Repeat on opposite side. Useful for preventing some cases of dysmenorrhea.

10. Spine Twist

This exercise stretches the trunk rotators and lateral rotators of the thighs. Start in hook-lying position, arms extended at shoulder level. Cross left knee over right; keep arms and shoulders on floor while touching knees to floor on left. Stretch and hold. Reverse leg position and lower knees to right.

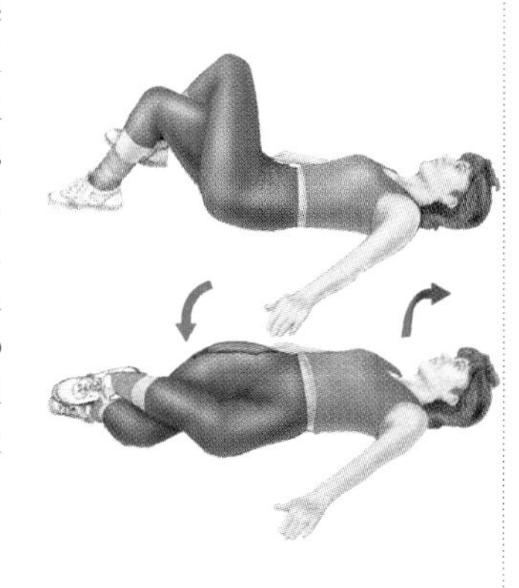

12. Two-Hand Ankle Wrap

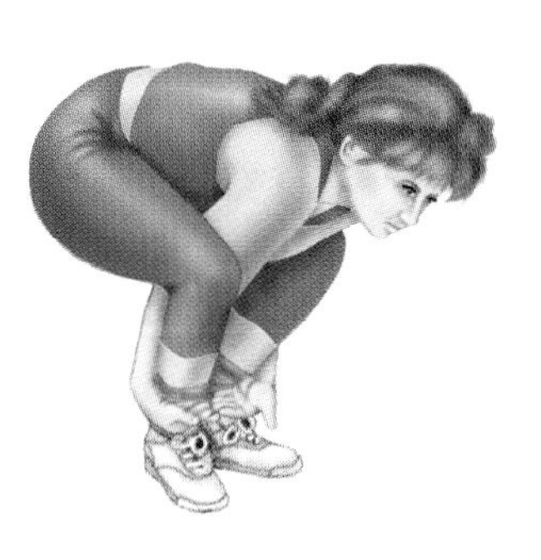

This exercise is most useful for athletes or people interested in performance. It should not be done until after individual muscles have been stretched using other exercises. It stretches multiple muscle groups including the back, shoulders, and legs. Stand with heels together. Bend forward and place arms between knees; bend knees and wrap arms around legs, attempting to touch fingers in front of ankles. Hold.

Lab Resource Materials: Flexibility Tests

Directions: It is impractical to test the flexibility of all joints. These tests are for joints used frequently. Follow instructions carefully.

Test

1. *Modified Sit-and-Reach* (Flexibility Test of Hamstrings)
   a. Remove shoes and sit on the floor. Place the sole of the foot of the extended leg flat against a box or bench, and place the head, back, and hips against a wall; 90-degree angle at the hips.
   b. Place one hand over the other and slowly reach forward as far as you can with arms fully extended; head and back remain in contact with the wall. A partner will slide the measuring stick on the bench until it touches the fingertips.
   c. With the measuring stick fixed in the new position, reach forward as far as possible, three times, holding the position on the third reach for at least 2 seconds while the partner reads the distance on the ruler. Keep the knee of the extended leg straight (see illustration).
   d. Repeat the test a second time and average the scores of the two trials.

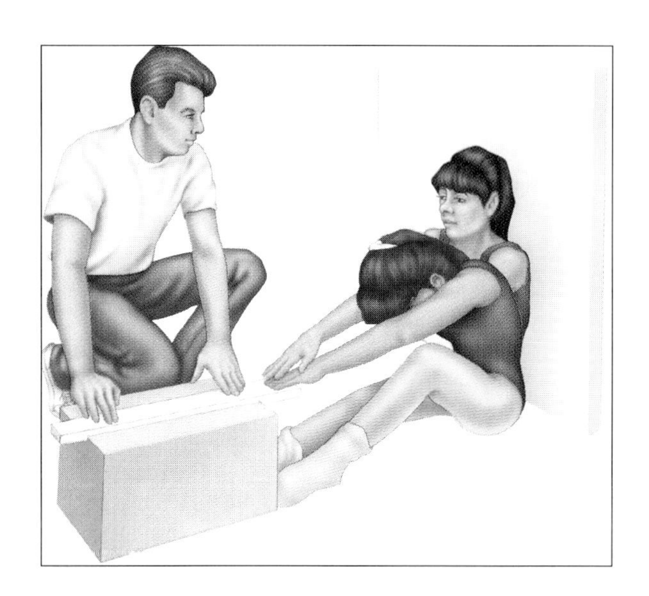

Test

2. *Shoulder Flexibility* ("Zipper" Test)
   a. Raise your arm, bend your elbow, and reach down across your back as far as possible.
   b. At the same time, extend your left arm down and behind your back, bend your elbow up across your back, and try to cross your fingers over those of your right hand as shown in the accompanying illustration.
   c. Measure the distance to the nearest half-inch. If your fingers overlap, score as a plus; if they fail to meet, score as a minus; use a zero if your fingertips just touch.
   d. Repeat with your arms crossed in the opposite direction (left arm up). Most people will find that they are more flexible on one side than the other.

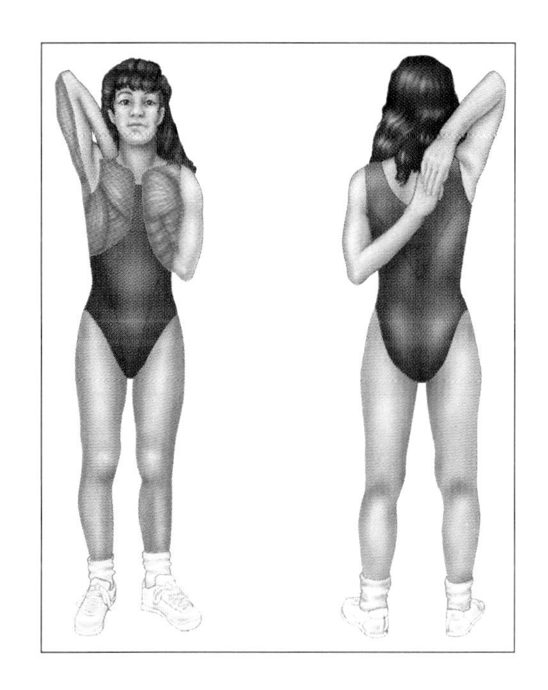

Test

3. *Hamstring and Hip Flexor Flexibility*

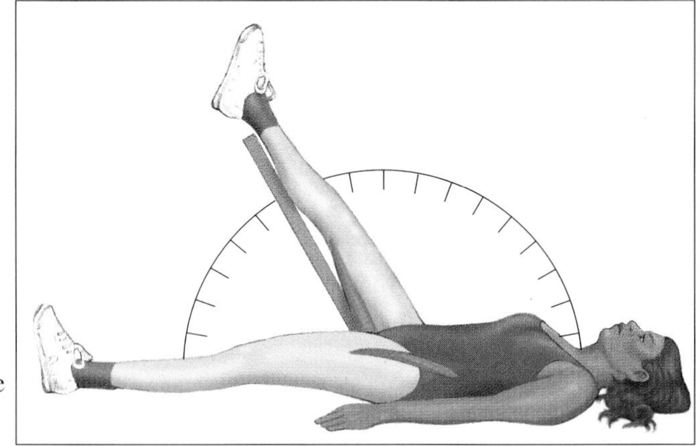

- **a.** Lie on your back on the floor beside a wall.
- **b.** Slowly lift one leg off the floor. Keep the other leg flat on the floor.
- **c.** Keep both legs straight.
- **d.** Continue to lift the leg until either leg begins to bend or the lower leg begins to lift off the floor.
- **e.** Place a yardstick against the wall and underneath the lifted leg.
- **f.** Hold the yardstick against the wall after the leg is lowered.
- **g.** Using a protractor, measure the angle created by the floor and the yardstick. The greater the angle, the better your score.
- **h.** Repeat with the other leg.*

*Note: For ease of testing, you may want to draw angles on a piece of posterboard as illustrated. If you have goniometers, you may be taught to use them instead.

Test

4. *Trunk Rotation*

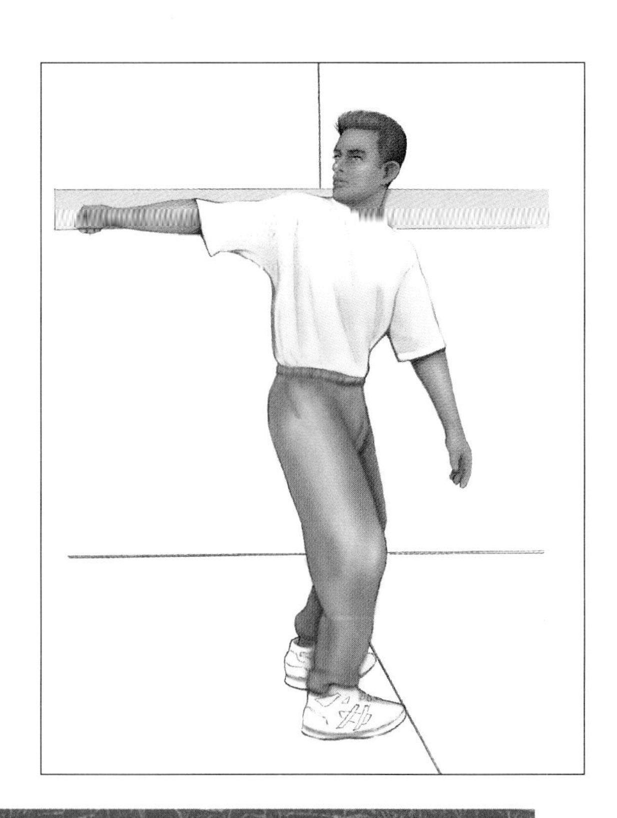

- **a.** Tape two yardsticks to the wall at shoulder height, one right side up and the other upside down.
- **b.** Stand with your left shoulder an arm's length (fist closed) from the wall. Toes should be on the line (which is perpendicular to the wall and even with the 15-inch mark on the yardstick).
- **c.** Drop the left arm and raise the right arm to the side, palm down, fist closed.
- **d.** Without moving your feet, rotate the trunk to the right as far as possible, reaching along the yardstick, and hold it 2 seconds. Do not move the feet nor bend the trunk. Your knees may bend slightly.
- **e.** A partner will read the distance reached to the nearest half-inch. Record your score. Repeat two times and average your two scores.
- **f.** Next, perform the test facing the opposite direction. Rotate to the left. For this test you will use the second yardstick (upside down) so that the greater the rotation, the higher the score. If you have only one yardstick, turn it right side up for the first test and upside down for the second test.

Chart 1 Flexibility Rating Scale for Tests 1–4

	Men					Women				
Classification	Test 1	Test 2		Test 3	Test 4	Test 1	Test 2		Test 3	Test 4
		Right Up	Left Up				Right Up	Left Up		
High-performance*	16+	5+	4+	111+	20+	17+	6+	5+	111+	20.5 or >
Good fitness zone	13–15	1–4	1–3	80–110	16–19.5	14–16	2–5	2–4	80–110	17–20
Marginal zone	10–12	0	0	60–79	13.5–15.5	11–13	1	1	60–79	14.5–16.5
Low zone	<9	<0	<0	<60	13 or less	<10	<1	<1	<60	14 or <

*Though performers need good flexibility, hypermobility may increase injury risk.

Lab 10B: Planning and Logging Stretching Exercises

Name	Section	Date

Purpose: To set one-week lifestyle goals for stretching exercises, to prepare a stretching for flexibility plan, and to self-monitor progress in your one-week plan.

Procedures:

1. On Chart 1 check the stretching exercises you plan to perform during the next week. Try to do at least eight exercises three times a week. The Basic 8 are listed. You may substitute other exercises by writing them in the "other" blank. See Table 5 for additional exercises.
2. Keep a one-week log of your actual participation using Chart 2. If possible, keep the log with you during the day. Place a check by each of the stretching exercises you perform each day—including ones that you didn't originally have planned. If you cannot keep the log with you, fill in the log at the end of the day. If you choose to keep a log for more than one week, make extra copies of the log before you begin.
3. Answer the questions in the results section.

Chart 1 Stretching Exercise Plan

Place a check beside the stretching exercises you plan to do and under the days you plan to do them.	Day 1 Date:	Day 2 Date:	Day 3 Date:	Day 4 Date:	Day 5 Date:	Day 6 Date:	Day 7 Date:
1. Calf stretcher							
2. Hip and thigh stretcher							
3. Sitting stretcher							
4. Hamstring stretcher							
5. Back stretcher (leg hug)							
6. Trunk twister							
7. Pectoral stretcher							
8. Arm stretcher							
Other:							
Other:							
Other:							
Other:							

Results:

	Yes	No
Did you do eight exercises at least three days in the week?	○	○
Did you do eight exercises more than three days in the week ?	○	○

Chart 2 Stretching Exercise Log

Place a check beside the stretching exercises you actually performed and the days on which you performed them.	Day 1 Date:	Day 2 Date:	Day 3 Date:	Day 4 Date:	Day 5 Date:	Day 6 Date:	Day 7 Date:
1. Calf stretcher							
2. Hip and thigh stretcher							
3. Sitting stretcher							
4. Hamstring stretcher							
5. Back stretcher (leg hug)							
6. Trunk twister							
7. Pectoral stretcher							
8. Arm stretcher							
Other:							
Other:							
Other:							
Other:							

Conclusions and Interpretations:

1. Do you feel that you will use stretching exercises as part of your regular lifetime physical activity plan, either now or in the future? Use several sentences to explain your answer.

2. Discuss the exercises you feel benefited you and the ones that did not. What exercises would you continue to do and which ones would you change? Use several sentences to explain your answer.

3. Did the logging of your stretching exercise help you to adhere to your program? In several sentences, explain why or why not.

Concept 11

Muscle Fitness

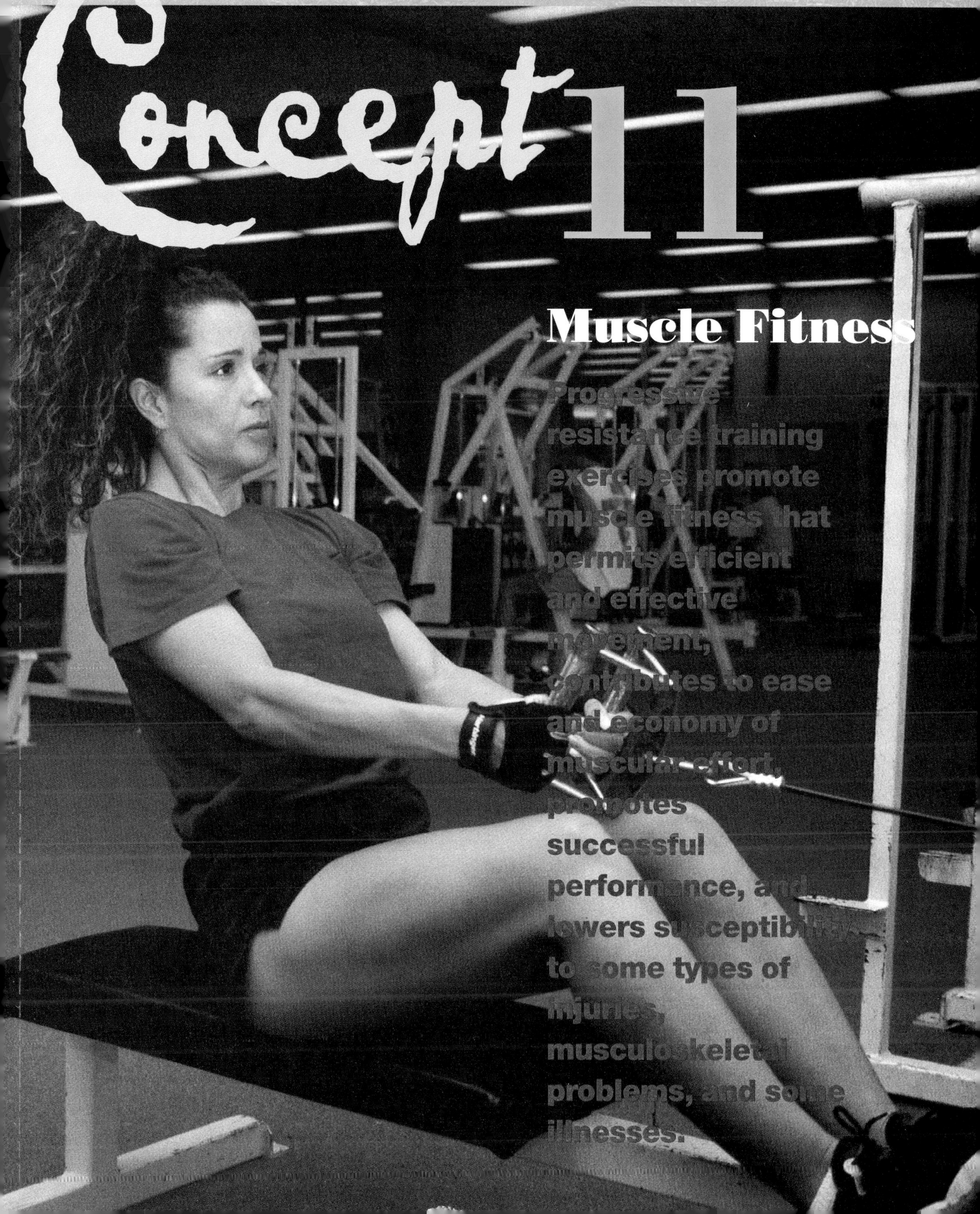

Progressive resistance training exercises promote muscle fitness that permits efficient and effective movement, contributes to ease and economy of muscular effort, promotes successful performance, and lowers susceptibility to some types of injuries, musculoskeletal problems, and some illnesses.

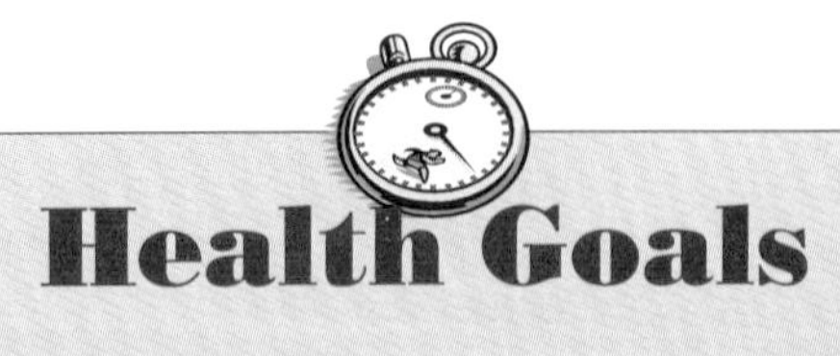

for year 2010

Increase proportion of people who regularly perform exercises for strength and muscular endurance.

Reduce steroid use especially among youth.

Increase screening and reduce incidence of osteoporosis.

Reduce activity limitation due to chronic back pain.

Introduction

There are two components of muscle fitness: strength and muscular endurance. Strength is the amount of force you can produce with a single maximal effort of a muscle group. Muscular endurance is the capacity of the skeletal muscles or group of muscles to continue contracting over a long period of time. You need both strength and muscular endurance to increase work capacity; to decrease the chance of injury; to prevent low back pain, poor posture, and other hypokinetic conditions; to improve athletic performance; and perhaps to save a life or property in an emergency. Muscle fitness training increases the fitness of the bones, tendons, and ligaments, as well as the muscles. It has been found to be therapeutic for patients with chronic pain.

Progressive resistance training is the type of physical activity done with the intent of improving muscle fitness. The many types of progressive resistance exercises designed to promote or maintain muscle fitness are described in this concept.

The Basic Facts about Strength and Muscular Endurance

There are three types of muscle tissue.

www.mhhe.com/phys_fit/webreview11 Click 01

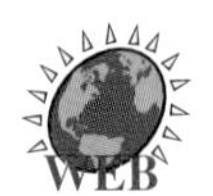

The three types of muscle tissue—smooth, cardiac, and skeletal—have different structures and functions. Smooth muscle tissue consists of long, spindle-shaped fibers with each fiber containing only one nucleus. The fibers are involuntary and are located in the walls of the esophagus, stomach, and intestines, where they function to move food and waste products through the digestive tract. Cardiac muscle tissue is also involuntary and, as its name implies, it is found only in the heart. These fibers contract in response to demands on the cardiovascular system. The heart muscle contracts at a slow steady rate at rest but contracts more frequently and forcefully during physical activity. Skeletal muscle tissues consist of long, cylindrical, multinucleated fibers. They provide the force needed to move the skeletal system and may be controlled voluntarily.

Skeletal muscle tissue consists of different types of fibers that respond and adapt differently to training.

There are three distinct types of muscle fibers, slow-twitch (Type I), fast-twitch (Type IIb) and an intermediate fiber type (Type IIa). The slow-twitch fibers are generally red in color and are well-suited to produce energy with aerobic metabolism. Slow-twitch fibers generate less tension but are more resistant to fatigue. Endurance training leads to adaptations in the slow-twitch fibers that allow them to produce energy more efficiently and better resist fatigue. Fast-twitch fibers are generally white in color and are well-suited to produce energy with anaerobic processes. They generate greater tension than slow-twitch fibers, but they fatigue more quickly. These fibers are particularly well suited to fast, high-force activities such as explosive weight-lifting movements, sprinting, and jumping. Progressive resistance exercise enhances strength primarily by increasing the size (muscle **hypertrophy**) of fast-twitch fibers but cellular adaptations also take place to enhance various metabolic properties. Intermediate fibers have biochemical and physiological properties that are between the slow- and fast-twitch fibers. A distinct property of these intermediate fibers is that they are highly adaptable depending on the type of training that is performed.

An example of fast-twitch muscle fiber in animals is the white meat in the flying muscles of a chicken. The chicken is heavy and must exert a powerful force to fly a few feet up to a perch. A wild duck that flies for hundreds of miles has dark meat (slow-twitch fibers) in the flying muscles for better endurance.

People who want large muscles will use progressive resistance exercises designed to build strength (fast-twitch fibers). People who want to be able to persist in activities for a long period of time without fatigue will want to use progressive resistance training programs designed to build muscular endurance (slow-twitch fibers). (See Figure 1.)

Genetics, gender, and age affect muscle fitness performance.

www.mhhe.com/phys_fit/webreview11 Click 02

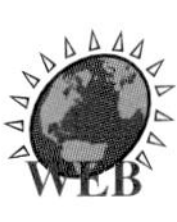

Each person inherits a certain percentage of fast-twitch and slow-twitch muscle fibers. This allocation influences the potential a person has for mus-

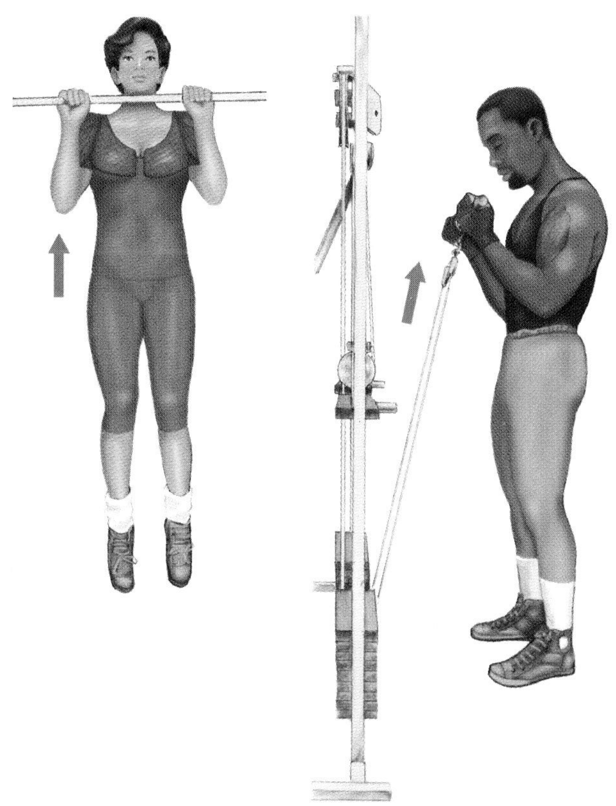

Figure 1
Overcoming a heavy resistance one time requires strength. Repeating an activity with less resistance requires muscular endurance.

cle fitness activities. Individuals with a larger percentage of fast-twitch fibers will generally increase muscle size and strength more readily than individuals endowed with a larger percentage of slow-twitch fibers. People with a larger percentage of slow-twitch fibers have greater potential for muscular endurance performance. Regardless of genetics, all people can improve their strength and muscular endurance with proper training.

Women have smaller amounts of the anabolic hormone testosterone and therefore have less muscle mass than men. Because of this, women typically have 60 percent to 85 percent of the **absolute strength** of men. **Absolute muscular endurance** also favors men over women, though not as dramatically as for strength. When differences in size and muscle mass are taken into consideration, women have **relative strength** and **relative muscular endurance** similar to men.

Maximum strength is usually reached in the twenties and typically declines with age. Though muscular endurance declines with age, it is not as dramatic as decreases in absolute strength. As people grow older, regardless of gender, strength, and muscular endurance is better among people who train than people who do not. This suggests that progressive resistance training is one antidote to premature aging.

Some endurance tests penalize the weaker person.

If you are tested on absolute endurance (the number of times you can move a designated number of pounds), a stronger person has an advantage. However, if you are tested on relative muscular endurance (the number of times you can move a designated percentage of your maximum strength), the stronger person does not have an advantage. For this reason, men and women can compete more evenly in relative muscular endurance activities. In fact, on some endurance tasks women have done as well or better than men. For example, the women at the United States Military Academy do as well as the men on tests of abdominal muscular endurance.

Hypertrophy Increase in the size of muscles as the result of strength training; increase in bulk.

Absolute Strength The maximum amount of force one can exert (e.g., maximum number of pounds or kilograms that can be lifted on one attempt. (See Relative Strength.)

Absolute Muscular Endurance (Dynamic Type) Endurance measured by the maximum number of repetitions (muscle contractions) one can perform against a given resistance (e.g., the number of times you can bench press 50 pounds).

Relative Strength Amount of force that can be exerted in relation to one's body weight or per unit of muscle cross-section; that is, if a 100-pound person lifts 250 pounds, he or she has lifted 2.5 pounds per pound of body weight, and thus has more relative strength than a 250-pound person who lifts 500 pounds, or 2 pounds per pound of body weight. The latter has more absolute strength.

Relative Muscular Endurance (Dynamic Type) Endurance measured by the maximum number of repetitions one can perform against a resistance that is a given percentage of one's 1 RM (e.g., the number of times you can lift 50 percent of your 1 RM).

Muscular endurance is related to cardiovascular endurance, but it is not the same thing.

Cardiovascular endurance depends primarily upon the efficiency of the heart muscle, circulatory system, and respiratory system. It is developed with activities that stress these systems, such as running, cycling, and swimming. Muscular endurance depends upon the efficiency of the local skeletal muscles and the nerves that control them. Most forms of cardiovascular exercises such as running require good cardiovascular and muscular endurance. For example, if your legs lack the muscular endurance to continue contracting for a sustained period of time, it will be difficult to perform well in running or other aerobic activities.

The Facts about the Health Benefits of Muscle Fitness

Good muscle fitness is associated with reduced risk of injury.

www.mhhe.com/phys_fit/webreview11 Click 03

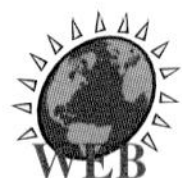

Experts believe that strong muscles with good endurance are able to resist various injuries. People with good muscle fitness are less likely to suffer joint injuries (e.g., neck, knee, ankle) than those with poor muscle fitness. Weak muscles are more likely to be involuntarily overstretched than are strong muscles.

Muscle balance is important in reducing the risk of injury. Resistance training should build both agonist and **antagonist muscles**. For example, if you do resistance exercise to build the quadriceps muscles (front of the thigh), you should also exercise the hamstring muscles (back of the thigh). In this instance, the quadriceps are the agonist (muscle being used), and the hamstrings are the antagonist. If the quadriceps become too strong relative to the antagonist hamstring muscles, the risk of injury increases (see Figure 2).

Good muscle fitness is associated with good posture and reduced risk of back problems.

www.mhhe.com/phys_fit/webreview11 Click 04

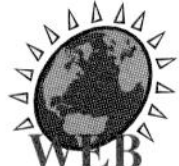

When muscles in specific body regions are weak or overdeveloped, poor posture can result. Lack of fitness of the abdominal and low back muscles is particularly related to poor posture and potential back problems. Excessively strong hip flexor muscles can lead to swayback. Poor balance in muscular development can also result in postural problems. For example, the muscles on the sides of the body must be balanced to maintain an erect posture.

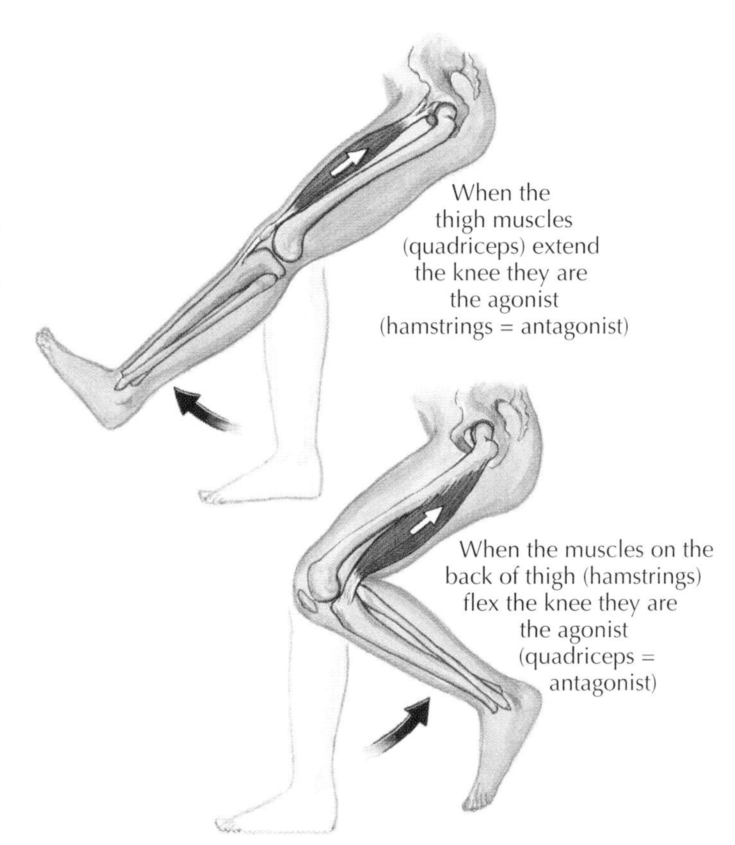

Figure 2
Agonist and antagonist muscles.

Good muscle fitness can bring about improved athletic performance.

Many sports depend on strength and muscular endurance. A football player must have good muscle strength to block and tackle effectively. A swimmer or a wrestler requires good muscular endurance to perform optimally. Athletes and people interested in jobs requiring high-level performance such as law enforcement and fire safety are especially likely to benefit from good muscle fitness.

Good muscular fitness is associated with wellness.

Wellness is reflected in quality of life and well-being. A person with muscle fitness is able to perform for long periods of time without undue fatigue. As a result, the person has energy to perform daily work efficiently and effectively and has reserve energy to enjoy leisure time. Among older people, maintenance of strength is associated with increased balance, less risk of falling, and greater ability to perform the tasks of daily living independently. Muscle fitness also contributes to looking one's best. Muscles can help the abdomen from protruding, and because people with more muscle burn more calories at rest, good muscle fitness helps in the maintenance of a healthy body weight.

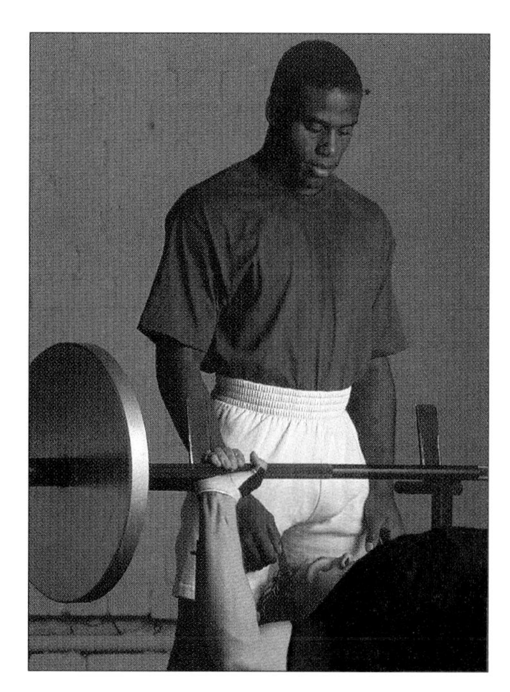

Progressive resistance exercises are methods of training designed to build muscle fitness.

The Facts about Progressive Resistance Exercise

The best type of training for muscle fitness is referred to as progressive resistance exercise.

The type of training most commonly used to promote muscle fitness is referred to as **progressive resistance exercise (PRE)**, or progressive resistance training (PRT). This name is used because the frequency, intensity, and length of time of muscle overload are progressively increased as muscle fitness increases. Progressive resistance exercises are typically done in one to three sets of three to 25 repetitions (also called reps). A set is a group of reps that are done in succession followed by a rest period.

Progressive resistance exercise is not the same thing as weight lifting, powerlifting, or bodybuilding.

Progressive resistance exercise is a method of training to build muscle fitness that provides health and performance benefits. It should not be confused with the following three competitive activities. Weight lifting is a competitive sport that involves two lifts: the snatch and the clean and jerk. Powerlifting is also a competitive sport that includes three lifts: the bench press, the squat, and the dead lift. Bodybuilding is a competition in which participants are judged on the size and **definition** of their muscles. All three of these competitive events rely on progressive resistance exercise to improve performance. Weight training is a form of PRE and is a method of improving muscle fitness that is different from weight lifting—the competitive event.

Progressive resistance exercise programs can be performed in a variety of ways and with different equipment.

Isotonic exercise (also called dynamic) refers to such activities as weight training, calisthenics, pulley weights, and resistance machine exercises. When performing isotonic exercise, both **concentric** (shortening) and **eccentric** (lengthening) **contractions** should be used. For example, in an overhead press exercise, the muscles on the back of the arm (triceps) shorten (contract concentrically) to lift the weight overhead (see Figure 3*a*). When the weight is lowered, the muscles lengthen (contract eccentrically) if the weight is lowered slowly. Both concentric and eccentric contractions build the

Antagonistic Muscles The muscles that have the opposite action from those that are contracting (agonists); normally, antagonists reflexively relax when agonists contract.

Progressive Resistance Exercise (PRE) Exercise done against a resistance; also referred to as progressive resistance training (PRT).

Definition (of Muscle) The detailed external appearance of a muscle.

Isotonic Type of muscle contraction in which the muscle changes length, either shortening (concentrically) or lengthening (eccentrically). Isotonic exercises are those in which a resistance is raised and then lowered, as in weight training and calisthenics (also called dynamic or phasic).

Concentric Contraction An isotonic muscle contraction in which the muscle gets shorter as it contracts, such as when a joint is bent and two body parts move closer together. An example is the biceps muscle contraction that occurs when pulling up on a chinning bar.

Eccentric Contraction An isotonic muscle contraction in which the muscle gets longer as it contracts; that is, when a weight is gradually lowered and the contracting muscle gets longer as it gives up tension. Lowering the body from a pull-up on a chinning bar is an example of eccentric contraction of the biceps muscle. Eccentric contractions are also called negative exercise.

muscle. Eccentric contractions, sometimes called negative contractions, are more likely to cause delayed-onset muscle soreness than concentric contractions. Typically, the stress on the muscle in either concentric or eccentric exercises varies with speed, joint position, and muscle length. Thus, the muscle may work harder at the beginning of a lift than it does near the end of the range of motion.

www.mhhe.com/phys_fit/webreview11 Click 05

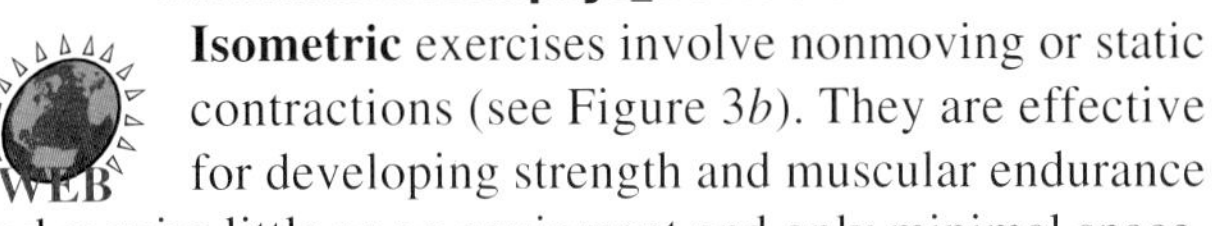

Isometric exercises involve nonmoving or static contractions (see Figure 3*b*). They are effective for developing strength and muscular endurance and require little or no equipment and only minimal space. Isometric exercises build **static strength** and **static muscular endurance** as opposed to **dynamic strength** or **dynamic muscular endurance**. They work the muscle only at the angle of the joint used in the exercise and promote less hypertrophy and strength than isotonic resistance exercise. Thus, isometric exercises are probably less effective as an overall training method than isotonic exercises. On the other hand, isometrics have been found to be quite useful for some athletes, such as wrestlers and gymnasts, and work especially well for people in the early stages of some rehabilitation programs. Research has shown that strength can be enhanced significantly by using isometric training at the **sticking points** of isotonic lifts.

Isometrics previously have been thought to be dangerous for people with high blood pressure or cardiovascular disease. Recent evidence suggests that may not be the case for all people with these cardiovascular problems. These people should consult a medical expert before using isometric techniques.

www.mhhe.com/phys_fit/webreview11 Click 06

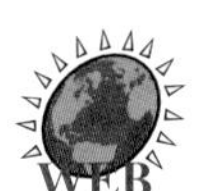

Isokinetic exercises are isotonic-concentric muscle contractions performed on devices such as the Apollo, Exer-Genie, Mini-Gym, Hydra-Fitness (hydraulic machine), or on electromechanical dynamometers, such as the Cybex II. These machines keep the velocity of the movement constant and match their resistance to the effort of the performer, permitting maximal tension to be exerted throughout the range of motion (see Figure 3*c*). For example, on the Cybex II, speeds range from 0 to 300 degrees per second. This rate-limiting mechanism prevents the performer from moving faster no matter how much force is exerted. Thus, isokinetic devices attempt to overcome the basic weakness of isotonics. On the other hand, these devices do not permit acceleration, so it is not possible to train specifically for sports skills, such as throwing or kicking, in which the limb is accelerated while applying maximum force. Another limitation is that some of these devices permit only concentric contractions. Isokinetic exercise has the advantage of being safer than most other forms of exercise and may be better for developing power (see concept on performance benefits of physical activity). It is not better for developing pure strength, however. More research is needed to determine the best training regimen for isokinetic exercise.

Some of the advantages and disadvantages of the various forms of progressive resistance exercises, not including plyometrics, are outlined in Table 1.

Plyometrics is a form of isotonic exercise that promotes athletic performance.

www.mhhe.com/phys_fit/webreview11 Click 07

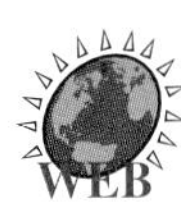

Plyometrics is a form of isotonic exercise that is especially useful for athletes training for power development. High jumpers, long jumpers, volleyball, and basketball players often use this technique, which includes jumping from boxes, hopping on one foot, and similar types of activities. For most people primarily interested in the health benefits of physical activity, plyometrics are not a

Isometric A type of muscle contraction in which the muscle remains the same length. Isometric exercises are those in which no movement takes place while a force is exerted against an immovable object (also known as static contraction).

Static Strength A muscle's ability to exert a force without changing length. It is also called isometric strength.

Static Muscular Endurance A muscle's ability to remain contracted for a long period. This is usually measured by the length of time you can hold a body position. It is also called isometric endurance.

Dynamic Strength A muscle's ability to exert force that results in movement. It is typically measured isotonically.

Dynamic Muscular Endurance A muscle's ability to contract and relax repeatedly. This is usually measured by the number of times (repetitions) you can perform a body movement in a given time period. It is also called isotonic endurance.

Sticking Point The point in the range of motion where the weight cannot be lifted any farther without extreme effort or assistance; the weakest point in the movement.

Isokinetic Isotonic concentric exercises done with a machine that regulates movement velocity and resistance.

Plyometrics A training technique used to develop explosive power. Referred to as speed-strength training in Eastern Europe and the former Soviet Union, where it originated. It consists of concentric isotonic muscle contractions performed after a prestretch or eccentric contraction of a muscle.

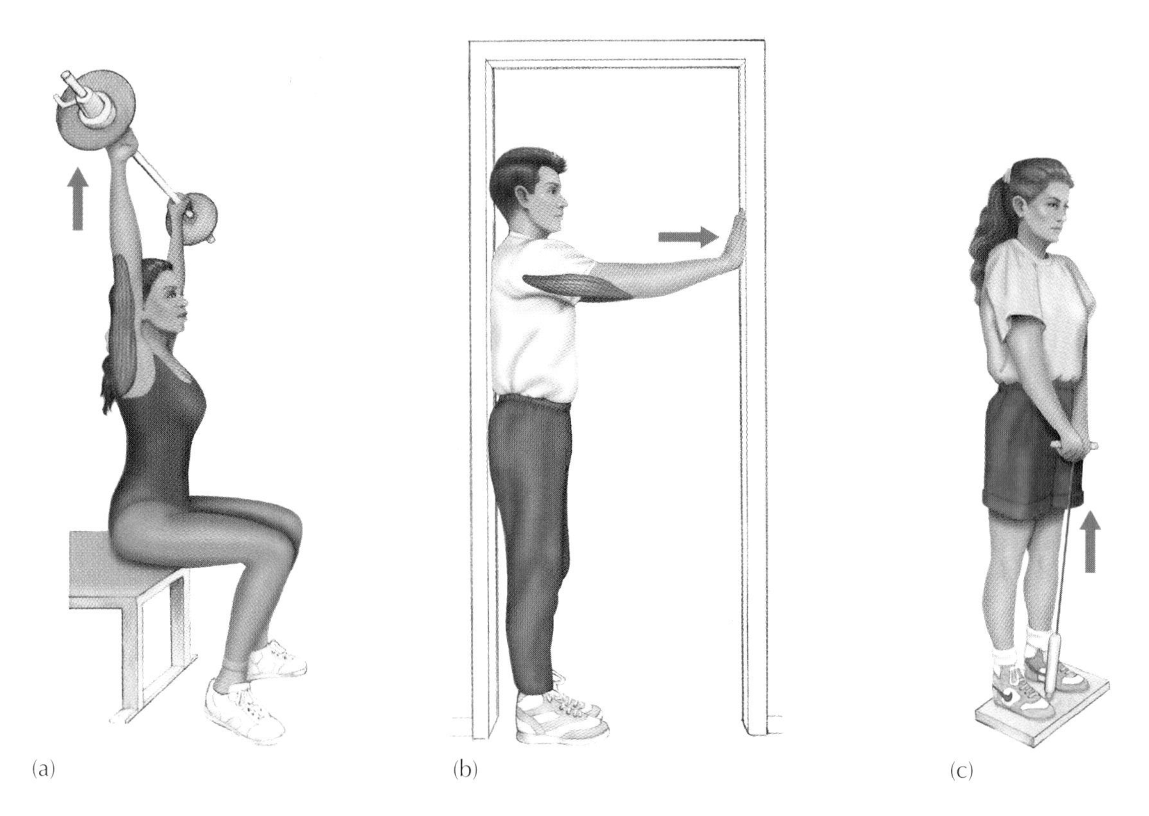

Figure 3
Examples of three types of muscle fitness exercises (*a*) isotonic, (*b*) isometric, and (*c*) isokinetic.

Table 1 Advantages and Disadvantages of Isometric, Isotonic, and Isokinetic Resistance Exercises*

	Isometrics (Statics)	Isotonics (Dynamics)	Isokinetics
In small space	E	F-G	F-G
No equipment or low-cost equipment	E	F-G	P
Provides feedback for motivation	P	E	F
Can rehabilitate immobilized joint	E	P	P
Builds strength through full range of motion	P	F-G	E
Less likely to cause soreness	E	F-G	E
Aids dynamic coordination	P	E	G
Safe for hypertensives	P	E	G-E
Amount of strength developed	F	E	E
Dynamic exercises and controlled testing	P	F-G	E
Hypertrophy	P	E	E
Power development	P	G	E
Rapid improvement in strength	E	F-G	F-G
Can accelerate to resemble sport skill	P	E	P

*Key: E = Excellent; G = Good; F = Fair; P = Poor

preferred type of exercise. In fact, they can increase risk of injury, especially among beginners. For more information on plyometrics, refer to the concept on the performance benefits of physical activity.

There are advantages of both free weights and machine weights.

Free weights are weights that are not attached to a machine or exercise device. Typically, they come in the form of a barbell or dumbbell that can be adjusted as necessary for different exercises to provide optimal resistance. Weight training with free weights is very popular because it can be done in the home with inexpensive equipment. Because free weights require balance and technique, they may be somewhat difficult for beginners to use, but competitive weight lifters generally prefer them because they can exercise muscle groups in a very specific way.

Resistance training machines can be effective in developing strength and muscular endurance if used properly. They can save time because, unlike free weights, the resistance can be changed easily and quickly. They may be safer because you are less likely to drop weights. A disadvantage is that the kinds of exercises that can be done on these machines are more limited than free-weight exercises. They also may not promote optimal balance in muscular development since a stronger muscle can often make up for a weaker muscle in the completion of a lift.

www.mhhe.com/phys_fit/webreview11 Click 08

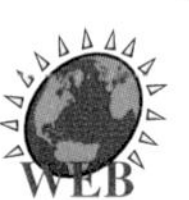

Some machines, such as Nautilus and Universal, offer what is called "variable" or "accommodating resistance." The Nautilus, for example, uses a cam to adapt the resistance as the performer moves through the range of motion. The Universal Trainer uses a rolling pivot to do the same thing. These adaptations attempt to compensate for an inherent weakness in isotonic constant-resistance exercises done with free weights and other machines. They are only partially successful, however, in adapting to the shapes, sizes, and torques of individual human bodies. There is no evidence that variable-resistance machines develop more strength or muscular endurance than other devices, although they may offer advantages in muscle fitness by allowing movement through an extended range of motion.

Table 2 provides a comparison of free weights with weight machines (for example, Nautilus, Universal, Marcy, Hydra-Gym, Dynacam, and Paramount). Free weights are compared with other resistance machines in Table 3.

Table 2 Advantages and Disadvantages of Free Weights and Resistance Machines

Free Weights	Resistance Machines
• Requires balance and coordination; uses more muscles for stabilization.	• Other body parts are stabilized; easier to isolate particular muscle group.
• Truer to real-life situation, so skills transfer to daily life.	• Controlled path of weight not true to life.
• Creates more possibility of injury.	• Safer because weight cannot fall on participant.
• Requires spotters for safety.	• No spotters required.
• Takes more time to change weights.	• Easy and quick to change weights.
• Unlimited number of exercises possible.	• Restricted to range and angle of movement permitted by the machine.
• Less expensive.	• Expensive; need to go to club if cannot afford equipment; need more than one machine for variety.
• Loose equipment clutters area and may get lost or stolen.	• Machines are stationary but occupy large space.

Many resistance training exercises can be done with little or no equipment.

Calisthenics are among the most popular forms of muscle fitness exercise among adults. Calisthenics, such as curl-ups and push-ups, are suitable for people of different ability levels, and can be used to improve both strength and muscular endurance. One disadvantage is that this type of exercise does little to increase strength unless resistance in addition to your body weight is added. For example, doing a push-up will build strength to a point. However, once you can do several, adding more repetitions will only build muscular endurance but not strength. To develop additional strength, you can add more weights to increase the resistance or change the body position so there is a greater gravitational effect or more torque. For example, you can elevate your feet or wear a weighted vest while doing push-ups.

Another alternative to expensive resistance training machines or commercially made free weights are homemade weights and elastic exercise bands. Homemade weights can be constructed from pieces of pipe or broom sticks and plastic milk jugs filled with water. Elastic tubes or bands available in varying strengths may be substituted for the weights and for the pulley device used in many resistance training machines to impart resistance.

Muscular endurance can be developed through activities such as running, swimming, circuit training, and aerobic dance if they are designed appropriately. Lifestlye activities such as gardening (e.g., raking, shoveling) or housework (lifting groceries) can also contribute to muscular endurance.

Table 3 Comparison of Selected Resistance Training Devices

	Free Weights	Weight-Stack Machine	Compressed Air Machine	Hydraulic Machine	Isokinetic Machine
Concentric resistance	+	+	+	+	+
Eccentric resistance	+	+	+	-	+-
Isometric resistance	+	+	+	+	-
Match resistance to effort through range of motion	-	+-	+	+	+
Isolation of all major muscle groups	-	+-	+	+	+
Safety features	-	+	+	+	+
Durability	+	+	+	+	+

From Wayne L. Westcott, "Strength Training" in *Sportcare & Fitness Magazine*, July/August 1988, page 62. Reprinted by permission of Wayne L. Westcott.

The Facts about How Much PRE Is Enough

> The overload principle must be applied using progressive resistance exercises such as those in the muscle fitness section of the physical activity pyramid if muscle fitness is to be developed and maintained.

It was in the area of muscle fitness development that the overload principle was first clearly outlined. Centuries ago, Milo of Crotona was said to have recognized the value of progressive overload. His strength increased as he repeatedly lifted a calf. As the calf grew into a bull, its weight increased, and Milo's strength increased as well. We now know that for most people, special exercises referred to as progressive resistance exercises are necessary if muscle fitness is to be developed and maintained (see Figure 4). Activities from other levels of the physical activity pyramid rarely promote adequate muscle fitness.

> The amount of overload for strength is different than for muscular endurance.

The stimulus for strength is maximal exertion. Strength training should therefore utilize high resistance overload with low repetitions. The stimulus for muscular endurance is repeated contractions with short rests. Muscular endurance exercises should be performed with a relatively high number of repetitions and lower resistance.

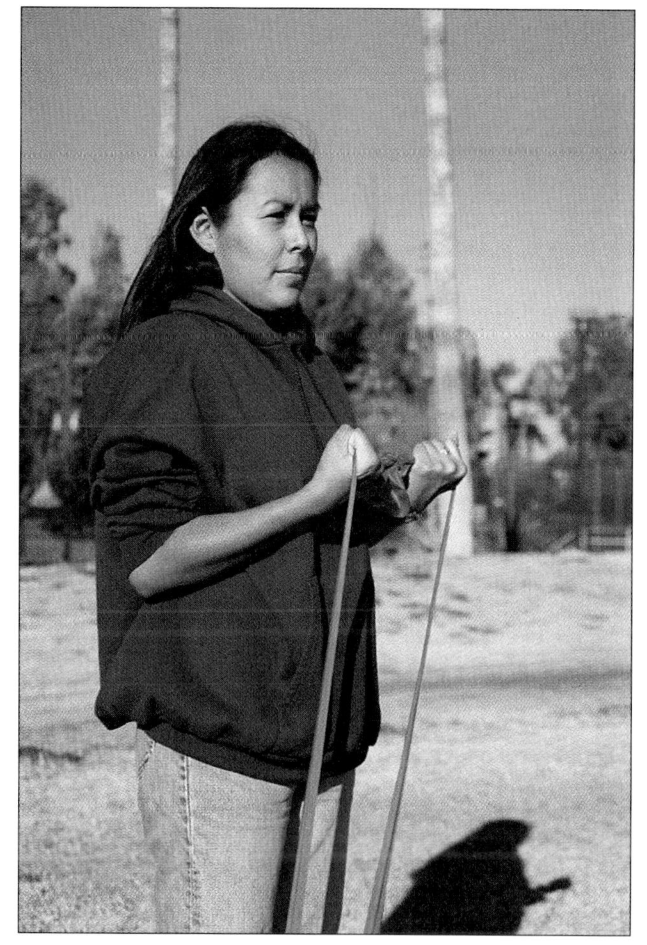

Elastic bands can provide resistance to build muscle fitness.

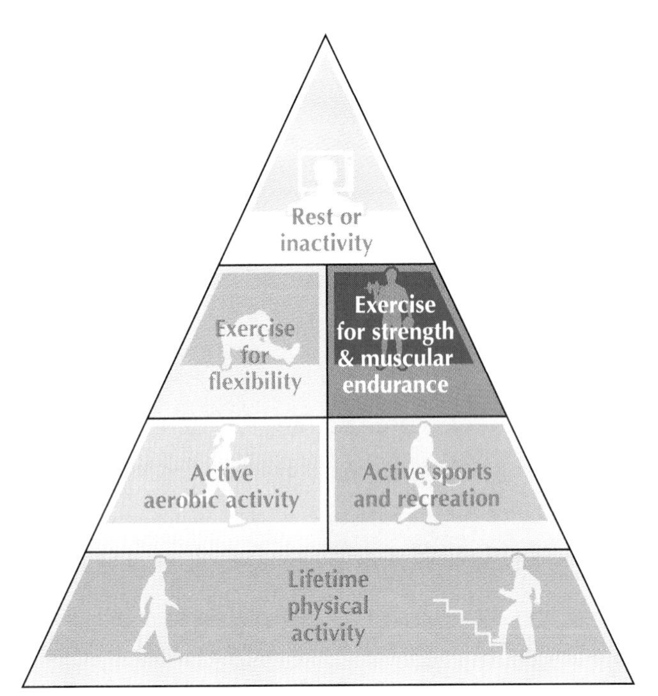

Figure 4
To build muscle fitness, activities should be selected from level 3 of the Physical Activity Pyramid.

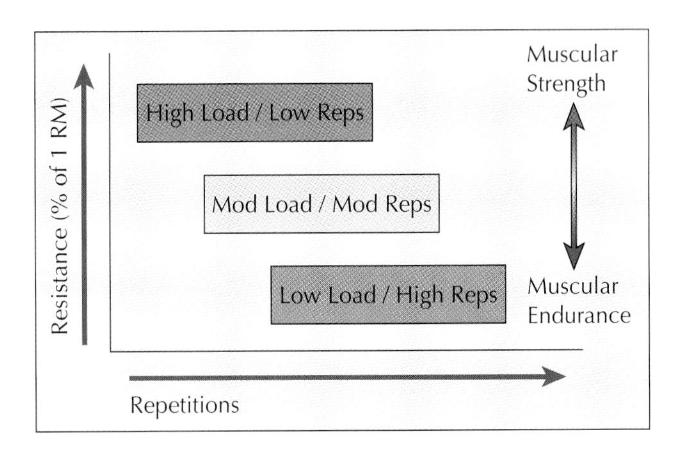

Figure 5
Comparison of muscular endurance to muscle strength developed by different repetitions and resistance.

The graph in Figure 5 illustrates the relationship between strength and muscular endurance. In *A*, the training program calls for a high number of repetitions and light resistance. This results in a small gain in strength (the area of the bar to the right of the line), and a large increase in absolute endurance (the area of the bar to the left of the line). In *B*, the training program calls for a moderate number of repetitions (less than in *A*), and a moderate resistance (more than in *A*). This results in slightly less absolute endurance and slightly more strength than in program *A*. Program *C* uses high resistance and low repetitions. This results in the least gain in endurance but the most gain in strength.

While strength training (program *C*) promotes strength, studies show that the person who is strength-trained will fatigue as much as four times faster than the person who is endurance-trained (program *A*). However, there is a modest correlation between strength and endurance because the person who trains for strength will develop some endurance, and the person who trains for muscular endurance will develop some strength.

Muscular endurance and strength are part of the same continuum.

Though strength and muscular endurance are developed in different ways, strength and muscular endurance are part of the same continuum (Figure 6). This has led some writers to refer to muscular endurance as strength endurance. "Pure" strength is approached as one nears the end (right) of the continuum, where only one maximum contraction is made. As the number of repetitions increases and the force of the contractions decreases, one nears the other end (left) of the continuum and approaches "pure" endurance. In between the two extremes, varying degrees of strength and endurance are combined. The activities listed along the continuum are examples that might represent points along the scale. You will note that most of the activities of daily living are at the middle of the continuum, indicating that they take a combination of strength and muscular endurance.

The intensity of muscle fitness training is determined using a percentage of the amount of weight you can lift one time (1 RM).

The maximum amount of resistance you can move (or weight you can lift) one time is called your one **repetition maximum (RM)**. The amount of resistance you use in a progressive resistance exercise program is based on a percentage of your 1 RM. The percentage of 1 RM used in a program depends on the program goals. For strength, the percentages vary from 60 to 80 percent depending on a person's current strength level. More experienced strength trainers often exercise at a higher percentage of 1 RM than beginners. For muscular endurance, the percentages vary from 20 to 40 percent. People interested in a combination of strength and muscular endurance should use 40 to 60 percent of 1 RM in their training.

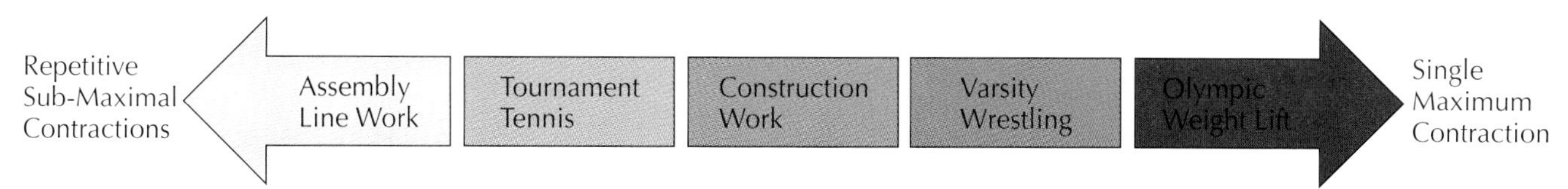

Figure 6
Muscle strength-endurance continuum.

The principle of specificity applies to progressive resistance exercise.

Depending on the specific muscle that you want to develop, you will use different types of resistance training programs. Factors that can be varied in your program are the type of muscle contraction (isometric or isotonic), the speed or cadence of the movement, and the amount of resistance being moved. For example, if you want strength in the elbow extensor muscles (e.g., triceps) so that you could more easily lift heavy boxes onto a shelf, you would train using isotonic contractions, at a relatively slow speed, with a relatively high resistance. If you want muscle fitness of the fingers to grip a heavy bowling ball, much of your training should be done isometrically using the fingers the same way you normally hold the ball. If you are training for a particular skill that requires explosive power, such as in throwing, striking, kicking, or jumping, your strength exercises should be done with less resistance and greater speed. If you are training for a skill that uses both concentric and eccentric contractions or is plyometric, you should perform strength exercises using these characteristics. More information on these techniques is included in the concept on the performance benefits of physical activity.

If you are not training for a specific task, but merely wish to develop muscle fitness for daily living, consider the advantages and disadvantages of isometrics, isotonics, and isokinetics listed in Table 1. You may wish to use a variety of methods.

The principle of diminishing returns applies to resistance training.

To get optimal strength gains from progressive resistance training, one or more sets of exercise repetitions is performed. Some high-level performers use as many as five sets of a particular exercise. Research indicates that most of the fitness and health benefits, however, are achieved in one set. As much as 80 to 90 percent of the benefits may result in the first set, with each additional set producing less and less benefit. Because compliance with resistance training programs is less likely as the time needed to complete the program increases, the American College of Sports Medicine recently recommended single-set programs for most adults. They acknowledge that additional benefits are likely with more multiset routines, but they believe that adults are more likely to participate if they can get most of the benefits in a relatively short amount of time. In sports or competition where very small performance differences make big differences, doing multiple sets is important.

The principle of rest and recovery especially applies to strength development.

Progressive resistance training for strength development done every day of the week does not allow enough rest and time for recovery. Recent studies have shown that the greatest proportion of strength is accomplished in two days of training per week. Exercise done on a third day does result in additional increases, but the amount of gain is relatively small compared to gains resulting from two days of training per week. For people interested in health benefits rather than performance benefits, two days a week saves time and may result in greater adherence to a strength-training program. For people interested in performance benefits, more frequent training may be warranted. Rotating exercises so that certain muscles are exercised on one day and other muscles are exercised the next allows for more frequent training

The amount of exercise necessary to maintain strength is less than the amount needed to develop it.

Recent evidence suggests that once strength is developed, it may be maintained by performing fewer sets or exercising fewer days per week. For example, if you have performed three sets of an exercise three days a week to build strength, you may be able to maintain current levels of strength with one set a week. Also you may be able to maintain strength by exercising one or two rather than three days per week. If schedules of fewer sets or fewer days per week result in strength loss, frequency must be increased.

Repetitions Maximum (RM) The maximum amount of resistance one can move a given number of times; for example: 1 RM = maximum weight lifted one time; 6 RM = maximum weight lifted six times.

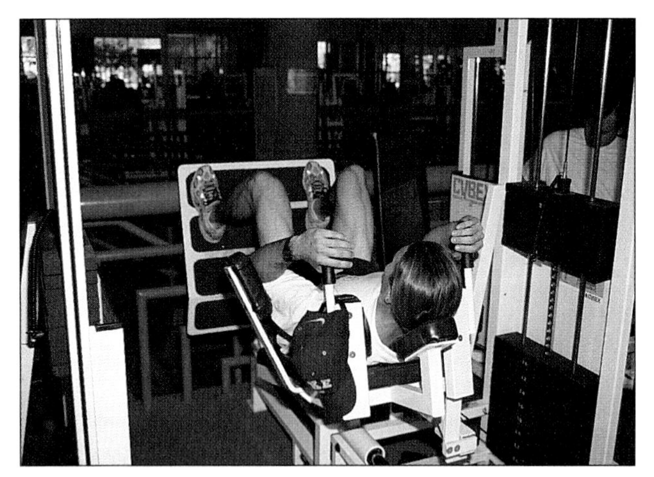

The repetition maximum (1 RM) is a good measure of strength.

Some muscle groups seem to need training less often to maintain strength levels. For example, evidence suggests that muscle fitness of the back can be maintained using one-day-a-week single-set exercises. Smaller muscles seem to need more frequent exercise.

There is a threshold of training and a target zone for strength development.

The FIT formula for strength defines the threshold and target values for strength development. Table 4 illustrates the FIT formula for isometrics, isotonics, and isokinetic resistance training for typical people. People interested in advanced progressive resistance training, such as body builders or competitive weight lifters, will need special training programs to excel at these activities (refer to the concept on the performance benefits of physical activity).

There is a threshold of training and a target zone for muscular endurance development.

There is a frequency, intensity, and time at which a training effect for muscular endurance will begin to take place (threshold). There is also an optimal range, or target zone, where the most effective and efficient improvement will occur (see Table 5). We do not know the exact range, but studies suggest that it has wide limits. Intensity of effort seems to be important and studies suggest that one set can be nearly as effective as three if done properly.

The Facts about Using PRE Effectively

The muscle fitness workout should be based on the principle of progression.

Many beginning resistance trainers experience extreme soreness after the first few days of training. The reason for the sore-

Table 4 Strength Threshold of Training and Fitness Target Zones

	Threshold of Training			Target Zone		
	Isometrics	Isotonics	Isokinetics	Isometrics	Isotonics	Isokinetics
Frequency	• 2 days a week for each muscle group.			• 2 to 3 days per week.		
Intensity	• Use 60–65% of maximum contraction (1 RM).	• 60–65% of 1 RM for every rep.	• 90% of 1 RM at set speed.	• Maximum contractions.	• 60–80% 1 RM (for number of reps on every set).	• Maximum effort at set speed.
Time	• 1 set. • 1 rep held for 2–5 seconds. • Repeat once a day.	• 1 set. • 3–8 reps.	• 2 sets. • 3 reps lasting 3–4 seconds (30–60 degrees per second). • Rest 1 minute between sets.	• 1 set. • 6 reps held 6–8 seconds (or 2 sets of 3 reps each). • Rest 30 seconds between reps.	• 1–3 sets. • 3–8 reps. • Rest 1 minute between sets.	• 3–5 sets. • 3–8 reps lasting 1–2 seconds (70–120 degrees per second). • Rest 1 minute between sets.

Table 5 Muscular Endurance Threshold of Training and Fitness Target Zones

	Threshold of Training	Target Zone
Dynamic Endurance		
Frequency	• 2 days per week.	• Every other day.
Intensity	• Move 20%–30% of the maximum resistance you can lift.	• Move 40%–60% of the maximum resistance you can lift.
Time	• One set of 9 repetitions of each exercise.	• 2–5 sets of 9–25 repetitions. • Rest 15–60 seconds between sets.
Static Endurance		
Frequency	• 3 days per week.	• Every other day.
Intensity	• Hold a resistance 50%–100% of the weight you ultimately will need to hold in your work or leisure activity.	• Hold a resistance equal to and up to 50% greater than the amount you will need to hold in your work or leisure activity.
Time	• Hold for lengths of time 10%–50% shorter than the time you plan to do the activity. Repeat 10–20 times. • Rest 30 seconds between reps.	• Hold for lengths of time equal to and up to 20% greater than the time you plan to do the activity. For longer times, use fewer repetitions (5–10). • Rest 30–60 seconds between reps.

ness is that the principle of progression has been violated. Soreness can occur with even modest amounts of training if the volume of training is considerably more than normal. In the first few days or weeks of training, the primary adaptations in the muscle are due to motor learning factors rather than to muscle growth. Because these adaptations occur no matter how much weight is used, it is prudent to start your program slowly with very light weights. After these adaptations occur and the rate of improvement slows down, it would be necessary to follow the appropriate target zone to achieve proper overload.

The most common progression used in resistance training is the double progressive system, so-called because this system periodically adjusts both the resistance and the number of repetitions of the exercise performed. For example, if you are training for strength, you may begin with three repetitions in one set. As the repetitions become easy, additional repetitions are added. When you have progressed to eight repetitions, increase the resistance and decrease the repetitions in each set back to three and begin the progression again.

There are various systems available regarding the order and progression of exercises in a workout.

www.mhhe.com/phys_fit/webreview11 Click 09

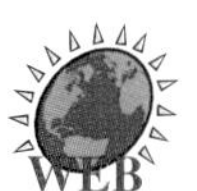

There are numerous variables that could be manipulated within a training session to alter the training effect. Some recommend a "light to heavy" system (Delorme system) in which progressively heavier weights are lifted with each set. Others recommend the "heavy to light" system (Oxford system) in which the heaviest weight is used on the first set when the muscles are most rested. Still others advocate a pre-exhaust routine in which small accessory muscle groups are fatigued before the exercises for major muscle groups are performed. Various other systems are covered in the performance concept.

Circuit resistance training (CRT) is an effective way to build muscular endurance and cardiovascular endurance.

Circuit resistance training consists of the performance of high repetitions of an exercise with low to moderate resistance, progressing from one station to another, performing a different exercise at each station. The stations are usually placed in a circle to facilitate movement. CRT typically employs about 20 to 25 reps against a resistance that is 30 to 40 percent of 1 RM for 45 seconds. Fifteen seconds of rest is provided while changing stations. Approximately 10 exercise stations are used, and the participant repeats the circuit two to three times (sets). Because of the short rest periods, significant cardiovascular benefits have been reported, in addition to muscular endurance gains.

Circuit training on weight or hydraulic machines has been found to be more effective than standard set weight training for caloric consumption during and after exercise and for improving cardiovascular endurance, although it is not as effective as aerobic exercises, such as cycling or bench stepping.

Programs intended to slim the figure/physique should be of the muscular endurance type.

Many men and women are interested in exercises designed to decrease girth measurements. High-repetition, low-resistance exercise is suitable for this because it usually brings about some strengthening and may decrease body fatness, which in turn, changes body contour. Exercises do not spot-reduce fat but they do speed up metabolism so more calories are burned. However, if weight or fat reduction is desired, aerobic (cardiovascular) exercises are best. To increase girth, use strength exercises.

> Endurance training may have a negative effect on strength and power.

Some studies have shown that for athletes who rely primarily on strength and power in their sports event, too much endurance training can cause a loss of strength and power because of modification of different muscle fibers. Strength and power athletes need some endurance training, but not too much, just as endurance athletes need some strength and power training, but not too much.

Is There Strength in a Bottle? The Facts

> Anabolic steroids are used by some athletes and a significant number of nonathletes to enhance performance and build muscular bodies.

Anabolic steroids are a synthetic reproduction of the male hormone testosterone. Physicians prescribe them to treat such conditions as muscle diseases, breast cancer, severe burns, rare types of anemia, and kidney disease. Steroids have also been used to help people with AIDS and muscle-wasting diseases retain muscle mass. Because of their dangerous side effects, doctors prescribe minimal doses. At first, research showed steroids to be ineffective in promoting muscle gain. This was because the doses used in the studies were much smaller than those taken today for performance enhancement. Many athletes and people interested in muscle development have reportedly taken massive doses 20 to 100 times the normal therapeutic dose used for medical conditions. Studies now show that when taken in large doses by people doing regular strength training, gains in muscle mass and strength can be considerable. The best evidence indicates that steroids allow the muscles to recover faster, allowing more frequent training. Taking anabolic steroids without doing progressive resistance training would be ineffective.

Anabolic steroids are typically obtained on the black market or illegally from unethical physicians, coaches, trainers, body builders, athletes, and other entrepreneurs. While athletes use the drugs in an attempt to enhance performance, an increasing number of nonathletes use steroids to enhance their strength or improve their physique or appearance. Two million people are estimated to be using "roids." Steroid use has leveled off among males, but the levels among females has increased dramatically.

A popular product in recent years is androstenedione, also called "andro." This product causes the body to produce testosterone and has similar effects as taking artificial testosterone. It is controversial because it has not been banned by all athletic governmental groups and can be purchased legally. Androstenedione gained instant notoriety when baseball slugger Mark McGwire reported using it during his assault on the season home run record. Many people assumed that his success was due, at least in part, to the use of the supplement. However, a highly publicized study in the *JAMA* recently documented that andro had little or no effect on muscle adaptations from resistance training. This study also indicated a number of negative health effects associated with its use.

> Taking anabolic steroids is illegal and a dangerous way to build muscle fitness.

There are a number of significant side effects associated with steroid use. In women, unlike men, some of these effects are irreversible (see Table 6). As can be seen in the table, steroids (like all drugs) are dangerous. They can be addictive and produce more than 70 serious side effects, some of which may be fatal. More than a few deaths have been attributed to their use. Twenty-five athletes from the former Soviet Union who competed in the 1980 Olympics died because of conditions attributed to steroid use, and the deaths of several American professional athletes have also been attributed to anabolic steroid use. The death of Lyle Alzado, a former professional football star, was one of those attributed to steroid use. Unfortunately, some studies show that many athletes who use anabolic steroids are familiar with the adverse effects, but say, "I don't care, I will use them anyway."

Steroids have also been linked to other dangerous and unhealthy behaviors. Violent behavior, sometimes referred to as "roid rage," has been found to accompany steroid use. Recent research suggests that "roid rage" is most likely to result in people who are mentally unstable prior to use. Evidence indicates that steroid users are at greater risk of hepatitis or HIV/AIDS infections from shared needles.

Steroids taken in pill form are especially dangerous to the kidneys and other organs of the body. This is one reason why many medical experts are especially concerned about "andro," which is sometimes taken in pill form.

> Injuries happen more easily and last longer in people who use steroids.

Though steroids may make muscles stronger, tendons and ligaments do not proportionately increase in strength. Therefore, a strong muscle contraction can tear a tendon and/or a ligament. This is made more serious because steroids make the injury heal more slowly. When steroids increase muscle

Table 6 Adverse Effects of Anabolic Steroids

Gender	Physical	Psychological
M/F	• Cancer of liver	• Total personality changes
M/F	• Cardiac disease/early heart attacks	• Hostile and aggressive; violent behavior; sexual crimes
M/F	• Hypertension and increased risk of strokes	• Addiction (both psychological and physiological)
M/F	• Edema (puffy face)	• Inability to accept failure
M/F	• Scalp hair loss** (baldness in men)	• Sleep disturbance (when cycled off drug)
M/F	• Nosebleeds	• Depression
M/F	• Premature closure of growth plates of long bones	• Apathy
M/F	• Immune system may be suppressed	• Wide mood swings
M/F	• Decreased HDL	• "Reverse anorexia" (eating compulsion)
M/F	• Decreased aerobic capacity	
M/F	• Altered glucose tolerance	
M/F	• Severe acne (face, chest, upper back, and thighs)*	
M/F	• Oily skin*	
M/F	• Muscle or bone injuries	
M/F	• Injuries take longer to heal	
M/F	• Fever	
M/F	• Frequent headaches	
M/F	• Sterility	
M/F	• Death	
M	• Testicular atrophy	
M	• Prostate enlargement	
M	• Decreased sperm count	
M	• Impotence	
M	• Feminine breast characteristics	
F	• Uterine atrophy	
F	• Decreased breast size	
F	• Menstrual irregularities	
F	• Clitoral enlargement	
F	• Deepening voice**	
F	• Dark facial hair**	

Key: M = Males; F = Females

*In women, only partially reversible when drug is stopped.

**In women, irreversible when drug is stopped.

size, the extra muscle can grow around the bones and joints, causing them to break more easily.

> Human growth hormone (HGH), taken to increase strength, may be even more dangerous than anabolic steroids.

HGH is produced by the pituitary gland but is made synthetically. Some athletes are taking it in addition to anabolic

Anabolic Steroid A synthetic hormone similar to the male sex hormone testosterone. It functions androgenically to stimulate male characteristics and anabolically to increase muscle mass, weight, bone maturation, and virility.

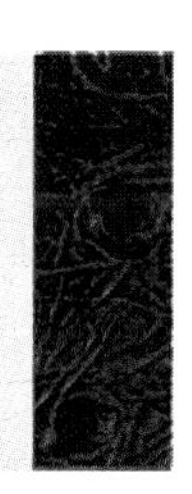

steroids or in place of anabolic steroids because it is difficult to detect in urine tests of competitors. It is believed to increase muscle mass and bone growth and hasten healing of tendons and cartilage; however, its adverse effects can be deforming and life-threatening. They include the danger of irreversible acromegaly (giantism) and gross deformities, cardiovascular disease, goiter, menstrual disorder, excessive sweating, lax muscles and ligaments, premature bone closure, decreased sexual desire, and impotence. In addition, the life span can be shortened by as much as 20 years. Like steroids, there are some medical uses for HGH. People deficient in HGH can benefit from it, though a recent well-controlled study shows that many of the health benefits for HGH were overstated and that side effects such as swelling of the ankles and legs as well as aching of the joints and hands were common.

Another hormone being used by some male athletes is human chorionic gonadotropin (HCG), a substance found in the urine of pregnant women. It is being used to stimulate testosterone production before competition. The International Olympic Committee (IOC) has banned its use, but no test has been developed to detect it.

> Creatine use is becoming increasingly popular among people training for strength development.

www.mhhe.com/phys_fit/webreview11 Click 10

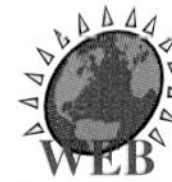

Creatine is produced naturally by your body from foods containing protein such as meat and fish. It is stored in the muscles and helps supply energy for muscle contraction. Because it is classified as a food supplement and not a drug, it is legal for people in competition. Users typically consume creatine as a powder that is dissolved in a liquid. Creatine supplements increase the creatine level in the muscle above the amount possible from normal food intake. The theory is that extra creatine in the muscle will allow quicker recovery from intense exercise such as vigorous strength training and sprinting. A review of many studies indicates that creatine supplements can keep muscle creatine levels higher than normal, and this may result in faster recovery from vigorous short-duration exercise bouts. This, in turn, may allow more intense workouts.

An important point is that strength gains resulting from creatine supplementation occur as a result of the increased training stimulus and not from the supplement itself. Results indicate that creatine causes relatively immediate increases in body weight, but it is mostly a result of water retention. The ability to train harder may benefit strength trainers and people interested in very short intense performances such as sprinting, but few benefits would occur for those who do not do this type of intense training. There is no evidence of muscular endurance benefits or benefits to performance in swimming and distance running events. In fact, the extra weight resulting from water retention may actually impair endurance performance and may also negatively affect sports such as high jumping because the body has to lift the extra weight over the bar.

Recently, the deaths of three college wrestlers led the FDA to study creatine to determine if it was in some way associated with these deaths. No evidence of creatine involvement was found, though the various organizations have warned that creatine supplementation may precipitate dehydration. This could be a problem among athletes who are trying to lose weight by losing body water. The long-term effects of creatine supplementation are unknown, and public health officials are concerned. Short-term side effects include stomach distress and cramping. Many people using the supplement take doses far in excess of those recommended for optimal saturation in the muscles. A recent position statement by the American College of Sports Medicine suggests that doses of 20–25 grams per day for five days followed by much smaller doses of 3 to 5 grams per day will result in maximal muscle saturation. Though not recommended for most people, if you are going to take creatine, it should not be taken in doses greater than those listed above. Further, changes in the law in 1994 leave quality-control issues up to the manufacturer rather than the government. For this reason, the quality of any food supplement (which creatine is considered) is only as good as the integrity of the supplier.

> Some people have turned to other dietary supplements and glandular extracts, which have been promoted as substitutes for anabolic steroids.

In an effort to avoid the undesirable side effects of anabolic steroids or the detection of its use by sports-governing bodies who have banned it, some athletes or body builders are taking chemicals and supplements such as boron, chromium picolinate, gamma oryzanol, and L-carnitine (see concept on quackery). There is also a considerable market for "glandulars" such as ground-up bull testes, hypothalamus and pituitary glands, hearts, livers, spleens, and brains. These products have been advertised as "steroid alternatives." Dietitians, the FDA, and the National Council for Reliable Health Information are alarmed and consider these products potentially dangerous because they have not been tested on humans or animals for safety and effectiveness. Very little is known about some of them. There is no published scientific evidence to substantiate claims for improved human performance. An article in the *Journal of the American Medical Association* has cautioned people concerning the use of such "body-building" supplements.

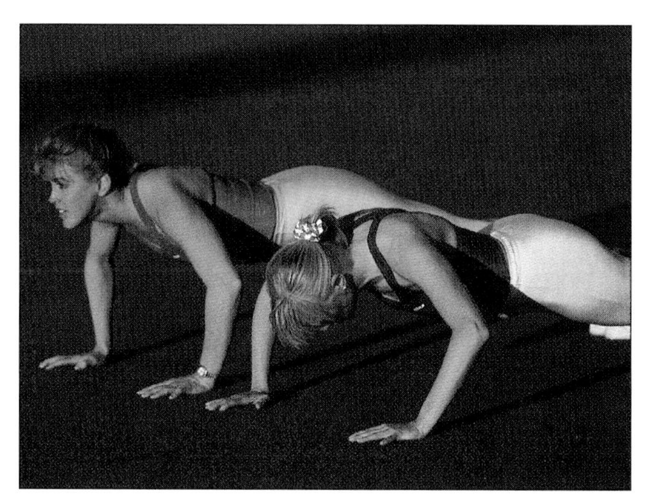

Resistance training can reduce the risk of osteoporosis.

The Facts about the Health Benefits of PRE

PRE is associated with reduced risk of osteoporosis.

Progressive resistance exercises provide a positive stress on the bones. Together with good diet, including adequate calcium intake, this stress on the bones reduces the risk of osteoporosis. Evidence suggests that young people who do PRE develop a high bone density. As we grow older, bone mass decreases, so people who have a high bone density when they are young have a "bank account" from which to draw as they grow older. These people have bones that are less likely to fracture or be injured. Injuries to the bones, particularly the hip and back, are common among older adults. Regular PRE can reduce the risk of these conditions. For postmenopausal women, adequate estrogen is important in preventing osteoporosis.

PRE contributes to weight control and looking your best.

Regular PRE results in muscle mass increases. Muscle or lean body mass takes up less space than fat, contributing to attractive appearance. Further, muscle burns calories at rest so extra muscle built through PRE can contribute to increased resting and basal metabolism. Recent studies indicate that muscle mass decreases as people grow older, resulting in lower metabolism and gradual increase in body fatness. PRE can help people retain muscle mass as they grow older.

A combined strength/muscular endurance program provides most of the health benefits associated with PRE.

Recent research has shown that for healthy adults most health benefits can be achieved using a combined strength/muscular endurance program. The American College of Sports Medicine current guidelines suggest the following. For young adults, one set of eight to 12 repetitions performed two days a week provides most of the health benefits of PRE. For older adults (50 and older), less intense exercises performed 10–15 times appears to be most effective. For both age groups, eight to 10 basic exercises are recommended so that muscle fitness of the total body is accomplished. Those who want pure strength or high-level muscular endurance for performance will benefit from extra sets and from the specific protocols outlined in Tables 4 and 5. For people interested primarily in health benefits, the FIT formula outlined in Table 7 is recommended.

The Facts about PRE Methods

There is a proper way to perform resistance training.

While weight training offers considerable health benefits, there are also some risks if the exercises are not performed correctly or if safety procedures are not followed. A recent survey published in the *Physician and Sports Medicine* estimated that there were over 1 million emergency room visits in the U.S. attributed to weight training during the 20-year period from 1978 to 1998. The leading predictor of injury identified in this survey was improper use of equipment. If you are unfamiliar with how to operate weight-training equipment, be sure to follow printed guidelines on the equipment and/or ask for general instruction.

Table 7 The FIT Formula for PRE Designed to Achieve Health Benefits

Frequency	Young adults	2 to 3 days a week
	Adults over 50	2 to 3 days a week
Intensity	Young adults	40 to 60% of 1 RM
	Adults over 50	30 to 50% of 1 RM
Time	Young adults	1 set of 8 to 12 reps
	Adults over 50	1 set of 10 to 15 reps

The following are some guidelines for safe and effective strength training for beginners:

- When beginning a weight program, start with weights that are too light so you can learn proper technique and avoid soreness and injury. Novices might, for example, start with one-fourth of their body weight for the military press; and half of the body weight for back and leg exercises.
- Progress gradually. For strength training, use one set of three repetitions with a light weight to begin; add one or two repetitions when it gets easy, then another, until you reach eight repetitions; then drop back to three repetitions and add a second set. Repeat until you can do three sets.
- Beginning exercisers should probably begin with endurance training. For example, a reasonable goal might be 10 to 15 repetitions at 20 to 40 percent of the maximum amount of weight they can lift for one repetition.
- Beginners should not attempt to use advanced techniques. After training for several months, you may wish to experiment with such things as supersets, split routines, and plateau systems used by advanced trainers.
- To ensure overall development, include all body parts and balance the strength of antagonistic muscles. For example, the ratio of quadriceps strength to hamstring strength should be 60:40. Exercise large muscles before small muscles.
- Athletes should train muscles the way they will be used in their skill, employing similar patterns, range of motion, and speed (the principle of specificity). This applies to anyone who knows the precise skill for which he or she is training.
- If you wish to develop a particular group of muscles, remember that the muscle group can be worked harder when isolated than when worked in combination with other muscle groups.
- Sports participants should include some eccentric training, such as plyometrics, to prevent injury to decelerating muscles during sports events and to develop power in accelerating muscles. Choose an exercise sequence that alternates muscle groups so muscles have a rest period before being used in another exercise.
- Make all movements through the full range of motion.
- To avoid boredom, especially when you reach a plateau or sticking point, use such motivating techniques as music, record keeping, partners, competition, and variation in routine.
- To avoid overtraining, take a break by resting or choosing some other activity after eight to 10 weeks. Also, try varying your training days so one is light, one is medium, and one is heavy. It has been estimated that motivation can account for 10 to 15 percent of the score on a strength test. Varying the routine helps motivation.
- Lifters may reduce spinal and abdominal injury by using a belt that supports the back and abdomen.

There are many fallacies, myths, and superstitions associated with strength training.

Some common misconceptions about strength training are described below:

- It is *not* true that you will become muscle-bound and lose flexibility just because you do strength training. This could only happen if you train improperly. It has been found, however, that powerlifters are less flexible than other weight lifters.
- It is *not* true that women will become masculine looking if they develop strength. Contrary to popular belief, most women will not be able to develop as large and bulky muscles as men, nor will their muscles be as well defined. On a heavy resistance training program, women and men make about the same percentage change in strength and hypertrophy. The greater percentage of fat in most women prevents the muscle definition possible in men and camouflages the increase in bulk. (Until CAT scans were used in research studies, it was not evident that women achieved hypertrophy at the same rate as men.)
- Strength training does *not* make you move more slowly or make you more uncoordinated. Up to a point, increased strength may help to increase speed.
- The expression "*no pain, no gain*" is a fallacy. It may be helpful to strive for a burning sensation in the muscle, but this is not painful. If it hurts, you are probably harming yourself.
- Protein supplements are not ergogenic aids and do *not* benefit muscle mass or strength building. You do need a balanced diet, however.
- Drugs do *not* make you fit. Anabolic steroids, growth hormones, diuretics, narcotics, and other drugs taken to enhance performance are extremely dangerous and ultimately produce an unhealthy person rather than a fit one.
- Strength training is *not* effective in building cardiovascular fitness and flexibility. Gains in muscle mass do cause an increase in resting metabolism so muscle fitness training can aid in controlling body fatness.
- It does *not* require two hours to complete a workout in weight training—unless you are a competitive lifter or bodybuilder. If you are training for athletics, you will need 45 to 90 minutes; the beginner or the person training for fitness or recreation can complete a circuit in 30 to 45 minutes.
- It is *not* true that progressive resistance training is only for young people. Studies have shown that even people in the 80s and 90s can benefit from regular PRE training.

Table 8 How to Prevent Injury (for the Beginner)

- Warm up 10 minutes before the workout and stay warm during the workout.
- Do not hold your breath while lifting. This may cause blackout or hernia.
- Avoid hyperventilation before lifting a weight.
- Avoid dangerous or high-risk exercises.
- Progress slowly.
- Use good shoes with good traction.
- Avoid arching your back. Keep the pelvis in normal alignment.
- Keep the weight close to the body.
- Do not lift from a stoop (bent over with back rounded).
- When lifting from the floor, do not let the hips come up before your upper body.
- For bent-over rowing, lay your head on a table and bend the knees, or use one-arm rowing and support the trunk with the free hand.
- Stay in a squat as short a time as possible and do not do a full squat.
- Be sure collars on free weights are tight.
- Use a moderately slow, continuous, controlled movement and hold the final position a few seconds.
- Overload but don't overwhelm! A program that is too intense can cause injuries.
- Do not pause between repetitions.
- Try to keep a steady rhythm.
- Do not allow the weights to drop or bang.
- Do not train without medical supervision if you have a hernia, high blood pressure, fever, infection, recent surgery, heart disease, or back problems.
- Use chalk or a towel to keep hands dry when handling weights.

Most injuries can be prevented by using correct technique and proper care.

Refer to Table 8 for some tips on injury prevention.

Strategies for Action: The Facts

An important step in taking action for developing and maintaining muscle fitness is assessing your current status.

www.mhhe.com/phys_fit/webreview11 Click 11

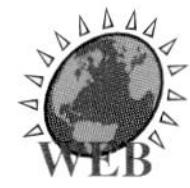

An important early step in taking action to improve fitness is self-assessment. There are many different tests of muscle fitness. A 1 RM test of isotonic strength is described in the lab resource materials. This test allows you to determine both absolute and relative strength for the arms and legs. In addition, the 1 RM values can be used to help you select the appropriate resistance for your muscle fitness training program. A grip strength test of isometric strength is also provided in the resource materials for Lab 11A. In addition to descriptions of the 1 RM test, a body weight test for isotonic strength is provided in the Web Review for people who do not have the equipment to perform the 1 RM assessment.

www.mhhe.com/phys_fit/webreview11 Click 12

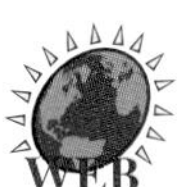

Three tests of muscular endurance are described in the lab resource materials for Lab 11B. It is recommended that you perform the assessments for both strength and muscular endurance before you begin your progressive resistance training program. Periodically reevaluate your muscle fitness using these assessments.

Many factors other than your own basic abilities affect muscle fitness test scores.

If muscles are warmed up before lifting, more force can be exerted, and heavier loads can be lifted. Muscle endurance performance may also be enhanced by a warm-up. It is important, however, not to perform your self-assessments after vigorous exercise because that exercise can cause fatigue and result in less-than-optimal test results. It is appropriate to practice the techniques involved in the various tests on days preceding the actual testing. People who have good technique achieve better scores than those who do not have good technique and are less likely to be injured when performing tests. It is best to perform the strength and muscular endurance tests on different days.

Choose exercises that build muscle fitness in the major muscle groups of the body.

www.mhhe.com/phys_fit/webreview11 Click 13

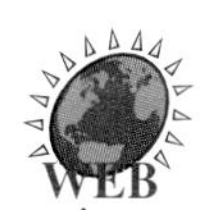

The American College of Sports Medicine recommends eight to ten basic exercises for muscle fitness. The Basic 8 exercises for free weights and resistance machines should be supplemented with one or both of the exercises presented in Table 9. To aid the reader, four different sets of basic exercises have been prepared for free weights (Table 10), resistance machines (Table 11), isometrics (Table 12), and calisthenics (Table 13). For most people performing the Basic 8, using any of the four types of exercises will produce the majority of benefits associated muscle fitness.

People interested in additional exercises that serve as alternates exercises or that focus on improving fitness in other muscle groups are referred to the supplemental exercises in Web Review. Web Review also includes eight basic exercises using elastic bands as well as many of the exercises described in Table 13.

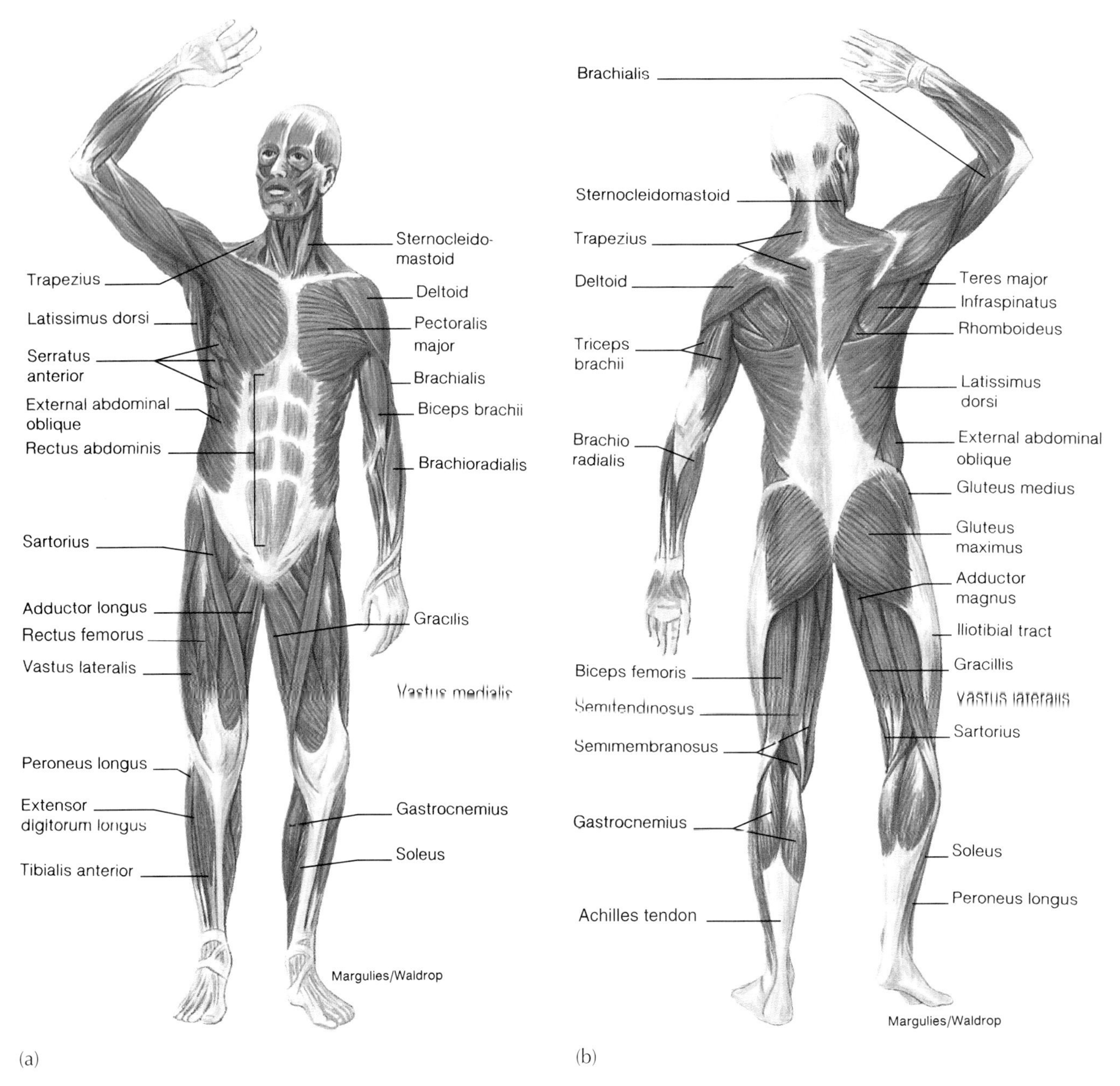

Figure 7
Muscles in the body.

Keeping records of progress is important to adhering to a PRE program.

An activity logging sheet is provided in Lab 11C to help you keep records of your progress as you regularly perform PRE to build and maintain good muscle fitness. A guide to the different muscles of the body is presented in Figure 7.

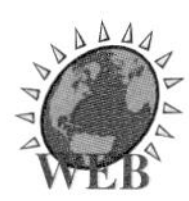

Web Review

Web review materials for Concept 11 are available at *www.mhhe.com/phys_fit/webreview11 Click 14.*

American College of Sports Medicine
www.acsm.org

Muscle Fitness Exercises
www.mhhe.com/phys_fit/webreview11 click 12

National Athletic Trainers Association
www.nata.org

National Strength and Conditioning Association
www.nsca-cc.org

The Physician and Sports Medicine Online
www.physsportsmed.com

Suggested Readings

American College of Sports Medicine. *ACSM's Guidelines for Exercise Testing and Prescription.* 6th ed. Philadelphia: Lippincott, Williams and Wilkins, 2000.

American College of Sports Medicine. "Creatine Supplementation: Current Content." (www.acsm.org).

Baechle, T. R., and Earle, R. W. eds. *Essentials of Strength Training and Conditioning.* 2nd ed. Champaign, IL: Human Kinetics, 2000.

Brandon, L. J. et. al. "Strength Training for Older Adults." *ACSM's Health and Fitness Journal.* 4(6)(2000): 13–28.

Ebbens, W. P., and Jensen, R. L. "Strength Training for Women." *The Physician and Sports Medicine.* 26(5)(1998):86.

Earnest, C. P. "Dietary Androgen Supplements." *The Physician and Sports Medicine.* 29(5)(2001): 63–79.

Francis, P. R. et al. "An Electromyographical Approach to the Evaluation of Abdominal Exercises." *ACSM's Health and Fitness Journal.* 5(4)(2001): 8+.

Hartgens, F. et al. "Androgenic-Anabolic Steroid-Induced Body Changes in Strength Athletes." *The Physician and Sports Medicine.* 29(1)(2001): 49–66.

Holt, S. "Mechanics of Machines: Selecting the Right Piece of Equipment." *Fitness Management.* July 2001, 56+

Jones, C. S., Christenson, C., and Young, M. "Weight Training Injury Trends: A 20-Year Survey." *The Physician and Sports Medicine.* 28(7)(2000): 61–72.

Pollock, M. L., and Vincent, K. R. "Resistance Training for Health." In Corbin, C. B., and Pangrezi, R. P. (eds.) *Toward a Better Understanding of Physical Fitness and Activity.* Scottsdale, AZ: Holcomb-Hathaway, 1999.

Schilling, B. K. et. al. "Creatine Supplementation and Health Variables." *Medicine and Science in Sports and Exercise.* 33(2)(2001): 183–188.

Volek, J. S. "Update: What We Know about Creatine." *ACSM's Health and Fitness Journal.* 3(3)(1999): 27–33.

Westcott, W. L., and Baechle, T. R. *Strength Training for Seniors.* Champaign, IL: Human Kinetics, 1999.

Yesalis, C. E., and Cowart, V. S. *The Steroids Game.* Champaign, IL: Human Kinetics, 1998.

Table 9

Exercise for the Abdominals

1. Crunch (Curl-Up)

This exercise develops the upper abdominal muscles. Lie on the floor with the knees bent and the arms extended or crossed with hands on shoulders or palms on ears. If desired, legs may rest on bench to increase difficulty. For less resistance, place hands at side of body (do not put hands behind neck). For more resistance, move hands higher. Curl up until shoulder blades leave floor, then roll down to the starting position. Repeat. Note: Twisting the trunk on the curl-up develops the oblique abdominals.

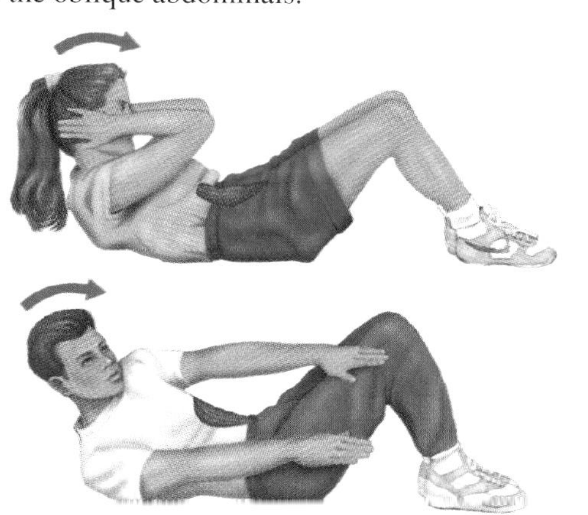

2. Reverse Curl

This exercise develops the lower abdominal muscles. Lie on the floor. Bend the knees, place the feet flat on the floor, and place arms at sides. Lift the knees to the chest, raising the hips off the floor; do not let the knees go past the shoulders. Return to the starting position. Repeat.

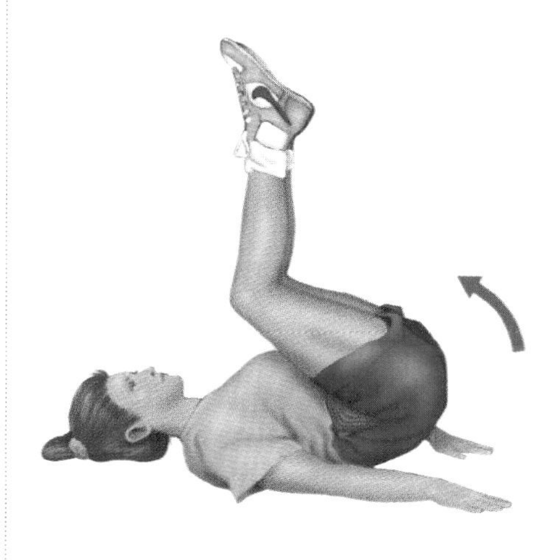

Table 10
The Basic 8 for Free Weights

1. Bench Press

This exercise develops the chest (pectoral) and triceps muscles. Lie supine on bench with knees bent and feet flat on bench or flat on floor in stride position. Grasp bar at shoulder level. Push bar up until arms are straight. Return; repeat; do not arch lower back. Note: Feet may be placed on floor if lower back can be kept flattened. Do not put feet on the bench if it is unstable.

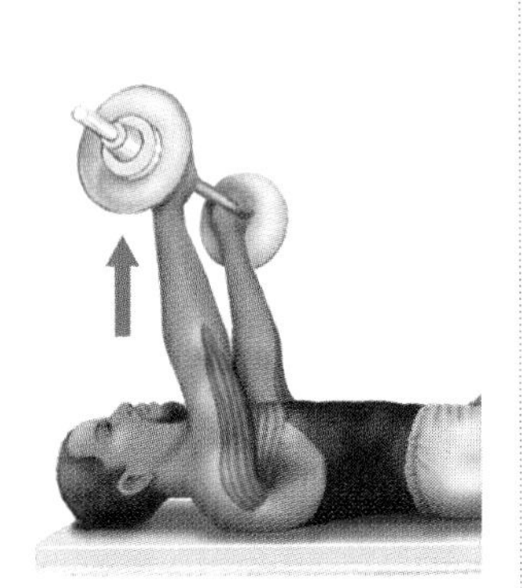

2. Overhead (Military Press)

This exercise develops the muscles of the shoulders and arms. Sit erect, bend elbows, palms facing forward at chest level, hands spread (slightly more than shoulder width). Have bar touching chest, spread feet (comfortable distance). Tighten your abdominal and back muscles. Move bar to overhead position (arms straight). Lower bar to chest position. Repeat. Caution: Keep arms perpendicular and do not allow weight to move backward or wrists to bend backward. Spotters are needed.

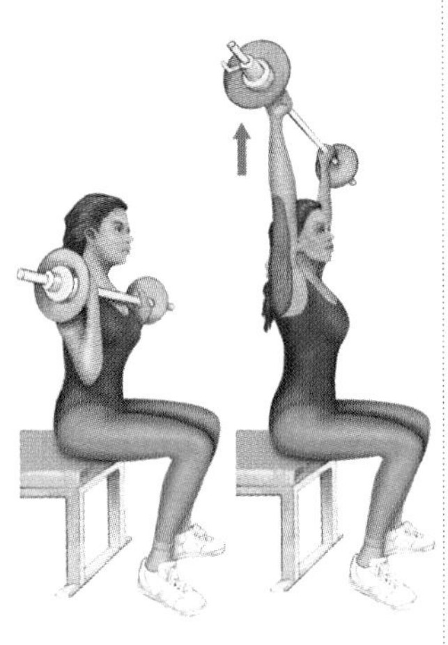

3. Biceps Curl

This exercise develops the muscles of the upper front part of the arms (biceps). Stand erect with back against a wall, palms forward, bar touching thighs. Spread feet in comfortable position. Tighten abdominals and back muscles. Do not lock knees. Move bar to chin, keeping body straight and elbows near the sides. Lower bar to original position. Do not allow back to arch. Repeat. Spotters are usually not needed. Variations: Use dumbbell and sit on end of bench with feet in stride position, work one arm at a time; or use dumbbell with the palm down or thumb up to emphasize other muscles.

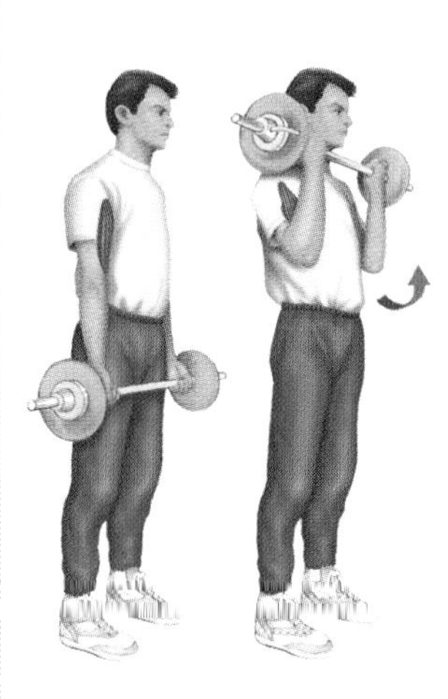

4. Triceps Curl

This exercise develops the muscles on the back of the upper arms (triceps). Sit erect, elbows and palms facing up, bar resting behind neck on shoulders, hands near center of bar, feet spread. Tighten abdominal and back muscles. Keep upper arms stationary. Raise weight overhead, return bar to original position. Repeat. Spotters are needed. Variation: Substitute dumbbells (one in each hand, or one held in both hands, or one in one hand at a time).

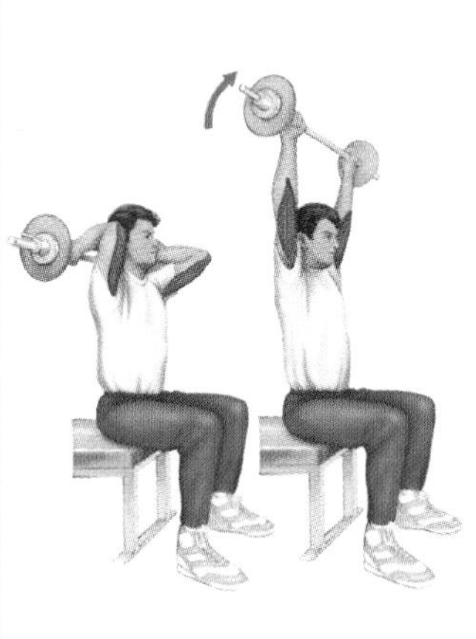

Table 10
The Basic 8 for Free Weights *(continued)*

5. Wrist Curl

This exercise develops the muscles of the fingers, wrist, and forearms. Sit astride a bench with the back of one forearm on the bench, wrist and hand hanging over the edge. Hold a dumbbell in the fingers of that hand with the palm facing forward. To develop the flexors, lift the weight by curling the fingers then the wrist through a full range of motion. Slowly lower and repeat. To strengthen the extensors, start with the palm down. Lift the weight by extending the wrist through a full range of motion. Slowly lower and repeat. Note: Both wrists may be exercised at the same time by substituting a barbell in place of the dumbbell.

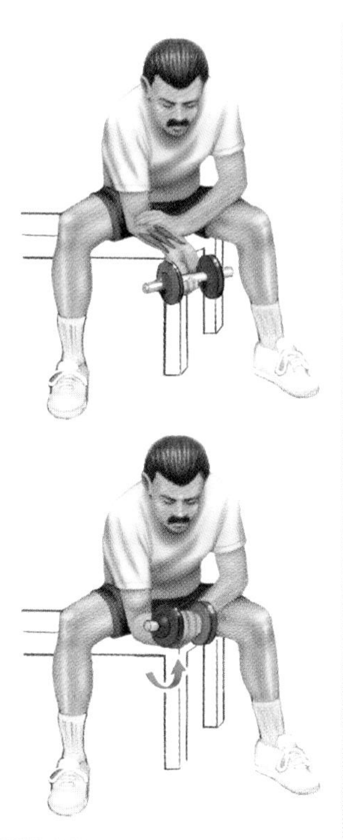

7. Lunge

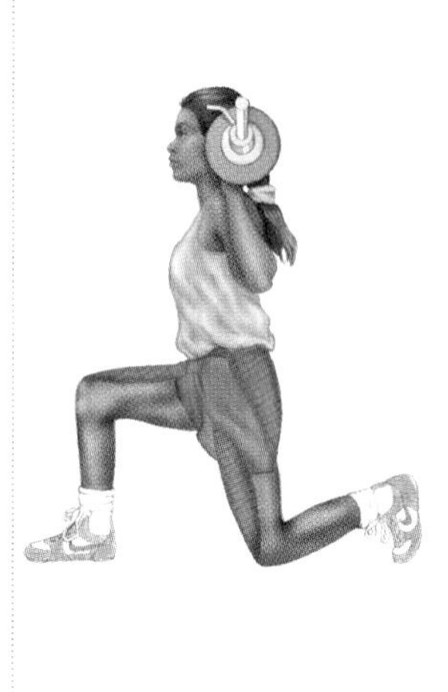

This exercise develops the thigh and gluteal muscles. Place a barbell (with or without weight) behind your head and support with hands placed slightly wider than shoulder-width apart. In a slow and controlled motion, take a step forward and allow the leading leg to drop so that it is nearly parallel with the ground. The lower part of the leg should be near vertical and the back should be maintained in an upright posture. Take stride with opposite leg to return to standing posture. Repeat with other leg, remaining stationary or moving slowly in a straight line with alternating steps.

6. Half-Squat

This exercise develops the muscles of the thighs and buttocks. Stand erect, feet turned out 45 degrees. Rest bar behind neck on shoulders. Spread hands in a comfortable position. Squat slowly, keeping back straight, eyes ahead. Bend knees to approximately 90 degrees; keep knees over feet. Pause, then stand. Repeat. Spotters are needed. Variations: Substitute dumbbell in each hand at sides.

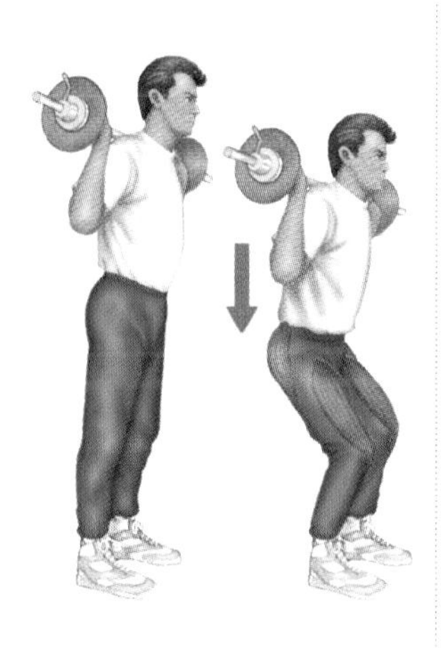

8. Heel Raise

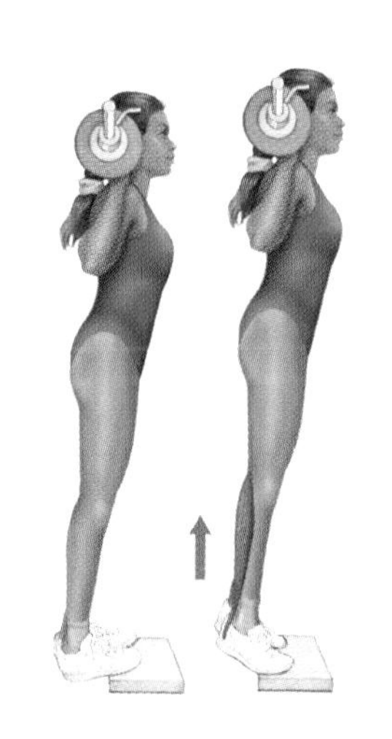

This exercise develops the muscles of the legs (calf). Stand erect with palms facing forward, hands wider than shoulder-width apart, bar resting behind neck on shoulders. Rest balls of feet on 2-inch block with heels on floor. Toes together, heels apart. Rise on toes quickly, hold for 1 second. Lower heels to floor. Repeat. Keep toes turned in slightly. Spotters are needed. Note: Some people do this with toes straight ahead or turned out; however, this tends to weaken the foot muscles.

Chart 4 Rating Scale for Dynamic Muscular Endurance

Age:	17–26		27–39		40–49		50–59		60+	
Classification	Curl-Up	Push-Ups	Curl-Up	Push-Ups	Curl-Up	Push-Ups	Curl-Up	Push-Ups	Curl-Up	Push-Ups
Men										
High-performance zone	35+	29+	34+	27+	33+	26+	32+	24+	31+	22+
Good fitness zone	24–34	20–28	23–33	18–26	22–32	17–25	21–31	15–23	20–30	13–21
Marginal zone	15–23	16–19	14–22	15–17	13–21	14–16	12–20	12–14	11–19	10–12
Low zone	<15	<16	<14	<15	<13	<14	<12	<12	<11	<10
Women										
High-performance zone	25+	17+	24+	16+	23+	15+	22+	14+	21+	13+
Good fitness zone	18–24	12–16	17–23	11–15	16–22	10–14	15–21	9–13	14–20	8–12
Marginal zone	10–17	8–11	9–16	7–10	8–15	6–9	7–14	5–8	6–13	4–7
Low zone	<10	<8	<9	<7	<8	<6	<7	<5	<6	<4

Chart 5 Rating Scale for Static Endurance (Flexed-Arm Support)

Classification	Score in Seconds
High-performance zone	30+
Good fitness zone	20–29
Marginal zone	10–19
Low zone	10

Lab 11A: Evaluating Muscle Strength: 1 RM and Grip Strength

Name	Section	Date

Purpose: To evaluate your muscle strength using 1 RM and to determine the best amount of weight to use for various strength exercises.

Procedure: 1 RM refers to the maximum amount of weight you can lift for a specific exercise. Testing yourself to determine how much you can lift only one time using traditional methods can be fatiguing and even dangerous. The procedure you will perform here allows you to estimate 1 RM based on the number of times you can lift a weight that is less than 1 RM.

Evaluating Strength Using Estimated 1 RM

1. Use a resistance machine for the leg press and arm or bench press for the evaluation part of this lab.
2. Estimate how much weight you can lift two or three times. Be conservative; it is better to start with too little weight than too much. If you lift a weight more than 10 times, the procedure should be done again on another day when you are rested.
3. Using correct form, perform a leg press with the weight you have chosen. Perform as many times as you can up to 10.
4. Use Chart 1 to determine your 1 RM for the leg press. Find the weight used in the left-hand column and then find the number of repetitions you performed across the top of the chart.
5. Your 1 RM score is the value where the weight row and the repetitions column intersect.
6. Repeat this procedure for the arm or bench press using the same technique.
7. Record your 1 RM scores for the leg press and bench press in the Results section.
8. Next divide your 1 RM scores by your body weight in pounds to get a "strength per pound of body weight" (str/lb/body wt.) score for each of the two exercises.
9. Determine your strength rating for your upper body strength (arm press) and lower body (leg press) using Chart 2 in the lab resource materials. Record in the Results section. If time allows, assess 1 RM for other exercises you choose to perform (see Lab 3).
10. If a grip dynamometer is available, determine your right- and left-hand grip strength using the procedures in the lab resource materials. Use chart 3 to rate your grip (isometric) strength.

Results:

Arm press (or bench press): Wt. selected [ ] Reps [ ] Estimated 1 RM [ ] (Chart 1, lab resource materials)

Strength per lb. body weight [ ] (1 RM ÷ body weight) Rating [ ] (Chart 2, lab resource materials)

Leg press: Wt. selected [ ] Reps [ ] Estimated 1 RM [ ] (Chart 1, lab resource materials)

Strength per lb. body weight [ ] (1 RM ÷ body weight) Rating [ ] (Chart 2, lab resource materials)

Grip strength: Right grip score [ ] Right grip rating [ ]

Left grip score [ ] Left grip rating [ ]

Total score [ ] Total rating [ ]

Conclusion and Implications: In several sentences, discuss your current strength, whether you believe it is adequate for good health, and whether you think that your "strength per pound of body weight" scores are really representative of your true strength.

Lab 11C: Planning and Logging Muscle Fitness Exercises: Free Weights or Resistance Machines

Name	Section	Date

Purpose: To set lifestyle goals for muscle fitness exercise, to prepare a muscle fitness exercise plan, and to self-monitor progress for the one-week plan.

Procedures:

1. The Basic 8 exercises are listed for free weights and resistance machines. Use Chart 1 to select 8 exercises to represent your Basic 8 exercises. If you would like to add other exercises to your program, then list them on the lines at the bottom of the chart. Descriptions of the exercises are provided in Tables 10 and 11.
2. In Chart 1, also indicate the days of the week that you plan on performing the exercises and the number of reps and the number of sets. Be sure to base your program on your goals (strength/endurance). If you are just starting out it is best to start with one set of 12–15 repetitions. Use the 1 RM procedure described in Lab 11A, to help you determine the amount of weight or resistance to use. Plan to do at least eight exercises, two or three times a week. Note: All exercises do not have to be performed on the same day, but many people find this more convenient.
3. Though abdominal exercises are not typically done using free weights or resistance machines, an abdominal exercise is recommended as part of a resistance exercise program. Two abdominal exercises are provided in the "other" category for you to consider (see Table 9).
4. In Chart 2, keep a one-week log of your actual participation. For best results, keep the log with you during your workout session. Indicate the exercises you performed, including any that you didn't plan on performing when you developed your schedule. If you would like to keep a log for more than one week, make extra copies of the log before you begin.
5. Answer the questions in the Results section.

Chart 1 Muscle Fitness Exercise Plan

What is your goal? Check one or more: Strength ❑ Endurance ❑ General Fitness ❑
Check boxes beside at least 8 exercises, note days, reps, sets, and resistance to be used.

Primary Body Parts to Be Exercised	Free Weight Exercises (Basic 8)		Machine Weight Exercises (Basic 8)		Day 1 Date	Day 2 Date	Day 3 Date	How Many Reps?	How Many Sets?	Weight or Setting
Chest	Bench press		Chest press							
Shoulder	Overhead press		Seated press							
Arm (bicep)	Bicep curl		Bicep curl							
Arm (tricep)	Tricep curl		Tricep press							
Arm (wrist)	Wrist curl		(No equivalent*)							
Back	(No equivalent*)		Lat pull down							
Back (lower)	(No equivalent*)		Seated rowing							
Hip/leg (thigh)	Lunge		(No equivalent*)							
Leg (thigh)	Half squat		Knee extension							
Leg (hamstring)	(No equivalent*)		Hamstring curl							
Leg (calf)	Heel raise		(No equivalent*)							
Other exercises										
Abdominal	Crunch		Reverse curl							

*Note: Some free weight and machine exercises do not have equivalents.

Chart 2 Muscle Fitness Exercise Log

Check the exercises you performed and the days you performed them.

Primary Body Parts to Be Exercised	Free Weight Exercises (Basic 8)		Machine Weight Exercises (Basic 8)		Day 1 Date	Day 2 Date	Day 3 Date
Chest	Bench press		Chest press				
Shoulder	Overhead press		Seated press				
Arm (bicep)	Bicep curl		Bicep curl				
Arm (tricep)	Tricep curl		Tricep press				
Arm (wrist)	Wrist curl		(No equivalent*)				
Back	(No equivalent*)		Lat pull down				
Back (lower)	(No equivalent*)		Seated rowing				
Hip/leg (thigh)	Lunge		(No equivalent*)				
Leg (thigh)	Half squat		Knee extension				
Leg (hamstring)	(No equivalent*)		Hamstring curl				
Leg (calf)	Heel raise		(No equivalent*)				
Other exercises							
Abdominal	Crunch		Reverse curl				

*Note: Some free weight and machine exercises do not have equivalents.

Results:

Were you able to do your Basic 8 exercises at least two days in the week? ◯ Yes ◯ No

Conclusions and Implications:

1. Do you feel that you will use muscle fitness exercises as part of your regular lifetime physical activity plan, either now or in the future? Use several sentences to answer.

2. Discuss the exercises you feel benefited you and the ones that did not. What modifications would you make in your program for it to work better for you? Use several sentences to answer.

Lab 11D: Planning and Logging Muscle Fitness Exercises: Calisthenics or Isometric Exercises

Name	Section	Date

Purpose: To set lifestyle goals for muscle fitness exercises that can easily be performed at home, to prepare a muscle fitness exercise plan, and to self-monitor progress for a one-week plan.

Procedures:

1. The Basic 8 exercises are listed for calisthenics and isometric exercises. Use Chart 1 to select eight exercises to represent your Basic 8. If you would like to add other exercises to your program, then list them on the lines at the bottom of the chart. Descriptions of the exercises are provided in Tables 12 and 13.
2. In Chart 1, indicate the days of the week that you plan to perform the exercises and the number of reps and the number of sets. Plan to do at least eight exercises, two or three times a week. Note: All exercises do not have to be performed on the same day, but many people find this more convenient. Do what is best for your schedule.
3. In Chart 2, keep a one-week log of your actual participation. For best results, keep the log with you during your workout session. Indicate the exercises you performed, including any that you didn't plan on. If you would like to keep a log for more than one week, make extra copies of the log before you begin.
4. Answer the questions in the Results section.

Chart 1 Muscle Fitness Exercise Log

What is your goal? Check one or more: Strength ❑ Endurance ❑ General Fitness ❑
Check boxes beside at least 8 exercises, note days, reps, sets, and resistance to be used.

Primary Body Parts to Be Exercised	Calisthenic Exercises (Basic 8)		Isometric Exercises (Basic 8)		Day 1 Date	Day 2 Date	Day 3 Date	How Many Reps?	How Many Sets?
Chest	Knee pushup		Arm press in door						
Shoulder	(No equivalent*)		Overhead press in door						
Arm (bicep)	Modified pullup		Bicep curl						
Arm (tricep)	Dips		Tricep press						
Trunk/back	Trunk lift		(No equivalent*)						
Abdominals	Crunch		Pelvic tilt						
Leg (outer)	Side leg raise		(No equivalent*)						
Leg (inner)	Lower leg lift		(No equivalent*)						
Leg (thigh)	Leg kneel		Leg press						
Leg (thigh)	(No equivalent*)		Wall seat						
Leg (hamstring)	(No equivalent*)		Hamstring exercise						
Other									

*Note: Calisthenics and isometric exercises may not have exact equivalents.

Chart 2 Muscle Fitness Exercise Log

Check the exercises you performed and the days you performed them.

Primary Body Parts to Be Exercised	Calisthenic Exercises (Basic 8)		Isometric Exercises (Basic 8)		Day 1 Date	Day 2 Date	Day 3 Date
Chest	Knee pushup		Arm press in door				
Shoulder	(No equivalent*)		Overhead press in door				
Arm (bicep)	Modified pullup		Bicep curl				
Arm (tricep)	Dips		Tricep press				
Trunk/back	Trunk lift		(No equivalent*)				
Abdominals	Crunch		Pelvic tilt				
Leg (outer)	Side leg raise		(No equivalent*)				
Leg (inner)	Lower leg lift		(No equivalent*)				
Leg (thigh)	Leg kneel		Leg press				
Leg (thigh)	(No equivalent*)		Wall seat				
Leg (hamstring)	(No equivalent*)		Hamstring exercise				
Other							

*Note: Calisthenics and isometric exercises may not have exact equivalents.

Results:

Were you able to do your Basic 8 exercises at least two days in the week? ◯ Yes ◯ No

Conclusions and Implications:

1. Do you feel that you will use these muscle fitness exercises as part of your regular lifetime physical activity plan, either now or in the future? Would the convenience of being able to do these exercises anywhere make it easier for you to stick with your program? Use several sentences to answer.

2. Discuss the exercises you feel benefited you and the ones that did not. What modifications would you make in your program for it to work better for you? Use several sentences to answer.

Section IV

Physical Activity: Special Considerations

Concept 12

Safe Physical Activity and Exercises

There are safe exercises that can be used as alternatives to questionable exercises that may cause more harm than good.

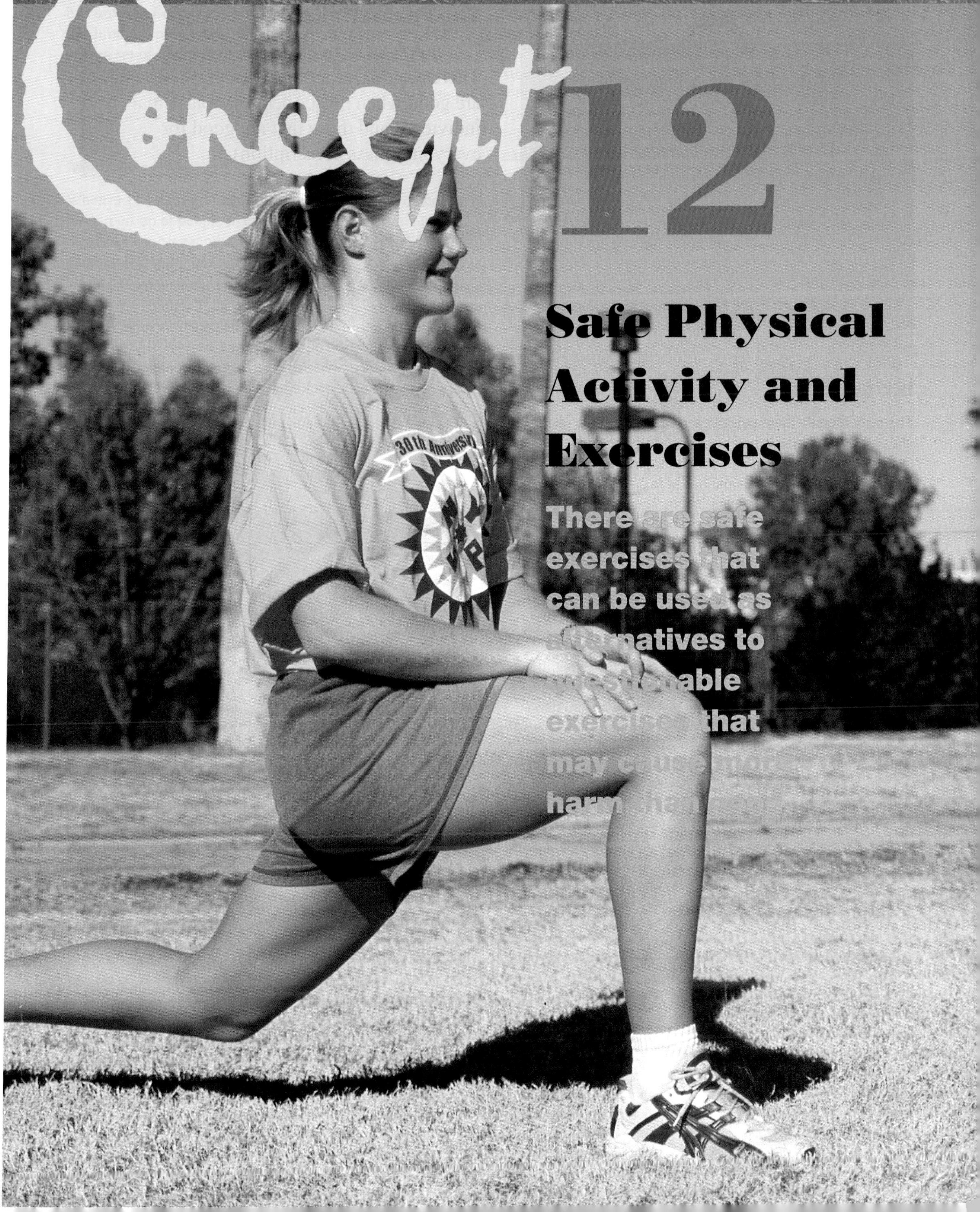

Conclusions and Interpretations:

1. In most cases, it takes a considerable amount of time for a questionable exercise and the microtrauma they cause to result in noticeable damage to the body. To what extent do you think that you might be effected by questionable exercises you have done in the past? Use several sentences to explain.

2. Will you change your way of exercising as a result of learning about questionable exercises and safe alternatives? Use several sentences to explain your answer.

Concept 13

Body Mechanics: Posture and Care of the Back and Neck

Proper body mechanics should be employed for both static and dynamic postures to ensure the health, integrity, and function of the back and the neck.

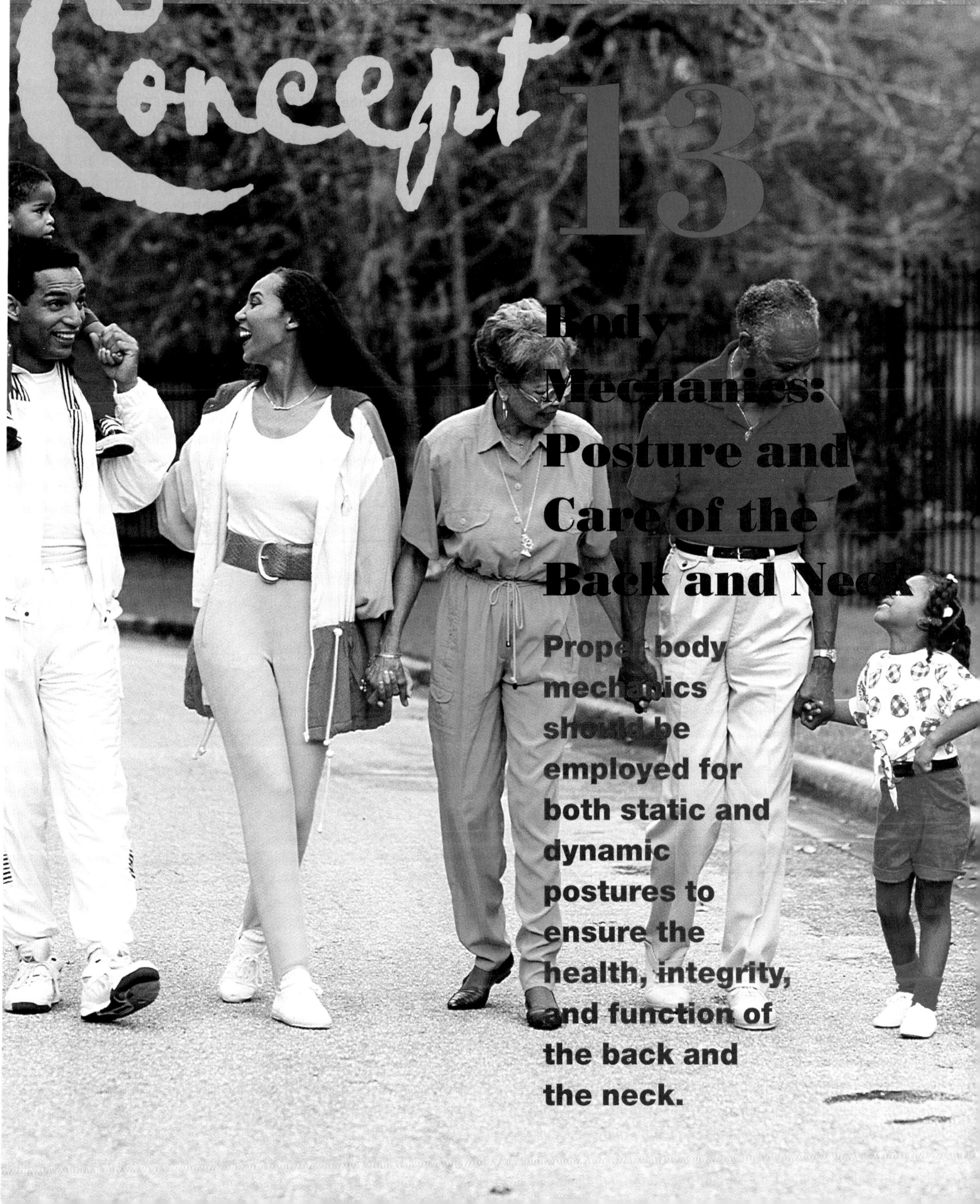

Chart 1 Healthy Back Tests (*Continued*)

Test 5—Ober's Test

Lie on left side with left leg flexed 90 degrees at the hip and 90 degrees at the knee. Partner places right hip in neutral position (no flexion) and right knee in 90-degree flexion; partner then allows the weight of the leg to lower it toward the floor.

- If there is no tightness in the iliotibial band (fascia and muscles on lateral side of leg), the knee touches the floor without pain and the test is passed. Repeat on the other side. (Both sides must pass in order to pass the test.)

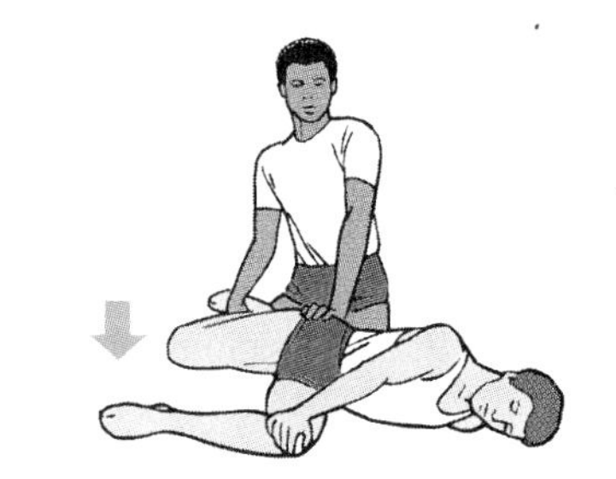

Test 6—Press-Up (Straight Arm)

Perform the press-up.

- If you can press to a straight-arm position, keeping your pubis in contact with the floor, and if your partner determines that the arch in your back is a continuous curve (not just a sharp angle at the lumbosacral joint), then there is adequate flexibility in spinal extension.

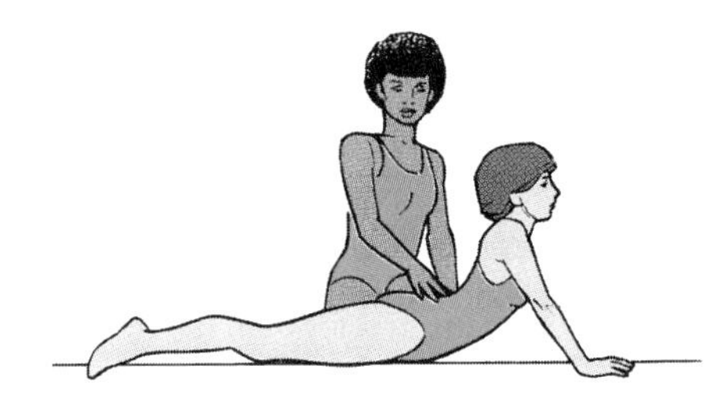

Test 7—Knee Roll

Lie supine with both knees and hips flexed 90 degrees, arms extended to the sides at shoulder level. Keep the knees and hips in that position and lower them to the floor on the right and then on the left.

- If you can accomplish this and still keep your shoulders in contact with the floor, then you have adequate rotation in the spine, especially at the lumbar and thoracic junction. (Both sides must pass in order to pass the test.)

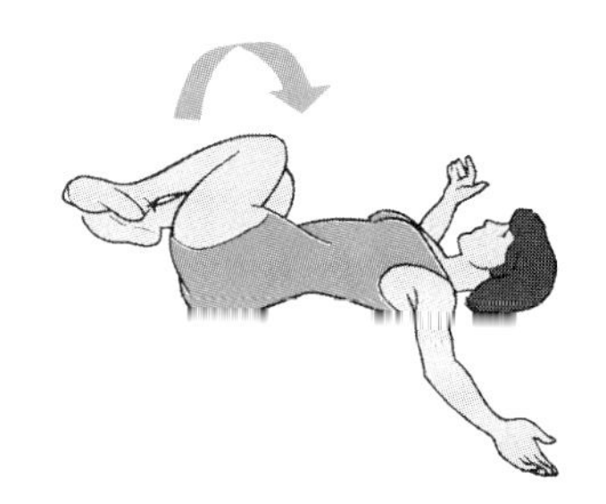

Test 8—Leg Drop Test*

Lie on your back on a table or on the floor with both legs extended overhead. Flatten the low back against the table or floor. Slowly lower legs while keeping the back flat.

- If your back arches before you reach a 45-degree angle, the abdominal muscles are too weak. A partner should be ready to support your legs if needed to prevent lower back arching or strain to the back muscles.

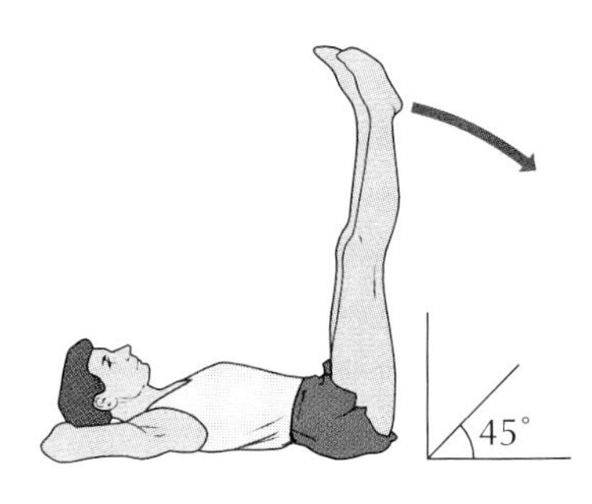

*The double leg drop is suitable as a diagnostic test when performed one time. It is not a good exercise to be performed regularly by most people. If it casuses pain, stop the test.

Chart 2 Healthy Back Test Ratings

Classification	Number of Tests Passed
Excellent	~~7–8~~ 4
Very good	~~6~~ 3
Good	~~5~~ 2
Fair	~~4~~ 1
Poor	~~1–3~~ 0

Lab 13C: Planning and Logging Exercises: Care of the Back and Neck

Name	Section	Date

Purpose: To select several exercises for the back and neck that meet your personal needs and to self-monitor progress for one of these.

Procedures:

1. On Chart 1 check the tests from the Healthy Back Test that you did *not* pass. Select at least one exercise from the group associated with those items. In addition, select several more exercises (a total of 8 to 10) that you think will best meet your personal needs. If you passed all of the items, select 8 to 10 exercises that you think will best prevent future back and neck problems. Check the exercises you plan to perform in Chart 1.
2. Perform each of the exercises you select three days in one week.
3. Keep a one-week log of your actual participation using the last 3 columns in Chart 1. If possible, keep the log with you during the day. Place a check by each of the exercises you perform for each day—including ones that you didn't originally have planned. If you cannot keep the log with you, fill in the log at the end of the day. If you choose to keep a log for more than one week, make extra copies of the log before you begin.
4. Answer the questions in the Results section.

Chart 1 Back and Neck Exercise Plan

Check the tests you failed:	√	Place a check beside the exercises you plan to do. In the last 3 columns, check the exercises done and the days done.	√	Day 1 Date:	Day 2 Date:	Day 3 Date:
1. Back to wall		Pelvic tilt				
		Bridging				
		Wall slide				
		Pelvic stabilizer				
2. Straight-Leg lift		Back-Saver hamstring stretch				
		Calf stretcher				
3. Thomas test		Hip and thigh stretcher				
4. Ely's test		Single knee-to-chest				
5. Ober's test		Lateral hip and thigh stretcher				
6. Press-up		Upper trunk lift				
		Trunk lift				
7. Knee roll		Side bender				
		Supine trunk twist				
8. Leg drop		Reverse curl				
		Crunch				
Choose other exercises for the neck and shoulders:		Chin tuck				
		Neck rotation				
		Arm lift				
		Pectoral stretch				

Results:

Did you do 8 to 10 exercises at least three days in the week? Yes ◯ No ◯

Conclusion and Interpretations:

1. Do you feel that you will use back and neck exercises as part of your regular lifetime physical activity plan, either now or in the future? Use several sentences to explain your answer.

2. Discuss the exercises you did. What exercises would you continue to do and which ones would you change? Use several sentences to explain your answer.

Concept 14

Performance Benefits of Physical Activity

Physical activity provides performance benefits above and beyond the benefits to health. These performance benefits can promote quality of life for the typical person and enhance the abilities of athletes and people in jobs requiring high levels of performance.

Lab Resource Materials

Important Note: Because skill-related physical fitness does not relate to good health, the rating charts used in this section differ from those used for health-related fitness. The rating charts that follow can be used to compare your scores to those of other people. You *do not* need exceptional scores on skill-related fitness to be able to enjoy sports and other types of physical activity; however, it is necessary for high-level performance. After the age of 30, you should adjust ratings by 1 percent per year.

Evaluating Skill-Related Physical Fitness

I. Evaluating agility: The Illinois agility run

An agility course using four chairs 10 feet apart, and a 30-foot running area will be set up as depicted in this illustration. The test is performed as follows:

1. Lie prone with your hands by your shoulders and your head at the starting line. On the signal to begin, get on your feet and run the course as fast as possible.
2. Your score is the time required to complete the course.

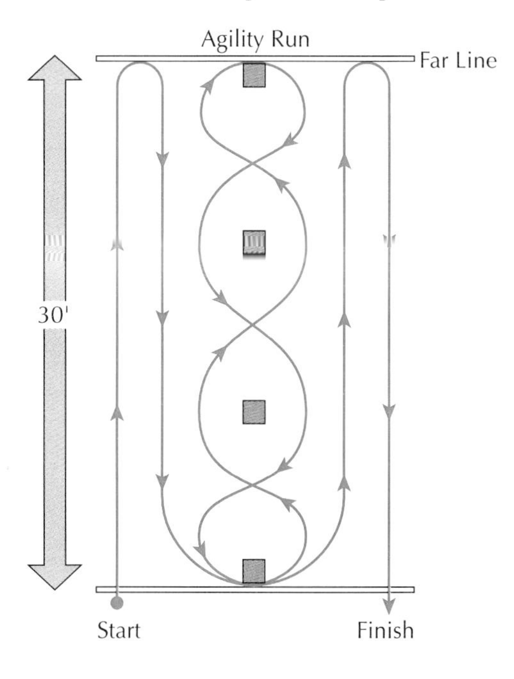

Chart 1 Agility Rating Scale

Classification	Men	Women
Excellent	15.8 or faster	17.4 or faster
Very good	16.7–15.9	18.6–17.5
Good	18.6–16.8	22.3–18.7
Fair	18.8–18.7	23.4–22.4
Poor	18.9 or slower	23.5 or slower

SOURCE: Data from Adams, et al., *Foundations of Physical Activity*, 1965, p. 111.

II. Evaluating balance: The Bass test of dynamic balance

Eleven circles (9 1/2-inch) are drawn on the floor as shown in the illustration. The test is performed as follows:

1. Stand on the right foot in circle X. *Leap* forward to circle 1, then circle 2 through 10, alternating feet with each leap.
2. The feet must leave the floor on each leap and the heel may not touch. Only the ball of the foot and toes may land on the floor.
3. Remain in each circle for 5 seconds before leaping to the next circle. (A count of five will be made for you aloud.)
4. Practice trials are allowed.
5. The score is 50, plus the number of seconds taken to complete the test, minus the number of errors.
6. For every error, deduct three points each. Errors include touching the heel, moving the supporting foot, touching outside a circle, or touching any body part to the floor other than the supporting foot.

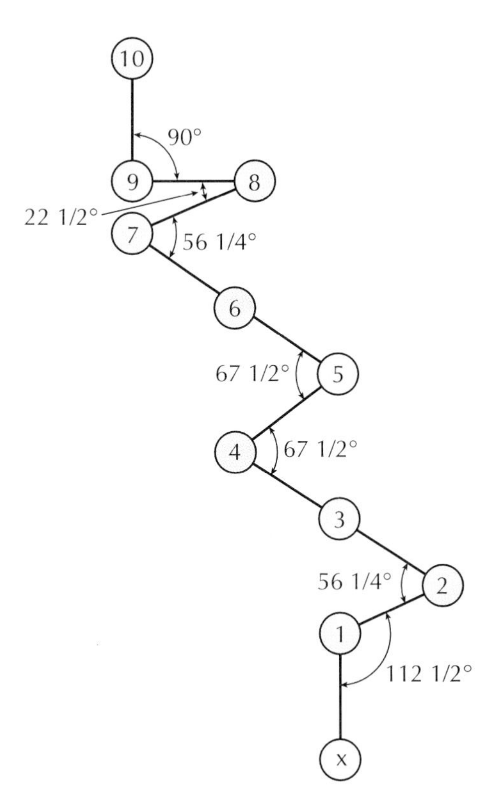

Strategies for Action: The Facts

> You can maximize your chances for success by selecting activities that match your abilities.

Whether your goal is high-level performance or finding an activity that you can enjoy during your leisure time, your choice of activity is important. To give yourself the best chance of being successful, you should consider choosing an activity that matches your abilities. Assessing your skill-related physical fitness abilities can help you determine your areas of strength. In Lab 14A, you have the opportunity to assess your skill-related fitness and build a fitness profile. Using Table 6, you can determine the sports and activities that best match your individual abilities.

It should be noted that the assessments provided in Lab 14A are but a few of the many tests that can be done for each of the skill-related fitness parts. You may want to try other tests if you want more information about your abilities. If you have a personal desire to train for a specific sport or activity, but do not have a fitness profile that predicts success, you should not be deterred. Lab 14A will help you find an activity that you will enjoy and in which you have a good chance of success. People with good motivation, who persist in training, can often excel over others with greater ability. Lab 14B will provide an assessment of overtraining for individuals who may be pursuing some type of high-level training or competitive sport.

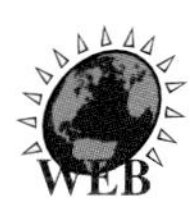

Web Review

Web review materials for Concept 14 are available at *www.mhhe.com/phys_fit/webreview14 Click 09.*

Gatorade Sports Science Institute
www.gssiweb.com

National Athletic Trainers Association
www.nata.org

National Collegiate Athletic Association
www.ncaa.org

National Strength and Conditioning Association
www.nsca-cc.org

Special Olympics International
www.specialolympics.org

United States Olympic Committee
www.usoc.org

Women's Sports Foundation
www.womenssportsfoundation.org

Suggested Readings

ACSM. (1997). "Position Stand on the Female Athlete Triad." *Medicine and Science in Sports and Exercise.* 29(5)(1997):i.

Albert, C. M. et al. "Triggering of Sudden Death from Cardiac Causes by Vigorous Exertion." *New England Journal of Medicine.* 243(19)(2000): 1355–1361.

Baechle, T. R., and Earle, R. W. eds. *Essentials of Strength Training and Conditioning.* 2nd ed. Champaign, IL: Human Kinetics, 2000.

Chu, D. A. *Jumping Into Plyometrics.* Champaign, IL: Human Kinetics, 1998.

Hill, K. L. *Frameworks for Sports Psychologists: Enhancing Sports Performance.* Champaign, IL: Human Kinetics, 2000.

Kraus, D. *Mastering Your Inner Game.* Champaign, IL: Human Kinetics, 2000.

Manore, M., and Thompson, J. *Sport Nutrition for Health and Performance.* Champaign, IL: Human Kinetics, 2000.

Moran, G. T., and McGlynn, G. H. *Cross-Training for Sports.* Champaign, IL: Human Kinetics, 1997.

Otis, C. "Too Slim, Amenorrheic, Fracture Prone: The Female Athlete Triad." *ACSM's Health and Fitness Journal.* 2(1)(1998):20.

Radcliffe, J., and Farentinos, R. *High-Powered Plyometics.* Champaign, IL: Human Kinetics, 1999.

Raglin, J., and Barzdukas, A. "Overtraining in Athletes: The Challenge of Prevention—A Consensus Statement." *ACSM's Health and Fitness Journal.* 3(2)(1999):27–31.

Uusitalo, A. L. "Overtraining." *The Physician and Sports Medicine.* 29(5)(2001): 35–50.

Volek, J. S. "Update: What We Know about Creatine." *ACSM's Health and Fitness Journal.* 3(3)(1999):27–33.

Williams, M. H. "Nutritional Ergogenics and Sports Performance." *PCPFS Research Digest.* (10)(1998):1.

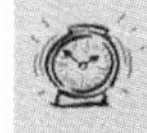

Physical Fitness News Update

The United States Olympic Committee and the American College of Sports Medicine have jointly developed a consensus statement on "overtraining syndrome." Overtraining syndrome refers to "untreated overreaching that results in chronic decreases in performance and impaired ability to train." Other health problems may be associated with the syndrome and may require medical attention. Those interested in training for high-level performance should be aware of the symptoms, causes, and treatments for the syndrome, as well as the methods of prevention. The key seems to be a well-conceived training program that does not "overreach." If you plan to begin training for high-level performance, you should seek more information about the overtraining syndrome (see suggested readings, Raglin and Barzdukas). Lab 14B will help you identify some of the symptoms of overtraining.

Lab Resource Materials

Important Note: Because skill-related physical fitness does not relate to good health, the rating charts used in this section differ from those used for health-related fitness. The rating charts that follow can be used to compare your scores to those of other people. You *do not* need exceptional scores on skill-related fitness to be able to enjoy sports and other types of physical activity; however, it is necessary for high-level performance. After the age of 30, you should adjust ratings by 1 percent per year.

Evaluating Skill-Related Physical Fitness

I. Evaluating agility: The Illinois agility run

An agility course using four chairs 10 feet apart, and a 30-foot running area will be set up as depicted in this illustration. The test is performed as follows:

1. Lie prone with your hands by your shoulders and your head at the starting line. On the signal to begin, get on your feet and run the course as fast as possible.
2. Your score is the time required to complete the course.

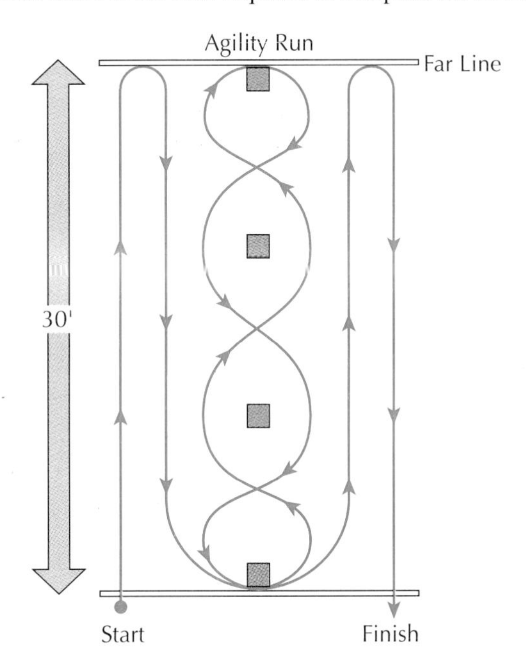

Chart 1 Agility Rating Scale

Classification	Men	Women
Excellent	15.8 or faster	17.4 or faster
Very good	16.7–15.9	18.6–17.5
Good	18.6–16.8	22.3–18.7
Fair	18.8–18.7	23.4–22.4
Poor	18.9 or slower	23.5 or slower

Source: Data from Adams, et al., *Foundations of Physical Activity*, 1965, p. 111.

II. Evaluating balance: The Bass test of dynamic balance

Eleven circles (9 1/2-inch) are drawn on the floor as shown in the illustration. The test is performed as follows:

1. Stand on the right foot in circle X. *Leap* forward to circle 1, then circle 2 through 10, alternating feet with each leap.
2. The feet must leave the floor on each leap and the heel may not touch. Only the ball of the foot and toes may land on the floor.
3. Remain in each circle for 5 seconds before leaping to the next circle. (A count of five will be made for you aloud.)
4. Practice trials are allowed.
5. The score is 50, plus the number of seconds taken to complete the test, minus the number of errors.
6. For every error, deduct three points each. Errors include touching the heel, moving the supporting foot, touching outside a circle, or touching any body part to the floor other than the supporting foot.

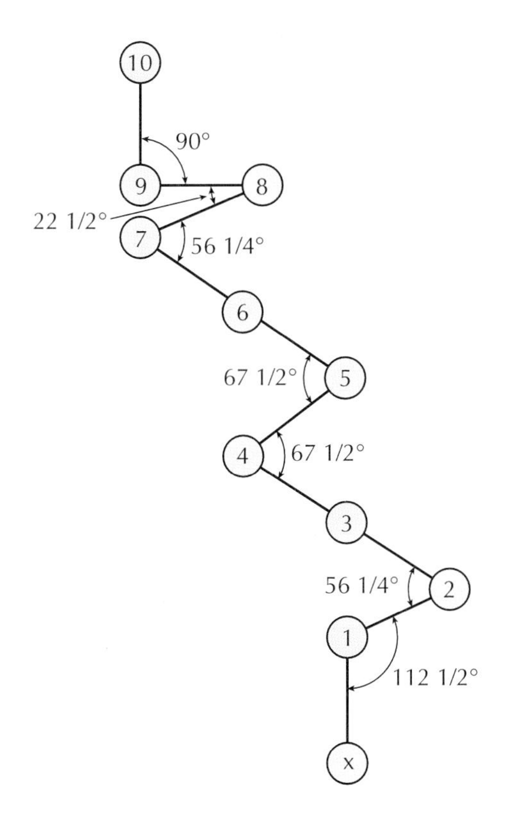

Chart 2 Balance Test Rating Scale

Rating	Score
Excellent	90–100
Very good	80–89
Good	60–79
Fair	30–59
Poor	0–29

III. Evaluating coordination: The stick test of coordination

The stick test of coordination requires you to juggle three wooden sticks. The sticks are used to perform a one-half flip and a full flip as shown in the illustrations.

1. *One-half flip*—Hold two 24-inch (one-half inch in diameter) dowel rods, one in each hand. Support a third rod of the same size across the other two. Toss the supported rod in the air so that it makes a half turn. Catch the thrown rod with the two held rods.
2. *Full flip*—Perform the preceding task, letting the supported rod turn a full flip.

The test is performed as follows:

1. Practice the half-flip and full flip several times before taking the test.
2. When you are ready, attempt a half-flip five times. Score one point for each successful attempt.
3. When you are ready, attempt the full flip five times. Score two points for each successful attempt.

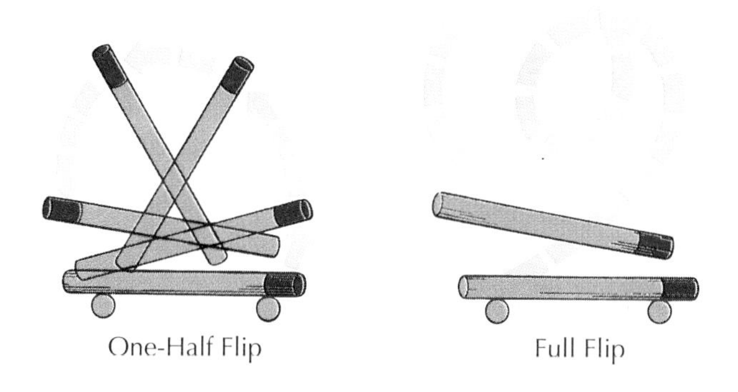

One-Half Flip Full Flip

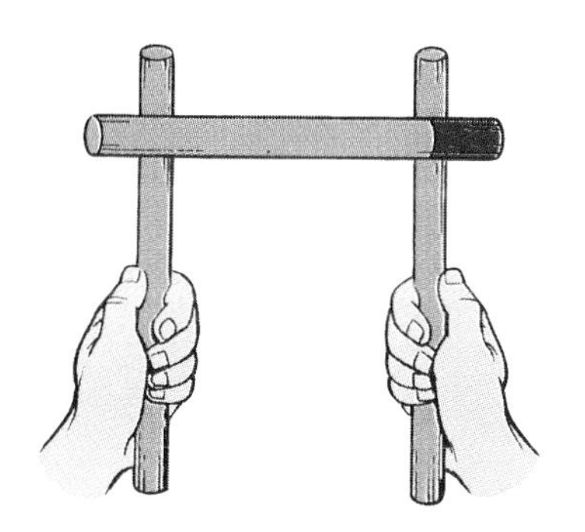

Hand Position

Chart 3 Coordination Rating Scale

Classification	Men	Women
Excellent	14–15	13–15
Very good	11–13	10–12
Good	5–10	4–9
Fair	3–4	2–3
Poor	0–2	0–1

IV. Evaluating power: The vertical jump test

The test is performed as follows:

1. Hold a piece of chalk so its end is even with your fingertips.
2. Stand with both feet on the floor and your side to the wall and reach and mark as high as possible.
3. Jump upward with both feet as high as possible. Swing arms upward and make a chalk mark on a 5′ × 1′ wall chart marked off in half-inch horizontal lines placed 6 feet from the floor.
4. Measure the distance between the reaching height and the jumping height.
5. Your score is the best of three jumps.

Chart 4 Power Rating Scale

Classification	Men	Women
Excellent	25 1/2" or more	23 1/2" or more
Very good	21"–25"	19"–23"
Good	16 1/2"–20 1/2"	14 1/2"–18 1/2"
Fair	12 1/2"–16"	10 1/2"–14"
Poor	12" or less	10" or less

Metric conversions for this chart appear in Appendix B.

V. Evaluating reaction time: The stick drop test

To perform the stick drop test of reaction time, you will need a yardstick, a table, a chair, and a partner to help with the test. To perform the test, follow these procedures:

1. Sit in the chair next to the table so that your elbow and lower arm rest on the table comfortably. The heel of your hand should rest on the table so that only your fingers and thumb extend beyond the edge of the table.
2. Your partner holds a yardstick at the very top, allowing it to dangle between your thumb and fingers.
3. The yardstick should be held so that the 24-inch-mark is even with your thumb and index finger. No part of your hand should touch the yardstick.
4. Without warning, your partner will drop the stick, and you will catch it with your thumb and index finger.

5. Your score is the number of inches read on the yardstick just above the thumb and index finger after you catch the yardstick.
6. Try the test three times. Your partner should be careful not to drop the stick at predictable time intervals so that you cannot guess when it will be dropped. It is important that you react only to the dropping of the stick.
7. Use the middle of your three scores (example: if your scores are 21, 18, and 19, your middle score is 19). The higher your score, the faster your reaction time.

Chart 5 Reaction Time Rating Scale

Classification		Score
Excellent		More than 21"
Very good		19"–21"
Good		16"–18 3/4"
Fair		13"–15 3/4"
Poor		Below 13"

Metric conversions for this chart appear in Appendix B.

VI. Evaluating speed: Running test of speed

To perform the running test of speed, it will be necessary to have a specially marked running course, a stopwatch, a whistle, and a partner to help you with the test. To perform the test, follow this procedure:

1. Mark a running course on a hard surface so that there is a starting line and a series of nine additional lines, each 2 yards apart, the first marked at a distance 10 yards from the starting line.
2. From a distance 1 or 2 yards behind the starting line, begin to run as fast as you can. As you cross the starting line, your partner starts a stopwatch.
3. Run as fast as you can until you hear the whistle that your partner will blow exactly 3 seconds after the stopwatch was started. Your partner marks your location at the time when the whistle was blown.
4. Your score is the distance you were able to cover in 3 seconds. You may practice the test and take more than one trial if time allows. Use the better of your distances on the last two trials as your score.

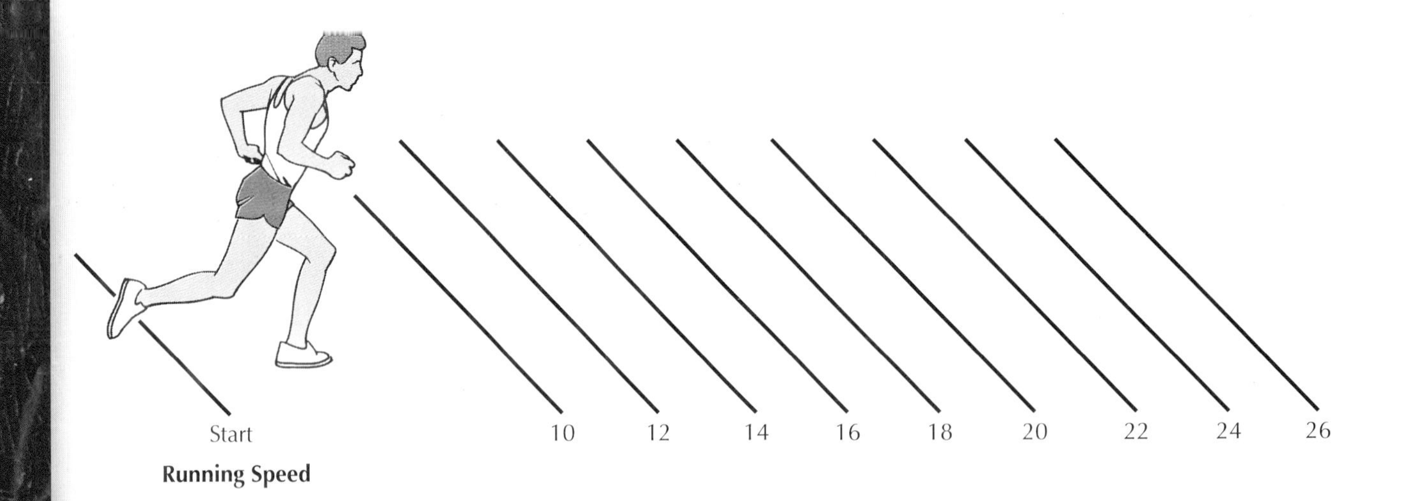

Running Speed

Chart 6 Speed Rating Scale

Classification	Men	Women
Excellent	24–26 yards	22–26 yards
Very good	22–23 yards	20–21 yards
Good	18–21 yards	16–19 yards
Fair	16–17 yards	14–15 yards
Poor	Less than 16 yards	Less than 14 yards

Metric conversions for this chart appear in Appendix B.

Lab 14B: Identifying Symptoms of Overtraining

Name	**Section**	**Date**

Purpose: To help you identify symptoms associated with overtraining.

Procedures:

1. Answer the questions concerning overtraining syndrome in the results section. If you are in training, rate yourself; if not, evaluate a person you know who is in training. As an alternative you may evaluate a person you know who was formerly in training (and who experienced symptoms) or evaluate yourself when you were in training (if you trained for performance in the past).
2. Use Chart 1 to rate the person (yourself or another person) who is (or was) in training.
3. Use Chart 2 to identify some steps that you might take to treat or prevent overtraining syndrome.
4. Answer the questions in the conclusions section.

Results:

Place a check in the circle by any of the overtraining symptoms you (or the person you are evaluating) experienced.

○ 1. Has performance decreased dramatically in the last week or two?

○ 2. Is there evidence of depression?

○ 3. Is there evidence of atypical anger?

○ 4. Is there evidence of atypical anxiety?

○ 5. Is there evidence of general fatigue that is not typical?

○ 6. Is there general lack of vigor or loss of energy?

○ 7. Have sleeping patterns changed (inability to sleep well)?

○ 8. Is there evidence of heaviness of the arms and/or legs?

○ 9. Is there evidence of loss of appetite?

○ 10. Is there a lack of interest in training?

Chart 1 Ratings for Overtraining Syndrome

Number of Yes Answers	Rating
9–10	Overtraining syndrome is very likely present. Seek help.
6–8	Person is at risk of overtraining syndrome if it is not already present. Seek help to prevent additional symptoms.
3–5	Some signs of overtraining syndrome are present. Consider methods of preventing further symptoms.
0–2	Overtraining syndrome is not present, but attention should be paid to the few symptoms that do exist.

Conclusions:
Chart 2 lists some of the steps that may be taken to help eliminate or prevent overtraining syndrome. Check the steps that you think would be (or would have been) most useful to the person you evaluated.

Chart 2 Steps for Treating or Preventing Overtraining Syndrome

○ 1. Consider a break from training.
○ 2. Taper the program to help reduce symptoms.
○ 3. Seek help to redesign the training program.
○ 4. Alter your diet.
○ 5. Evaluate other stressors that may be producing symptoms.
○ 6. Reset performance goals.
○ 7. Talk to someone about problems.
○ 8. Have a medical check-up to be sure there is no medical problem.
○ 9. If you have a coach, consider a talk with him/her.
○ 10. Add fluids to help prevent performance problems from dehydration.

Discuss overtraining syndrome in general. Elaborate on one or two of the steps in Chart 2 that you think would be (or would have been) most effective in treating or preventing overtraining syndrome for the person you evaluated.

Concept 15

Body Composition

Possessing an optimal amount of body fat contributes to health and wellness.

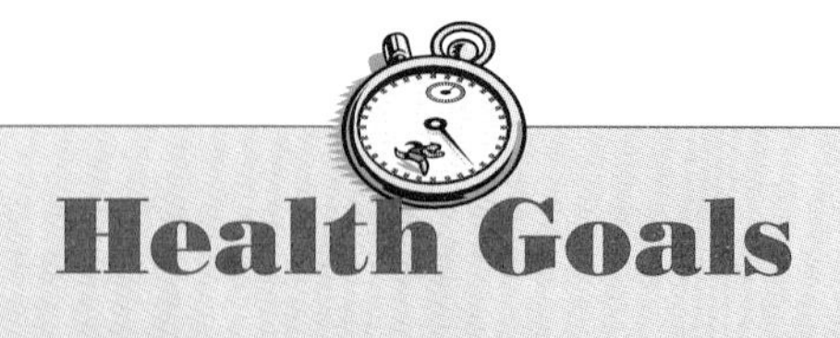

Increase the proportion of adults who are at a healthy weight.

Reduce the proportion of adults who are obese.

Reduce the proportion of children and adolescents who are overweight or obese.

Introduction

Body composition refers to the relative percentage of muscle, fat, bone, and other tissue of the body. Of primary concern, because of its association with various health problems, is body fatness. Being overfat or underfat can result in health concerns.

Despite general public awareness and concerns about weight control, the prevalence of obesity has continued to rise. A highly publicized article in The Journal of the American Medical Association revealed that the prevalence of obesity in the United States has increased from 12 percent to 18 percent in the last decade. The patterns are similar for both sexes and all ages and socioeconomic classes. Similar trends are occurring in nearly all industrialized countries and many developing nations. The World Health Organization recently concluded that "obesity's impact is so diverse and extreme that it should now be regarded as one of the greatest neglected public health problems of our time with an impact on health which may well prove to be as great as that of smoking." Since eating disorders such as anorexia nervosa and bulimia are also a significant health concern, especially among teens, the national goal is to keep the percentage of overfat teens from increasing while at the same time reducing the incidence of those who have too little fat associated with eating disorders.

The Facts about the Meaning and Measurement of Fatness

> There are standards that can be used to determine how much body fat an individual should possess.

Every person should possess at least a minimal amount of fat (**percent body fat**) for good health. This fat is called **essential fat** and is necessary for temperature regulation, shock absorption, and regulation of essential body nutrients, including vitamins A, D, E, and K. The exact amount of fat considered essential to normal body functioning has been debated, but most experts agree that males should possess no less than 5 percent and females no less than 10 percent. For females, an exceptionally low body fat percentage (**underfat**) is especially of concern. **Amenorrhea** may occur at fat levels higher than 10 percent (11 to 16 percent for many women). Some people feel that amenorrhea, when associated with low body fat levels, is a reversible condition that is merely the body's method of preventing pregnancy. However, low body fat levels, accompanied by amenorrhea, places a woman at risk of bone loss (osteoporosis). A body fat level below 10 percent is one of the criteria often used by clinicians for diagnosing eating disorders such as anorexia nervosa.

Close inspection of Table 1 reveals an overlap between essential fat, borderline, and high-performance classifications for body fatness. As noted previously, essential fat levels are those necessary for normal body functioning. Because individuals differ in their response to low fatness, a borderline range is provided. There appear to be no particular health benefits associated with being in the borderline range, and for some people there are health risks. Even though low body fat levels (borderline range) are not generally recommended, there are some individuals who are interested in high-level performance and seek low body fatness in an attempt to enhance performance. Standards for high-level performers are typically lower than for normally active people primarily interested in good health. Performance levels considered to be in the borderline area for nonperformers can be acceptable if the performer eats well, avoids overtraining, and practices a healthy lifestyle. If symptoms such as amenorrhea, bone loss, and frequent injury occur, then levels of body fatness should be reconsidered, as should training tech-

Table 1 Standards for Body Fatness (Percent Body Fat)

Classification	Males	Females
Essential fat	No less than 5%	No less than 10%
Borderline	5%–9%	10%–16%
High performance	5%–15%	10%–23%
Good fitness (healthy)	10%–20%	17%–28%
Marginal	21%–25%	29%–35%
Overfat	25%+	35%+

niques and eating patterns. For many people in training, maintaining performance levels of body fatness is temporary, thus the risk of long-term health problems is diminished.

Nonessential fat is fat above essential fat levels that accumulates when you take in more calories than you expend. When nonessential fat accumulates in excessive amounts, **overfatness** or even **obesity** can occur. Just as the percent of body fat should not drop too low, it should not get too high either. There is a desirable range of fatness that is associated with good metabolic fitness, good health, and wellness. It is referred to as the good fitness or healthy fatness range. People with more than healthy fat levels but who are not considered obese have scores in the marginal zone. While it is desirable to reach the healthy fitness zone, it will be harder for some people. Most experts agree that fat levels in the marginal zone are healthier than those in the overfatness zone.

Decisions about body composition should be based on more than one measurement.

In Lab 15A, you will have the opportunity to do several different measurements of body composition. Using only one of the methods may result in misinformation and unrealistic goals, which is why it is wise to use several techniques when making decisions about personal body composition goals. As you read about the various ways to assess body composition, consider the strengths and weaknesses of each technique and learn to use the techniques that provide the most information to you personally.

Overfat is more important than overweight in making decisions about health and wellness.

Many of the measures described in the following sections of this concept are indicators of the amount of body fat a person possesses. Others focus primarily on body weight. People who do regular physical activity and possess a large muscle mass can be high in body weight without being too fat. This is one of the limitations of measures based primarily on weight. Also, weight measures vary greatly based on your state of hydration or dehydration. You can lose weight merely by losing body water (becoming dehydrated) or gain weight by gaining body water (becoming hydrated). For this reason, measures that use weight as the primary indicator of body composition should be viewed with caution.

There are many ways to assess body fatness.

www.mhhe.com/phys_fit/webreview15 Click 01

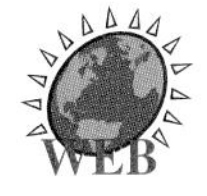

Underwater weighing, also referred to as "hydrostatic weighing," is considered the gold standard for assessing body fatness. In this laboratory procedure, a person is weighed underwater and out of the water. Corrections are made for the amount of air in the lungs when the underwater weight is measured. Using Archimedes' principle, the body's density can be determined. Because the density of various body tissues is known, the amount of the total body fat can be determined. Body fatness is usually expressed in terms of a percentage of the total body weight. Most of the other techniques for assessing body composition are based on predicting body fatness as assessed using underwater weighing.

Because underwater weighing takes considerable time, equipment, and specialized training, it is not practical for use except in well-equipped laboratories. Other methods of measuring body fatness or body weight are skinfold measurements, bioelectrical impedance, near-infrared interactance, X-ray absorptiometry, dual energy X-ray absorptiometry (DEXA) measurements, height/weight measurements, body mass index (BMI), and body circumference measurements. Table 2 presents a summary of the effectiveness of several of the more commonly used measures. Not all of these have been shown to be equally reliable and valid.

Skinfold measurements are a preferred, practical method of assessing body fatness.

Body fat is distributed throughout the body. About one-half of the body's fat is located around the various body organs and in the muscles. The other half of the body's fat is located just under the skin, or in skinfolds (Figure 1). A skinfold is two thicknesses of skin and the amount of fat that lies just under the skin. By measuring skinfold thicknesses of various sites around the body it is possible to estimate total body

Percent Body Fat The percentage of total body weight that is composed of fat.

Essential Fat The minimum amount of fat in the body necessary to maintain healthful living.

Underfat Too little of the body weight composed of fat (see Table 1).

Amenorrhea Absence of, or infrequent, menstruation.

Nonessential Fat Extra fat or fat reserves stored in the body.

Overfat Too much of the body weight composed of fat (see Table 1).

Obesity Extreme overfatness.

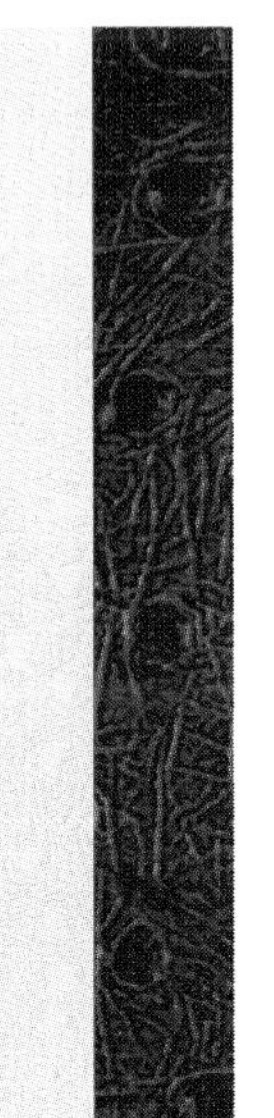

Table 2 Ratings of the Validity and Objectivity of Body Composition Methods

Method	Precise	Objective	Accurate	Valid Equations	Overall Rating
Skinfold measurement	4.0	3.5	3.5	3.5	3.5
Bioelectric impedance	4.0	4.0	3.5	3.5	3.5
Circumferences	4.0	4.0	3.0	3.0	3.0
Near-infrared interactance	5.0	4.5	2.0	2.0	2.5
Body mass index	5.0	5.0	1.5	1.5	2.0

Precise: Can the same person get the same results time after time?
Objective: Can two different people get the same results consistently?
Accurate: Do values compare favorably to underwater weighing?
Valid: Is the formula accurate for predicting fat from measurements?
5 = excellent; 4 = very good; 3 = good; 2 = fair; 1 = unacceptable.

Adapted from Lohman, T.G., Houtkooper, L.H., and Going, S.B. "Body Fat Measurement Goes Hi Tech." *ACSM's Health and Fitness Journal.* 1(1)(1998).

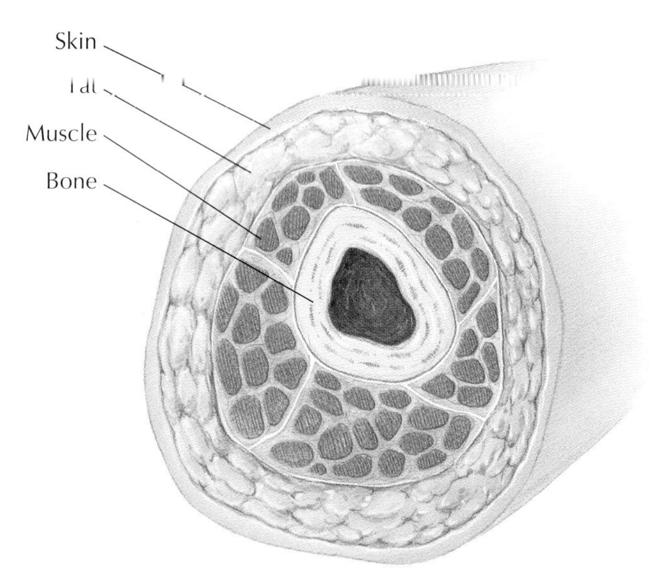

Figure 1
Location of body fat.

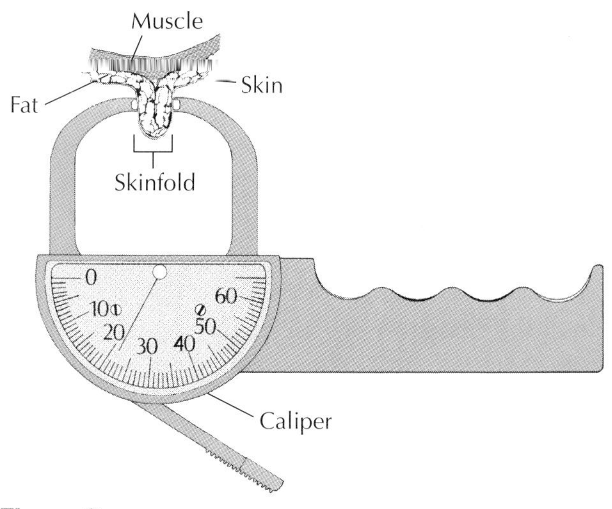

Figure 2
Measuring skinfold thickness.

fatness (Figure 2). Skinfold measurements are often used because they are relatively easy to do. They are not nearly as costly as underwater weighing and other methods that require expensive equipment. A set of calipers is used to make the measurements (Figure 3). The better, more accurate calipers cost several hundred dollars. However, considerably less expensive calipers are now available.

www.mhhe.com/phys_fit/webreview15 Click 02

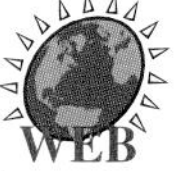

In general, the more skinfolds measured, the more accurate the body fatness estimate. However, measurements with two or three skinfolds have been shown to be reasonably accurate and can be done in a relatively short period. Two skinfold techniques are used in Lab 15A. You are encouraged to try both. With adequate training, most anyone can learn to use calipers to get a

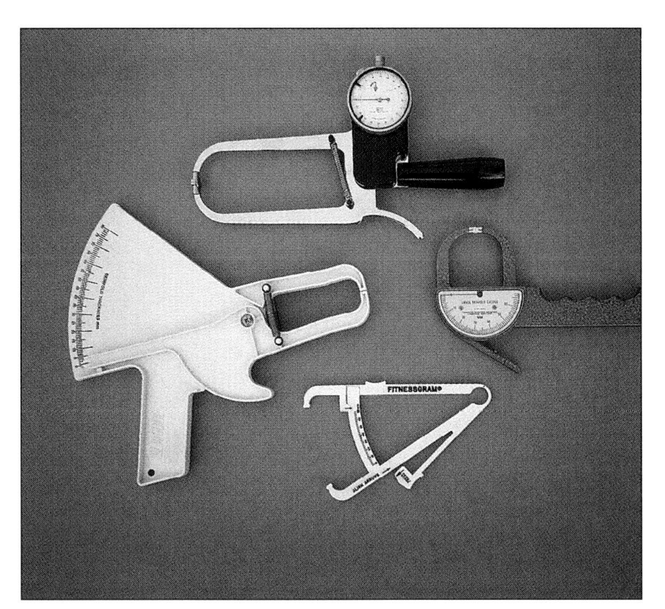

Figure 3
Skin-fold calipers.

good estimate of fatness. When performed by a trained person, skinfold techniques are rated very favorably by experts (see Table 2), but it is a skill that takes practice. Measurements made by an untrained person can be quite inaccurate.

Body circumference measures can be used to assess body fatness.

www.mhhe.com/phys_fit/webreview15 Click 03

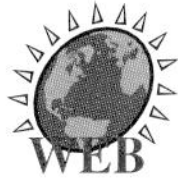

Body circumference, or girth measurements, can be used to determine body fatness using various weight, height, waist, thigh, hip, and other girth measurements. They are not rated as favorably as skinfold measurements (see Table 2), but they are easy to do. One weakness of circumference measures is they may misclassify people who have a large muscle mass. For this reason, they are not as useful as skinfold measures for active people who have a relatively large muscle mass compared to inactive people. As the sole measure of fatness, they should be used with caution. They can provide a useful second or third source of information about body fatness, however. Another technique that uses body circumferences—the waist-to-hip ratio—will be discussed in a later section.

A variety of technology-based assessments are available to estimate body fatness.

Recently, experts have rated the various techniques for assessing body fatness (see Table 2). Bioelectric impedance analysis ranks quite favorably for accuracy and has similar overall rankings to skinfold measurement techniques. The test can be performed quickly and is more effective for people high in body fatness (a limitation of skinfolds). The technique is based on measuring resistance to current flow. Electrodes are placed on the body and low doses of current are passed through the skin. Because muscle has greater water content than fat, it is a better conductor and has less resistance to current. The overall amount of resistance and body size are used to predict body fatness. Dehydration can bias the result and it is also critical to not have measures taken within three to four hours after a meal. Accurate measures require the use of high quality equipment but some commercially available "scales" now provide estimates of body fatness that are based on the same principles. Instead of electrodes, you simply stand on metal plates that measure the current flow.

Near infrared interactance machines use the absorption of light to estimate body fatness. The technique was originally developed to measure the fat content of meats. Commercially available units for humans have not been shown to be effective for estimating body fat. Various types of X-ray and magnetic resonance machines (MRI) have been used to assess body fatness. They can be quite useful, especially in determining body fatness in specific body locations. Unfortunately, these procedures require very expensive machines and are not practical for personal use. One relatively new procedure uses air displacement to assess fatness. Like X-ray and MRI, this technique requires special equipment, which makes it impractical for most people. One machine that uses this technique is called the BodPod. Preliminary evidence has shown it to be an acceptable alternative to underwater weighing, especially for special populations (obese, older people, and the physically challenged).

The body mass index (BMI) is considered to be a better measure than height-weight charts, but it has its limitations.

www.mhhe.com/phys_fit/webreview15 Click 04

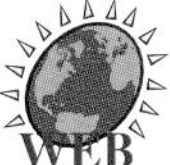

Individuals who are interested in controlling their weight often consult height-weight tables to determine their "desirable" weight. Being 20 percent or more above the recommended table weight is one commonly used indicator of obesity. New tables adopted by the federal government are now based on relative risk of health problems rather than normative comparisons to other people. A limitation of height and weight tables is that they don't take into account a person's degree of body fatness. A person who has a large muscle mass as a result of regular physical activity could appear to be

overweight using a height-weight table and still not be too fat. Some experts have criticized the new tables for not adjusting for age, sex, or fitness level. Others defend the fact that the tables encourage maintenance of weight over the lifespan rather than "allowing" weight gain with age.

The **body mass index (BMI)** is probably the best way to use height and weight to assess fatness. The BMI is calculated using a special formula and has a higher correlation with true body fatness than weights determined from height-weight tables. Nevertheless, the BMI may misclassify active people who have a large muscle mass. You can calculate your BMI using the procedures described in the lab resource materials. Just as height and weight standards have changed, the standards for BMI have also been modified recently. The National Institutes for Health now uses a BMI of 25 as the standard for overweight, 30 as the standard for obesity, and 40 as the standard for severe obesity. Prior to the establishment of these standards, different values for men and women were used and a value of approximately 27 was used as the indicator of overweight.

The revised standards are now consistent with those of the Department of Agriculture and the World Health Organization. These organizations have used the more stringent standards for a number of years. Consensus regarding the definition of these body composition categories now makes it easier to examine trends within the U.S. or to compare body composition levels and research results across countries. For example, BMI is the measure that public health officials have used to determine that over half of the U.S. population (52 percent) is either overweight or obese and to document increases in the past 10 years. Nearly all other developed countries are observing similar trends in the prevalence of obesity.

www.mhhe.com/phys_fit/webreview15 Click 05

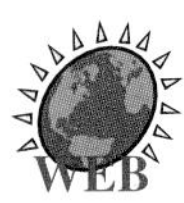

While the BMI is a useful indicator for large-scale research applications or to examine differences in groups, it is less valuable for making measurements for one specific individual at one particular point in time. Because the BMI is widely cited in news reports, it is important for all people to know how to calculate it and how to use it (and how not to misuse it). Plotting changes in BMI over time can be useful in tracking personal changes. Together with other techniques, the BMI can provide useful information, but the risk of misclassification is high among active people with a high amount of muscle if the BMI is used by itself.

The waist-to-hip ratio is a body circumference measurement technique that can be used in determining health risk.

www.mhhe.com/phys_fit/webreview15 Click 06

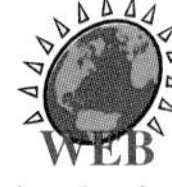

It has now been well established that the location of body fat can influence the health risks associated with obesity. Studies have shown that upper body fat poses a greater health risk than lower body fatness. For this reason, it is important to keep both your total and abdominal fat levels low, especially as you grow older. A useful indicator of fat distribution is the waist-to-hip circumference ratio. A high ratio between the waist and hip has been shown to be correlated with a high incidence of heart attack, stroke, chest pain, breast cancer, and death. Recent evidence indicates that people who exercise regularly accumulate less fat in the upper central regions of the body as they get older. This suggests that regular physical activity throughout life will result in a smaller waist-to-hip ratio and a reduced risk of various lifestyle diseases.

Body composition is considered a component of health-related fitness but can also be considered a component of metabolic fitness.

Body composition is generally considered to be a health-related component of physical fitness. Most national fitness tests include either a skinfold test or the BMI as an indicator of this component. Like the other parts of health-related physical fitness, body composition is related to good health.

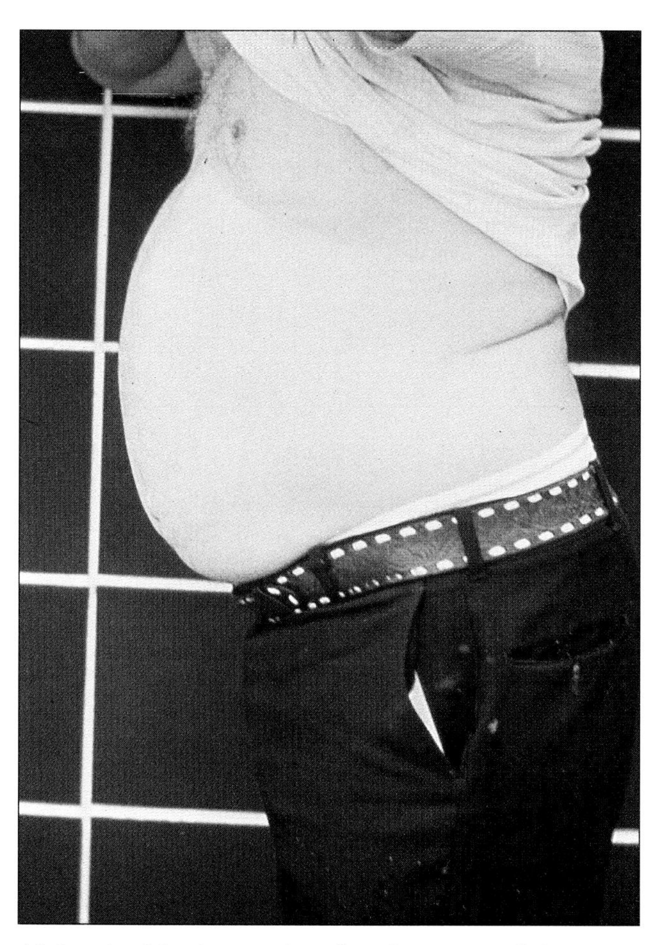

Abdominal fat is associated with increased disease risk.

However, body composition is unlike the other parts of health-related physical fitness in that it is not a performance measure. Cardiovascular fitness, strength, muscular endurance, and flexibility can be assessed using some type of movement or performance such as running, lifting, or stretching. Body composition requires no movement or performance. This is one reason why some experts prefer to consider body composition as a component of metabolic fitness.

Metabolic fitness includes other nonperformance measures associated with increased risk of health problems, such as high blood fat, high blood pressure, and high blood sugar levels. Some experts have hypothesized that metabolic fitness is really one syndrome that is characterized by body composition (body fatness) and the other highly related nonperformance measures described above. Whether you consider body composition to be a part of health-related or metabolic fitness, it is an important health-related factor.

Assessing body weight too frequently can result in making false assumptions about body composition changes.

Taking body weight measurements too frequently can provide incorrect information and lead to false assumptions. For example, people vary in body weight from day to day and even hour to hour based solely on their level of hydration. Short-term changes in weight are often due to water loss or gain, yet many people attribute the weight changes to their diet, a pill they have taken, or the exercise they are doing. In fact, short-term weight changes are more likely water changes than real body composition changes. We know this to be true because it takes a relatively long period of time for diet or exercise to affect weight changes. Monitoring your weight less frequently, once a week for example, is more useful than daily or multiple daily measures because it is more likely to represent real changes in body composition. Weighing at the same time of day, preferably early in the morning, is best because it reduces the chances that your weight variation will be a result of body water changes. Of course, it is best to use body composition assessments in addition to those based on body weight if accurate evaluations are expected.

Health Risks Associated with Overfatness: The Facts

Obesity has recently been elevated from a secondary to a primary risk factor for heart disease.

Prior to 1998, obesity was considered to be a secondary risk factor for heart disease. The reason for this was that the effects of obesity were thought to be mediated by other risk factors such as blood pressure and blood lipids. Because of the mounting evidence of the relationship of obesity to health risk, especially risk of heart disease, the American Heart Association now classifies obesity as a primary risk factor along with high blood lipids, high blood pressure, tobacco use, and sedentary living.

Overfatness or obesity can contribute to degenerative diseases, health problems, and even shortened life.

Some diseases and health problems are associated with overfatness and obesity. In addition to the higher incidence of certain diseases and health problems, there is evidence that people who are moderately overfat have a 40 percent higher than normal risk of shortening their lifespan. More severe obesity results in a 70 percent higher than normal death rate. This is evidenced by the exorbitant life insurance premiums paid by obese individuals.

Heart disease is not the only disease that is associated with obesity. Diabetes is another leading killer that is associated with all components of metabolic fitness including obesity. The incidence of diagnosis of this disease has increased sixfold in the last 40 years. Recent studies also indicate a significant increase in risk of breast cancer among the obese. High blood pressure and asthma are examples of other conditions associated with obesity.

It should be noted that statistics indicate that underweight people also have a higher than normal risk of premature death. Though there is adequate evidence that extreme leanness can be life threatening (e.g., anorexia nervosa), many underweight people included in these studies have lost weight because of a medical condition such as cancer. It appears that the medical problems are often the reason for low body weight rather than low body weight being the source of the medical problem. Most experts agree that people who are free from disease and who have lower than average amounts of body fat have a lower than average risk of premature death.

Excessive abdominal fat and excessive fatness of the upper body can increase the risk of various diseases.

As noted earlier, research studies have shown that a relationship exists between the amount of abdominal fat and various

Overweight Weight in excess of normal; not harmful unless it is accompanied by overfatness.

Body Mass Index (BMI) A measure of body composition using a height-weight formula. High BMI values have been related to increased disease risk.

health problems. Fat in the upper part of the body is sometimes called "Northern hemisphere" fat and is considered more risky than "Southern hemisphere" fat, such as in the hips and upper legs. People who have abdominal fatness are sometimes considered to have the "apple" fat pattern, while people with lower body fatness are considered to have the "pear" fat pattern. Regardless of the name used, it is clear that people who distribute fat around their middle as opposed to in the limbs are at greater risk of various health problems. The waist-to-hip ratio described in the previous section provides a means of assessing central body fatness. In general, men have higher waist-to-hip ration than women and postmenopausal women have higher ratios than premenopausal women. As you grow older, it is especially important to monitor your waist-to-hip ratio.

> High weight, and even relatively high body fat levels, may not increase risk of health problems if other indicators of poor health are not present.

www.mhhe.com/phys_fit/webreview15 Click 07

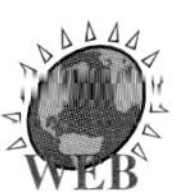

Recent research suggests that people who are above normal standards for BMI are not especially at risk if they participate in regular physical activity and possess relatively high levels of cardiovascular fitness. In fact, active people who have a high BMI are at less risk than inactive people with normal BMI levels. Even high levels of body fatness may not be especially likely to increase disease risk if a person has good metabolic fitness as indicated by healthy blood fat levels, normal blood pressure, and normal blood sugar levels. It is when several of these factors are present at the same time that risk levels increase dramatically. For this reason, it is important to consider your cardiovascular and metabolic fitness levels before drawing conclusions about the effects of high body weight or high body fat levels on health and wellness. This information also points out the importance of periodically assessing your cardiovascular and metabolic fitness levels.

Health Risks Associated with Excessively Low Body Fatness: The Facts

> Excessive desire to be thin or low in body weight can result in health problems.

In Western society, the near obsession with thinness has been, at least in part, responsible for health conditions now referred to as eating disorders. Eating disorders, or altered eating habits, involve extreme restriction of food intake and/or regurgitation of food to avoid digestion. The most common disorders are anorexia nervosa, bulimia, and anorexia athletica. All of these disorders are most common among highly achievement-oriented girls and young women, although they affect virtually all segments of the population.

Anorexia nervosa is the most severe of the three disorders. In fact, if not treated, it is life-threatening. Anorexics restrict food intake so severely that their bodies become emaciated. Among the many characteristics of the anorexic are fear of maturity and inaccurate body image. The anorexic starves herself/himself and may exercise compulsively or use laxatives to prevent the digestion of food in an attempt to attain excessive leanness. The anorexic's self-image is one of being too fat even when the person is too lean for good health. Assessing body fatness using procedures such as skinfolds and observation of the eating habits may help identify people with anorexia. Among anorexic girls and women, development of an adult figure is often feared. It is important that people with this disorder obtain medical and psychological help immediately, as the consequences are severe. People with anorexia may also have some of the characteristics of the person with bulimia. About 25 percent of those with anorexia do compulsive exercise in attempt to stay lean.

Bulimics may or may not be anorexic. It may not be possible to use measures of body fatness to identify bulimia, as the bulimic may be lean, normal, or excessively fat. The most common characteristics of bulimia are bingeing and purging. Bingeing means the periodic eating of large amounts of food at one time. A binge might occur after a relatively long period of dieting and often consists of junk foods containing empty calories. After a binge, the bulimic purges the body of the food by forced regurgitation or the use of laxatives. Another form of bulimia is bingeing on one day and starving on the next. The consequences of bulimia are not as severe as anorexia, but can result in serious mental, gastrointestinal, and dental problems.

Anorexia athletica is a recently identified eating disorder that appears to be related to participation in sports and activities, such as ballet, that emphasize excessive body leanness. Studies show that participants in sports such as gymnastics, wrestling, body building, and activities such as ballet and cheerleading are most likely to develop anorexia athletica. This disorder has many of the symptoms of anorexia nervosa, but not of the same severity. In some cases, anorexia athletica can lead to anorexia nervosa.

Female athlete triad is an increasingly common condition among female athletes. The three health concerns (the triad) that characterize the condition are eating disorders, amenorrhea, and osteoporosis. The disordered eating pat-

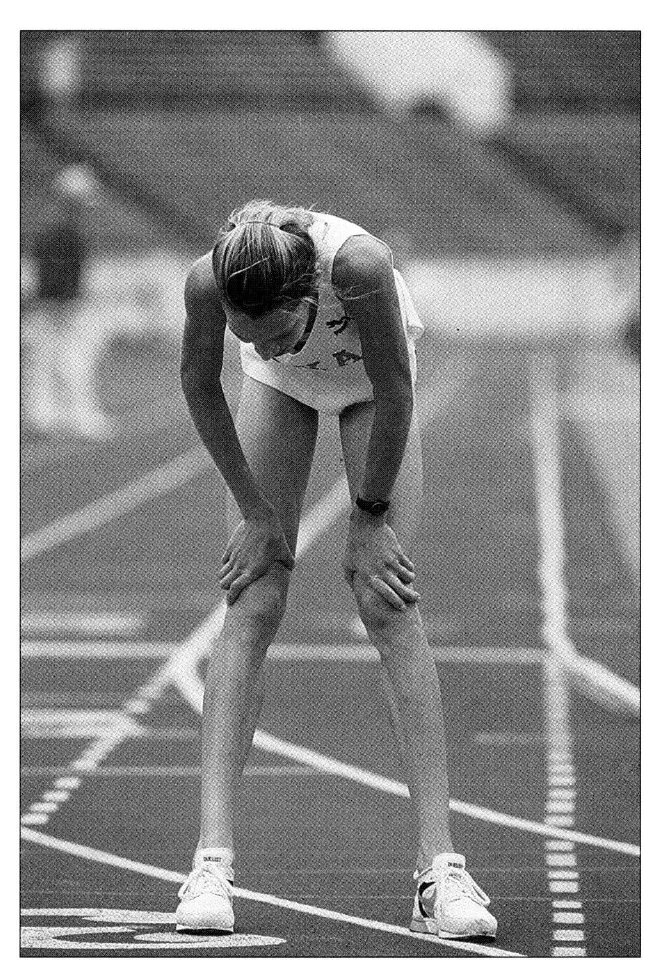

Excessively low levels of body fatness pose health problems.

terns may be extreme as in anorexia or bulimia, or less severe as evidenced by poor eating habits. Because they are athletes, females with this condition are very active. Together, the poor eating habits and high levels of activity typically result in low body fat levels. The triad of symptoms is often accompanied by considerable pressure to perform well, resulting in high stress levels. In addition to the triad of symptoms, the combination of poor eating, overexercise, and competitive stress can result in other problems, such as depression and anxiety, and even risk of suicide. Many female athletes train extensively and have relatively low body fat levels but experience none of the symptoms of the triad. Eating well, training properly, using stress-management techniques, and monitoring health symptoms are the keys to their success.

Fear of obesity is a less severe condition but it can still have negative health consequences. This condition is most common among achievement-oriented teenagers who impose a self-restriction on caloric intake because they fear obesity. Consequences include stunting of growth, delayed puberty, delayed sexual development, and decreased physical attractiveness. It is important to avoid excessive eating and inactivity to prevent the problems associated with overfatness and obesity; however, an excessive concern for leanness can also result in serious health problems.

Society can help reduce the incidence of the problems associated with disordered eating and desire to be thin by changing its image of attractiveness, especially among young women. Many of the models and movie stars who convey the "ideal" image are anorexic or are exceptionally thin. Teachers and athletic coaches can help by educating people about these disorders, by not placing too much emphasis on leanness, and by screening students for extreme leanness using procedures such as skinfolds and body mass index. Parents and friends can help by looking for excessive changes in body weight and lack of eating. Once an eating disorder is identified, it is important to help the individual obtain treatment for the problem. While regular physical activity is good, excessive activity can be harmful. It is important to help athletes learn not to overdo it and to keep competition in perspective so that it does not become excessively stressful.

Conflicting news reports should not deter efforts to maintain a healthy body fat level.

One recent headline said "Excess pounds deadly." One week later the headline read "It may be better to be a little fat." Adding to the confusion is that body mass index standards have been lowered in recent years so that more people are now classified as overweight using this measurement technique. At the same time, some of the standards for body fatness are now more lenient than they were in the past. In both cases, the changes are made based on new scientific evidence.

Sometimes people read conflicting headlines and adopt a defeatist attitude. It is important not to let one headline influence your overall plan of fat control. There will be a continuing debate in the years ahead as to just how much you should weigh or how much fat you should have for your good health and wellness. In the meantime, the message is clear! If possible, make several different assessments and consider all of the results before making decisions (see charts in lab resource materials). For some people, meeting the standards described in this book may be difficult. It is far better to be close to the standard than to say "I can't meet the standard, so I won't even try." Some experts feel that many people are overfat because they have repeatedly failed to meet unrealistic body fatness or weight goals. Adopting a realistic personal standard of fatness is very important. Using many different self-assessments and adopting realistic goals based on personal information rather than comparisons to others can help you make informed decisions about your body composition.

The Facts about the Origin of Fatness

Heredity plays a role in fatness.

Some people have suggested that every individual is born with a predetermined weight (sometimes called your set-point). This implies that you have little control over your weight or body fat levels. In fact, you do have considerable control over your weight and level of fatness as evidenced by the fact that calories taken in (diet) and calories expended (activity) are the two most important factors associated with fat control. Nevertheless, research suggests that people are born with a predisposition toward fatness or leanness. For years, some scholars have suggested that your body type, or **somatotype,** is inherited. Clearly, some people will have more difficulty than others controlling fatness because of their body types and because they come from families with a history of obesity. In fact, very recent research by a well-respected team of scholars indicates that the body has a "natural" fatness range, which is influenced by heredity. If you deviate more than 10 to 15 percent from this range, your body may actually alter its metabolism in an attempt to maintain your "natural" fatness level. But even these changes are temporary. If you continue the behavior that caused the weight gain (eating more or exercising less), after a period of time your body accepts your new weight as your "natural" level. Scientists caution people not to overgeneralize the importance of heredity to body fatness. Such overgeneralizations could lead to incorrect conclusions about regulation of body fat levels.

Recently the "ob-gene" (or gene responsible for obesity) was discovered. It is true that this is an important scientific discovery but it is unlikely that it will result in a "cure" for overfatness in the near future. In the meantime, more conventional methods of fat control must be used. Even if you come from a family with a history of obesity, you should not conclude that nothing can be done to prevent obesity. Virtually all people have a natural fatness below obese levels. Those with a predisposition to high fatness will have a harder time having a low body fatness level, but with healthy lifestyles, even these people can maintain body fat levels within normal ranges. Research shows that regular physical activity is especially effective in the control of genetically determined predispositions to fatness.

Glandular disorders are not a cause of overfatness for most people.

Glandular disorders can cause or contribute to overfatness. For example, thyroid problems can cause a low metabolic rate that results in fat gain. However, most experts suggest that only 1 to 2 percent of all overfatness is directly caused by problems of this type. Medical treatment is necessary for people suffering from these problems.

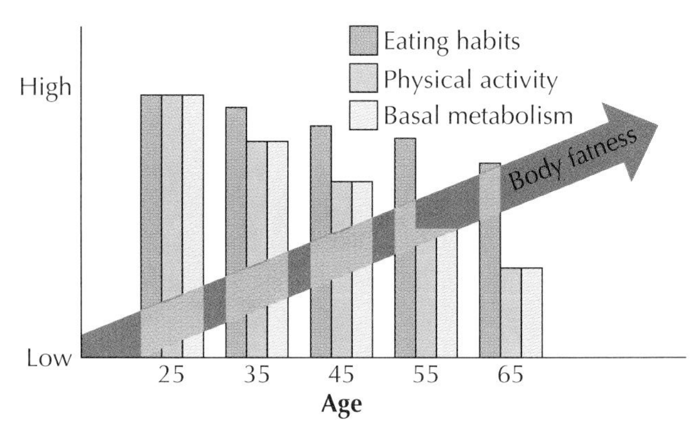

Figure 4
The creeping obesity.

Fatness early in life leads to adult fatness.

Retention of baby fat is not a sign of good health. On the contrary, excess body fat in the early years is a health problem of considerable concern. There is evidence that childhood overfatness results in hyperplasia, or an increased number of fat cells, and people with extra fat cells may have a greater tendency to become overfat. It was previously thought that only adult obesity was related to health problems. We now know that teens (ages 13–18) who are too fat are at greater risk of heart problems and cancer than their lean peers.

Changes in basal metabolic rate can be the cause of overfatness.

The amount of energy you expend each day must be balanced by your energy intake if you are to maintain your body fat and body weight over time. Your energy intake is determined by the calories you eat. Expenditure is determined by a combination of several factors. You expend calories just to exist—even when you are inactive. Your **basal metabolic rate** (**BMR**) is the indicator or your energy expenditure when your are totally inactive. You also expend calories digesting food and, of course, in the activities of daily living.

Basal metabolic rate is highest during the growing years. The amount of food eaten increases to support this increased energy expenditure. When growing ceases, if eating does not decrease or activity level increase, fatness can result. Basal metabolism also decreases gradually as you grow older. One major reason for this is the loss of muscle mass associated with inactivity. Regular physical activity throughout life helps keep the muscle mass higher, resulting in a higher BMR. Very recent evidence suggests that regular exercise can contribute in other ways to increased BMR. The higher BMR of active people helps them prevent overfatness, particularly in later life.

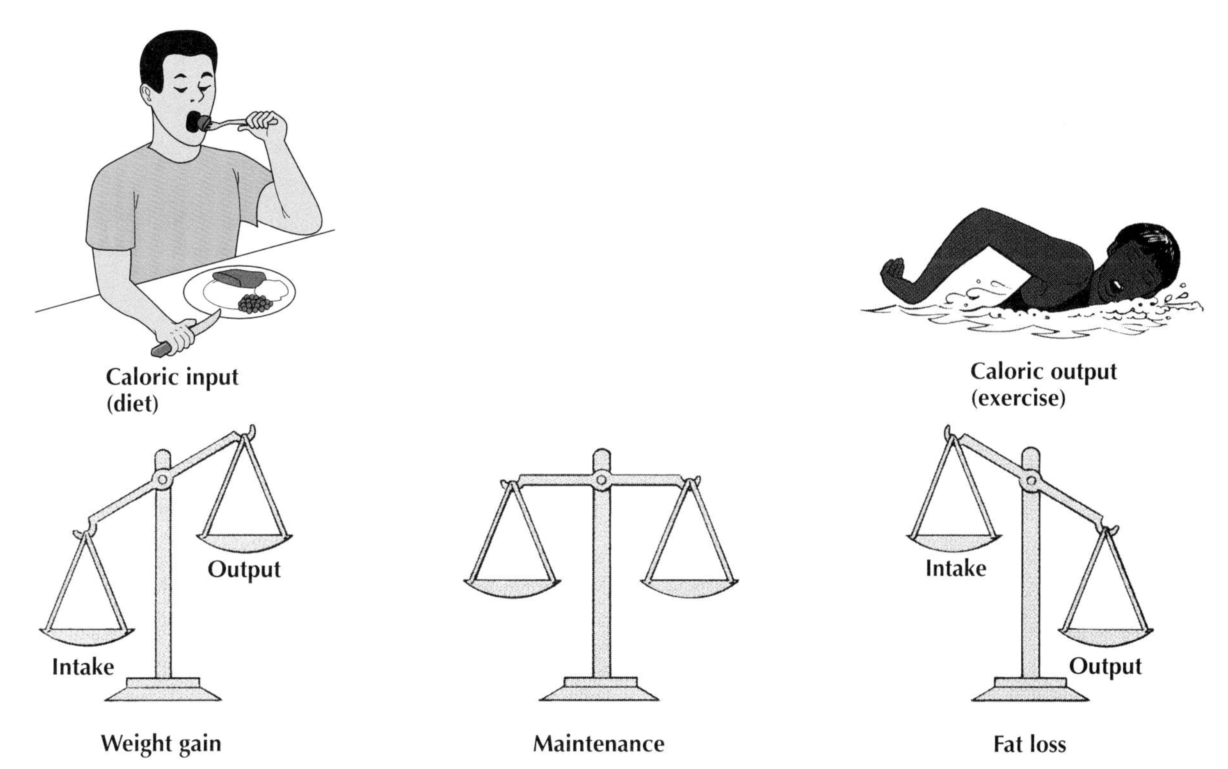

Figure 5
Balancing calorie input and output.

"Creeping obesity" is a problem as you grow older.

People become less active and their BMR gradually decreases with age. Calorie intake does seem to decrease somewhat with age, but the decrease does not adequately compensate for the decreases in BMR and activity levels. For this reason, body fat increases gradually for the typical person as he or she ages (see Figure 4). This increase in fatness over time is commonly referred to as "creeping obesity" because the increase in fatness is gradual. For a typical person, creeping obesity could result in a gain of one-half to one pound per year. People who stay active can keep muscle mass high and delay changes in BMR. For those who are not active, it is suggested that caloric intake should decrease by 3 percent each decade after 25 so that by age 65, caloric intake is at least 10 percent less than it was at age 25. The decrease in calorie intake for active people need not be as great.

The principal cause of most overfatness is the intake of more calories than are expended.

While obesity is clearly caused by multiple factors, an increased energy intake (food calories) and a reduced energy expenditure (physical inactivity) are the prime causes (see Figure 5). Results of several studies have suggested that the recent increases in obesity are more related to declines in physical activity than to systematic changes in eating patterns.

Excess caloric intake results in an increase in fat cell size.

Overfatness can result in an increase in the number of fat cells among children. For adults, overfatness is a result of the increase in size of fat cells (hypertrophy). When fat cells become excessively large, they can cause dimples or lumps under the skin. Some people refer to these large fat cells as cellulite. Quacks say that this type of fat is different from other types of fat and is removed from the body in different ways than regular fat. This is not true. All fatness among adults is a result of enlarged fat cells. All fat is lost as a result of reduction in fat cell size.

Somatotype Inherent body build: ectomorph (thin), mesomorph (muscular), and endomorph (fat).

Basal Metabolic Rate (BMR) Your energy expenditure in a basic or rested state.

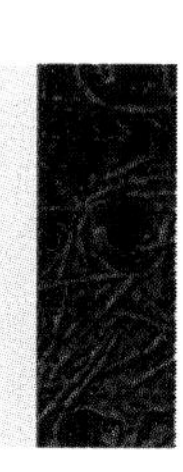

The Facts about Diet, Physical Activity, and Fatness

A combination of regular physical activity and dietary restriction is the most effective means of losing body fat.

Studies indicate that regular physical activity combined with dietary restriction is the most effective method of losing fat. One study of adult women indicated that diet alone resulted in loss of weight, but much of this loss was lean body tissue. Those who were dieting as well as exercising experienced similar weight losses, but this loss included more body fat. For optimal results, all weight loss programs should combine a lower caloric intake with a good physical exercise program. Thresholds of training and target zones for body fat reduction, including information for both physical activity and **diet** are presented in Table 3.

Good physical activity and diet habits can be useful in maintaining desirable body composition.

Table 3 illustrates how fat can be lost through regular physical activity and proper dieting. However, not all people want to lose fat. For those who wish to maintain their current body composition, a **caloric balance** between intake and output is effective. For people who want to increase their lean body weight, increased caloric intake with increased exercise can result in the desired changes.

Physical activity is one effective means of controlling body fat.

Though physical activity or exercise will not result in immediate and large decreases in body fat levels, there is increasing evidence that fat loss resulting from physical activity may be more lasting than fat loss from dieting. Vigorous exercise can increase the resting energy expenditure up to 13 times (13 **METs**).

Table 3 Threshold of Training and Target Zones for Body Fat Reduction

	Threshold of Training*		Target Zones*	
	Physical Activity	**Diet**	**Physical Activity**	**Diet**
Frequency	• To be effective, activity must be regular, preferably daily, though fat can be lost over the long term with almost any frequency that results in increased caloric expenditure.	• It is best to reduce caloric intake consistently and daily. To restrict calories only on certain days is *not* best, though fat can be lost over a period of time by reducing caloric intake at any time.	• Daily moderate activity is recommended. For people who do regular vigorous activity, 3 to 6 days per week may be best.	• It is best to diet consistently and daily.
Intensity	• To lose 1 pound of fat, you must expend 3,500 calories more than you normally expend.	• To lose 1 pound of fat, you must eat 3,500 calories fewer than you normally eat.	• Slow, low-intensity aerobic exercise that results in no more than 1–2 pounds of fat loss per week is best.	• Modest caloric restriction resulting in no more than 1–2 pounds of fat loss per week is best.
Time	• To be effective, exercise must be sustained long enough to expend a considerable number of calories. At least 15 minutes per exercise bout are necessary to result in consistent fat loss.	• Eating moderate meals is best. Do not skip meals.	• Exercise durations similar to those for achieving aerobic cardiovascular fitness seem best. An exercise duration of 30–60 minutes is recommended.	• Eating moderate meals is best. Skipping meals or fasting is *not* most effective.

**Note:* It is best to combine exercise and diet to achieve the 3,500 caloric imbalance necessary to lose a pound of fat. Using both exercise and diet in the target zone is most effective.

Inactivity is more often the cause of childhood obesity than overeating. Many fat children eat less but are considerably less active than their nonfat peers. Excessive television watching may be one reason for inactivity among children if the television viewing is done during daytime hours when children have the opportunity to be active. Studies show that adults who watch more than three hours of television per day are twice as likely to be obese as those who view television for less than one hour per day.

If you exercise moderately for an extra 15 minutes a day, you will lose up to 10 pounds in a year's time. Regular walking, jogging, swimming, or any type of sustained exercise can be effective in producing losses in body fat.

Physical activity that can be sustained for relatively long periods is considered the most effective for losing body fat.

Physical activities from virtually any level of the physical activity pyramid (see Figure 6) can be effective in controlling body fatness because all physical activities expend calories. Among the most effective activities are those in the aerobic activity section of the pyramid because they can be done for relatively long periods of time. Lifestyle activities are also effective, if performed regularly for extended periods of time. Table 4 shows the caloric expenditures for one hour of involvement in various physical activities. Heavier people expend more **calories** than lighter people because more work is required to move larger bodies.

Popular books have recently claimed that vigorous activities are not effective in helping with body fat loss because they say vigorous activities burn less fat than less intense activities. While this is true in theory, it has little practical meaning for most people. It is the total calories expended in your activity that counts. If you run for the same period of time that you walk, you will expend more calories in running.

Even though vigorous activity can be effective, it will not work if you do not do it regularly. For this reason, more vigorous activity may not be as effective as some less vigorous activities for certain people. For example, running at 10 miles per hour (a 6-minute mile) will cause a 150-pound person to expend 900 calories in one hour. Jogging about half as fast, or at 5 1/2 miles per hour (approximately an 11-minute mile), will result in an expenditure of about 650 calories in the same amount of time. At first glance, the more vigorous exercise seems to be a better choice. But how many people can continue to run at a 10-mile-per-hour pace for a full hour? Each mile run at 10 miles per hour results in an expenditure of 90 calories, while each mile run at 5 1/2 miles per hour results in an expenditure of 118 calories. Per mile, you expend more calories in slow running. It takes longer to run a mile, but by the same token, you can also persist longer. The key is to expend as many calories as possible during each regular exercise period. Doing less vigorous activity for longer periods is better for fat control than doing very vigorous activities that can be done only for short periods. Nevertheless, vigorous activity can be very effective for some people.

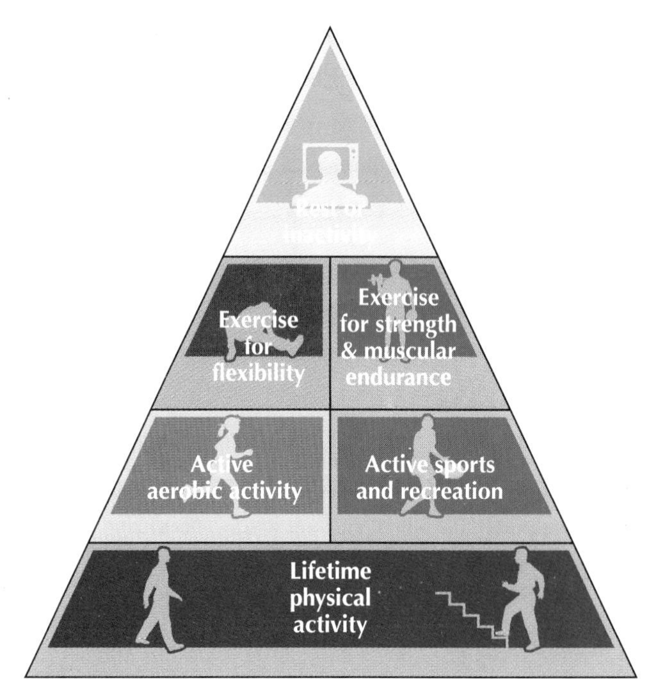

Figure 6
Activities from the lower three levels of the pyramid expend calories, but those from level 1 are especially effective in fat loss.

Strength training can be effective in maintaining a desirable body composition.

Performing exercises from the strength and muscular endurance level of the physical activity pyramid can be effective in maintaining desirable body fat levels. People who do strength training increase their muscle mass (lean body mass). This extra muscle mass expends extra calories at rest resulting

Diet The usual food and drink for a person or animal.

Caloric Balance Consuming calories in amounts equal to the number of calories expended.

MET METs are multiples of the amount of energy expended at rest, or approximately 1 calorie per kilogram (2.2 pounds) per hour.

Calorie A unit of energy supplied by food; the quantity of heat necessary to raise the temperature of a kilogram of water 1° C (actually a kilocalorie, but usually called a calorie for weight-control purposes).

5. Self-assessments require skill. With practice, you can become skillful in making measurements. Your first few attempts will no doubt lack accuracy.
6. Use the same measuring device each time you measure (scale, caliper, measuring tape, etc.). This will assure that any measurement error is constant and will allow you to track your progress over time. For example, your scale may be off by 2 pounds, but if you use the same scale every time you always know the amount of the error and you can correct for it. If you use a different scale each time you weigh, the error is variable. It is difficult to correct for variable errors.
7. Once you have tried all of the self-assessments in Lab 15A, choose the ones you want to continue to do and use the same measurement techniques each time you do the measurements.

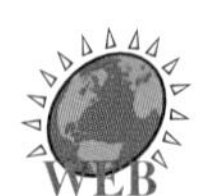

Web Review

Web review materials for Concept 15 are available at *www.mhhe.com/phys_fit/webreview15 Click 11.*

American Anorexia/Bulimia Association

www.aabainc.org

North American Association for the Study of Obesity (NAASO)

http://www.naaso.org

Shape up America

www.shapeup.org

Inexpensive Calipers (available from)

Fat Control Inc. Dept CC
19310 Dutton Rd.
Stewartstown, PA 17363
wellfarm@nfdc.net

Suggested Readings

Andersen, R.E. "Exercise, Active Lifestyle, and Obesity: Making an Exercise Prescription Work." *The Physician and Sports Medicine.* 27(10)(1999): 41–50.

Cataldo, D., and Heyward, V.H. "Pinch an Inch: A Comparison of Several High-Quality and Plastic Skinfold Calipers." *ACSM's Health and Fitness Journal.* 4(3)(2000):12–16.

Gaesser, G.A. "Thinness and Weight Loss: Beneficial or Detrimental to Longevity?" *Medicine and Science in Sports and Exercise.* 31(8)(1999): 1118–1128.

Lindeman, A.K. "Quest for Ideal Weight: Cost and Consequences." *Medicine and Science in Sports and Exercise.* 31(8)(1999): 1135–1140.

Lohman, T. G., Houtkooper, L. H., and Going, S. B. "Body Fat Measurement Goes Hi Tech." *ACSM's Health and Fitness Journal.* 1(1)(1998).

Manore, M. M., and Thompson, J. A. *Sport Nutrition for Health and Performance.* Champaign, IL: Human Kinetics, 2000.

Miller, W.C. "How Effective Are Traditional Dietary and Exercise Interventions for Weight Loss?" *Medicine and Science in Sports and Exercise.* 31(8)(1999): 1129–1134.

Mokdad, A. et al. "The Spread of the Obesity Epidemic in the United States." *Journal of the American Medical Association.* 282(1999): 1519–1522.

Newsweek. "Fat for Life." *Newsweek,* 3 July 2000. A series of articles on childhood obesity, pages 40–47.

Otis, C. L., Drinkwater, B., Johnson, M., Loucks, A., and Wilmore, J. "ACSM Position Stand on the Female Athlete Triad." *Medicine and Science in Sports and Exercise.* 29(5)(1997):i.

Thompson, S. R., Weber, M. M., and Brown, L. B. "The Relationship Between Health and Fitness Magazine Readings and Eating-Disordered Weight-Loss Methods Among High School Girls." *American Journal of Health Education.* [illegible]

U.S. Department of Health and Human Services, *Healthy People 2010.* (2nd ed.) With *Understanding and Improving Health* and *Objectives for Improving Health.* 2 vols. Washington, DC: U.S. Government Printing Office, November 2000, Chapter 19, "Nutrition and Overweight."

Wei, M. et al. "Relationship between Low Cardiorespiratory Fitness and Morbidity in Normal Weight, Overweight, and Obese Men," *Journal of the American Medical Association.* 282(1999):1547–1553.

Welk, G. J., and Blair, S. N. "Physical Activity Protects Against the Health Risk of Obesity." *President's Council on Physical Fitness and Sports Research Digest.* 3(12)(2000): 1–8.

World Health Organization. *Obesity: Preventing and Managing the Global Epidemic.* Geneva: World Health Organization, 2000.

Physical Fitness News Update

In our society we assume that if you are thin then you are likely to be fit and healthy and that if you are overweight then you are unfit and unhealthy. Recent studies from the Cooper Institute suggest that the health risks of body fatness are modified by fitness level. In one study, 21,925 men completed maximal treadmill tests and body composition assessments. The population was divided into Lean, Normal, and Obese groups and then subdivided by fitness level into Fit and Unfit categories based on established fitness standards. These individuals were then followed over an average of eight years to look at various health outcomes. Individuals in the Fit category had lower rates of death than individuals in the Unfit category and this relationship was consistent for all three body composition categories (see figure). This indicates that fatness is a risk only if a person is also unfit. It also indicates that if people are thin, they can still be at increased risk if they are not fit.

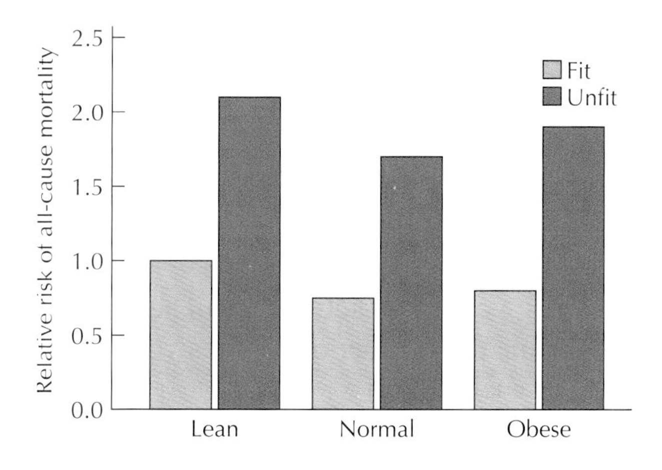

Lab Resource Materials: Evaluating Body Fatness

General Information about Skinfold Measurements

It is important to use a consistent procedure for "drawing up" or "pinching up" a skinfold and making the measurement with the caliper. The following procedures should be used for each skinfold site.

1. Lay the caliper down on a nearby table. Use the thumbs and index fingers of both hands to draw up a skinfold or layer of skin and fat. The fingers and thumbs of the two hands should be about 1 inch apart, or half an inch on either side of the location where the measurement is to be made.
2. The skinfolds are normally drawn up in a vertical line rather than a horizontal line. However, if the natural tendency of the skin aligns itself less than vertical, the measurement should be done on the natural line of the skinfold, rather than on the vertical.
3. Do not pinch the skinfold too hard. Draw it up so that your thumbs and fingers are not compressing the skinfold.
4. Once the skinfold is drawn up, let go with your right hand and pick up the caliper. Open the jaws of the caliper and place it over the location of the skinfold to be measured and one-half inch from your left index finger and thumb. Allow the tips, or jaw faces, of the caliper to close on the skinfold at a level about where the skin would be normally.
5. Let the reading on the caliper settle for 2 or 3 seconds, then note the thickness of the skinfold in millimeters.
6. Three measurements should be taken at each location. Use the middle of the three values to determine your measurement. For example, if you had values of 10, 11, and 9, your measurement for that location would be 10. If the three measures vary by more than 3 millimeters from the lowest to the highest, you may want to take additional measurements.

Skinfold Locations for Women

Triceps skinfold— Make a mark on the back of the right arm, one-half the distance between the tip of the shoulder and the tip of the elbow. Make the measurement at this location.

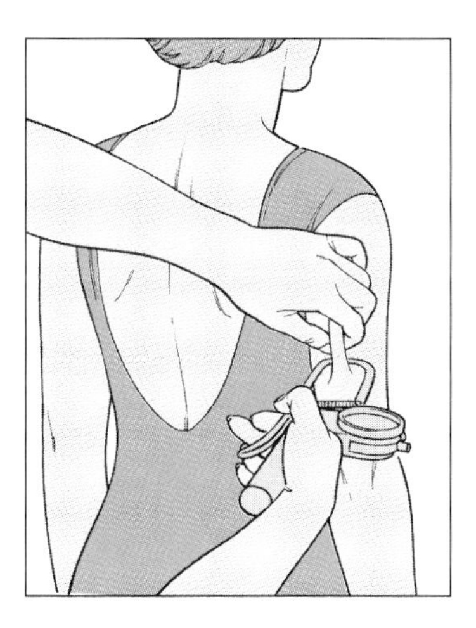

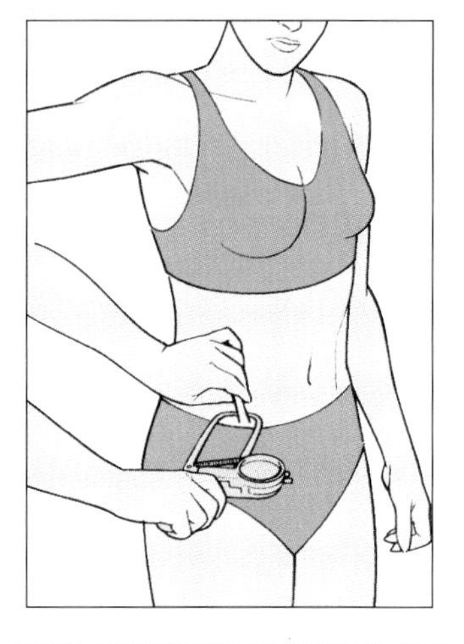

Iliac crest skinfold— Make a mark at the top front of the iliac crest. This skinfold is taken slightly diagonally because of the natural line of the skin.

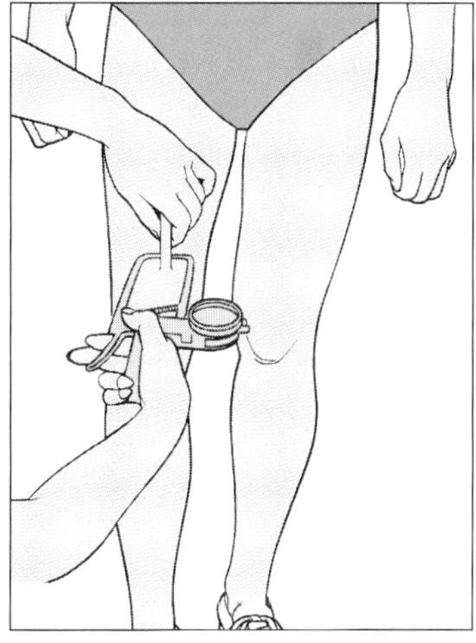

Thigh skinfold— Make a mark on the front of the thigh midway between the hip and the knee. Make the measurement vertically at this location.

Abdominal skinfold—Make a mark on the skin approximately one inch to the right of the navel. Make a horizontal measurement at this location for the Fitnessgram Method and a vertical measure for the Jackson-Pollock Method. (See page 290.)

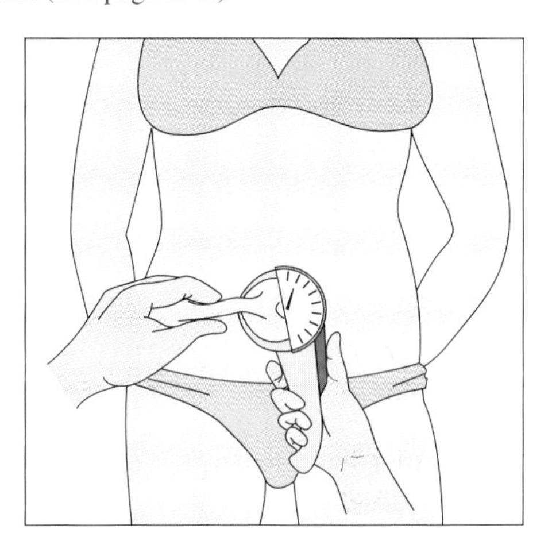

Calf skinfold—Same as for men.

Skinfold Locations for Men

Chest skinfold—Make a mark above and to the right of the right nipple (one-half the distance from the midline of the side and the nipple). The measurement at this location is often done on the diagonal because of the natural line of the skin.

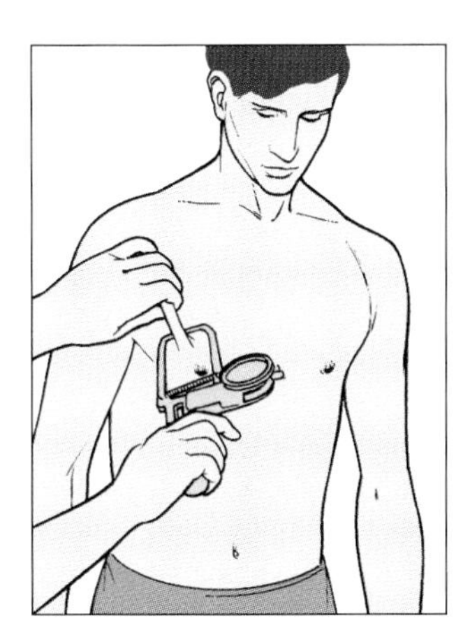

Abdominal skinfold—Make a mark on the skin approximately 1 inch to the right of the navel. Make a vertical measurement at that location for the Jackson-Pollock Method and horizontally for the Fitnessgram Method. (See page 289.)

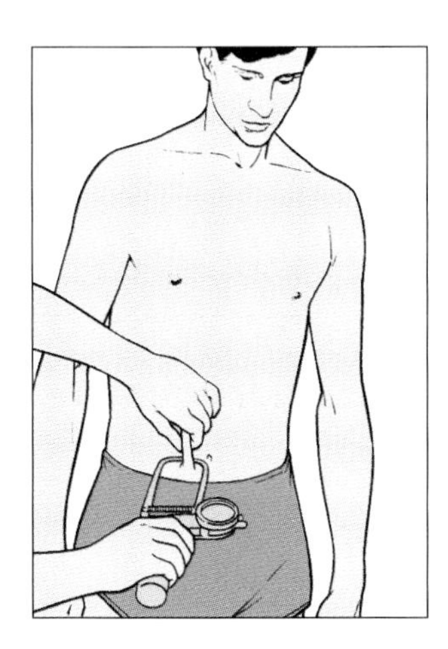

Thigh skinfold—Same as for women (see previous page).

Calf skinfold—Make a mark on the inside of the calf of the right leg at the level of the largest calf size (girth). Place the foot on a chair or other elevation so that the knee is kept at approximately 90 degrees. Make a vertical measurement at the mark.

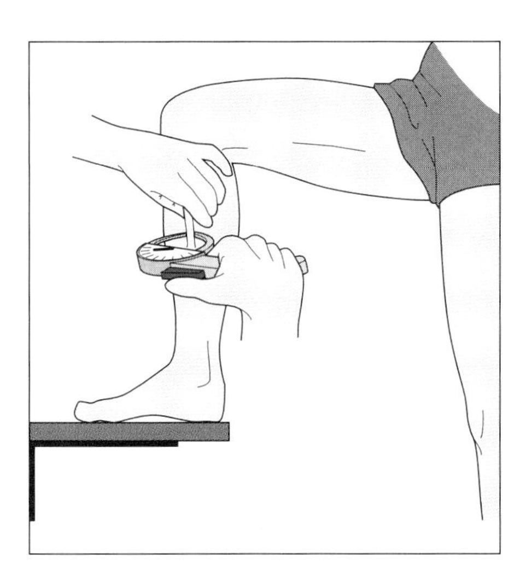

Self Measured Tricep Skinfold for Both Men and Women

This measurement is made on the left arm so that the caliper can easily be read. Hold the arm straight at shoulder height. Make a fist with the thumb faced upward. Place the fist against a wall. With the right hand place the caliper over the skinfold at it "hangs freely" on the back of the tricep (half way from the tip of the shoulder to the elbow).

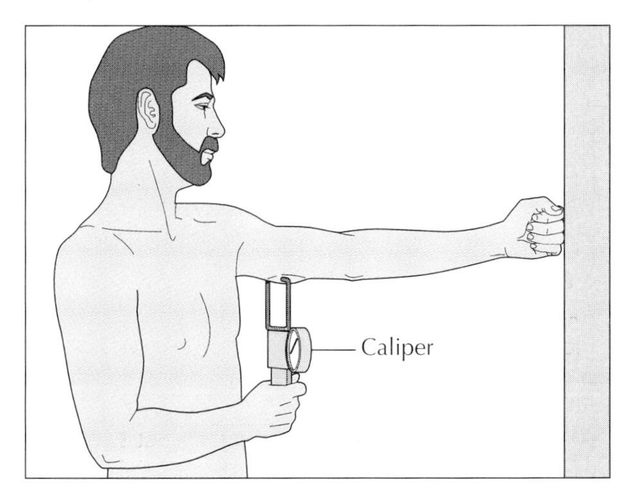

Calculating Fatness from Skinfolds (Jackson-Pollock Method)

1. Sum three skinfolds (triceps, iliac crest, and thigh for women; chest, abdominal (vertical), and thigh for men).
2. Use the skinfold sum and your age to determine your percent fat using Chart 1 for men and Chart 2 for women. Locate your sum of skinfold in the left column and your age at the top of the chart. Your estimated body fat percentage is located where the values intersect.
3. Use the Standards for Body Fatness (Chart 4) to determine your fatness rating.

Chart 1 Percent Fat Estimates for Men (Sum of Thigh, Chest, and Abdominal Skinfolds)

	Age to the Last Year								
Sum of Skinfolds (mm)	22 and Under	23 to 27	28 to 32	33 to 37	38 to 42	43 to 47	48 to 52	53 to 57	Over 58
8–10	1.3	1.8	2.3	2.9	3.4	3.9	4.5	5.0	5.5
11–13	2.2	2.8	3.3	3.9	4.4	4.9	5.5	6.0	6.5
14–16	3.2	3.8	4.3	4.8	5.4	5.9	6.4	7.0	7.5
17–19	4.2	4.7	5.3	5.8	6.3	6.9	7.4	8.0	8.5
20–22	5.1	5.7	6.2	6.8	7.3	7.9	8.4	8.9	9.5
23–25	6.1	6.6	7.2	7.7	8.3	8.8	9.4	9.9	10.5
26–28	7.0	7.6	8.1	8.7	9.2	9.8	10.3	10.9	11.4
29–31	8.0	8.5	9.1	9.6	10.2	10.7	11.3	11.8	12.4
32–34	8.9	9.4	10.0	10.5	11.1	11.6	12.2	12.8	13.3
35–37	9.8	10.4	10.9	11.5	12.0	12.6	13.1	13.7	14.3
38–40	10.7	11.3	11.8	12.4	12.9	13.5	14.1	14.6	15.2
41–43	11.6	12.2	12.7	13.3	13.8	14.4	15.0	15.5	16.1
44–46	12.5	13.1	13.6	14.2	14.7	15.3	15.9	16.4	17.0
47–49	13.4	13.9	14.5	15.1	15.6	16.2	16.8	17.3	17.9
50–52	14.3	14.8	15.4	15.9	16.5	17.1	17.6	18.1	18.8
53–55	15.1	15.7	16.2	16.8	17.4	17.9	18.5	18.2	19.7
56–58	16.0	16.5	17.1	17.7	18.2	18.8	19.4	20.0	20.5
59–61	16.9	17.4	17.9	18.5	19.1	19.7	20.2	20.8	21.4
62–64	17.6	18.2	18.8	19.4	19.9	20.5	21.1	21.7	22.2
65–67	18.5	19.0	19.6	20.2	20.8	21.3	21.9	22.5	23.1
68–70	19.3	19.9	20.4	21.0	21.6	22.2	22.7	23.3	23.9
71–73	20.1	20.7	21.2	21.8	22.4	23.0	23.6	24.1	24.7
74–76	20.9	21.5	22.0	22.6	23.2	23.8	24.4	25.0	25.5
77–79	21.7	22.2	22.8	23.4	24.0	24.6	25.2	25.8	26.3
80–82	22.4	23.0	23.6	24.2	24.8	25.4	25.9	26.5	27.1
83–85	23.2	23.8	24.4	25.0	25.5	26.1	26.7	27.3	27.9
86–88	24.0	24.5	25.1	25.5	26.3	26.9	27.5	28.1	28.7
89–91	24.7	25.3	25.9	25.7	27.1	27.6	28.2	28.8	29.4
92–94	25.4	26.0	26.6	27.2	27.8	28.4	29.0	29.6	30.2
95–97	26.1	26.7	27.3	27.9	28.5	29.1	29.7	30.3	30.9
98–100	26.9	27.4	28.0	28.6	29.2	29.8	30.4	31.0	31.6
101–103	27.5	28.1	28.7	29.3	29.9	30.5	31.1	31.7	32.3
104–106	28.2	28.8	29.4	30.0	30.6	31.2	31.8	32.4	33.0
107–109	28.9	29.5	30.1	30.7	31.3	31.9	32.5	33.1	33.7
110–112	29.6	30.2	30.8	31.4	32.0	32.6	33.2	33.8	34.4
113–115	30.2	30.8	31.4	32.0	32.6	33.2	33.8	34.5	35.1
116–118	30.9	31.5	32.1	32.7	33.3	33.9	34.5	35.1	35.7
119–121	31.5	32.1	32.7	33.3	33.9	34.5	35.1	35.7	36.4
122–124	32.1	32.7	33.3	33.9	34.5	35.1	35.8	36.4	37.0
125–127	32.7	33.3	33.9	34.5	35.1	35.8	36.4	37.0	37.6

*Percent fat calculated by the formula by Siri. Percent fat = [(4.95/BD) – 4.5] × 100, where BD = body density.

Chart 2 Percent Fat Estimates for Women (Sum of Triceps, Iliac Crest, and Thigh Skinfolds)

	Age to the Last Year								
Sum of Skinfolds (mm)	22 and Under	23 to 27	28 to 32	33 to 37	38 to 42	43 to 47	48 to 52	53 to 57	Over 58
23–25	9.7	9.9	10.2	10.4	10.7	10.9	11.2	11.4	11.7
26–28	11.0	11.2	11.5	11.7	12.0	12.3	12.5	12.7	13.0
29–31	12.3	12.5	12.8	13.0	13.3	13.5	13.8	14.0	14.3
32–34	13.6	13.8	14.0	14.3	14.5	14.8	15.0	15.3	15.5
35–37	14.8	15.0	15.3	15.5	15.8	16.0	16.3	16.5	16.8
38–40	16.0	16.3	16.5	16.7	17.0	17.2	17.5	17.7	18.0
41–43	17.2	17.4	17.7	17.9	18.2	18.4	18.7	18.9	19.2
44–46	18.3	18.6	18.8	19.1	19.3	19.6	19.8	20.1	20.3
47–49	19.5	19.7	20.0	20.2	20.5	20.7	21.0	21.2	21.5
50–52	20.6	20.8	21.1	21.3	21.6	21.8	22.1	22.3	22.6
53–55	21.7	21.9	22.1	22.4	22.6	22.9	23.1	23.4	23.6
56–58	22.7	23.0	23.2	23.4	23.7	23.9	24.2	24.4	24.7
59–61	23.7	24.0	24.2	24.5	24.7	25.0	25.2	25.5	25.7
62–64	24.7	25.0	25.2	25.5	25.7	26.0	26.2	26.4	26.7
65–67	25.7	25.9	26.2	26.4	26.7	26.9	27.2	27.4	27.7
68–70	26.6	26.9	27.1	27.4	27.6	27.9	28.1	28.4	28.6
71–73	27.5	27.8	28.0	28.3	28.5	28.8	28.0	29.3	29.5
74–76	28.4	28.7	28.9	29.2	29.4	29.7	29.9	30.2	30.4
77–79	29.3	29.5	29.8	30.0	30.3	30.5	30.8	31.0	31.3
80–82	30.1	30.4	30.6	30.9	31.1	31.4	31.6	31.9	32.1
83–85	30.9	31.2	31.4	31.7	31.9	32.2	32.4	32.7	32.9
86–88	31.7	32.0	32.2	32.5	32.7	32.9	33.2	33.4	33.7
89–91	32.5	32.7	33.0	33.2	33.5	33.7	33.9	34.2	34.4
92–94	33.2	33.4	33.7	33.9	34.2	34.4	34.7	34.9	35.2
95–97	33.9	34.1	34.4	34.6	34.9	35.1	35.4	35.6	35.9
98–100	34.6	34.8	35.21	35.3	35.5	35.8	36.0	36.3	36.5
101–103	35.3	35.4	35.7	35.9	36.2	36.4	36.7	36.9	37.2
104–106	35.8	36.1	36.3	36.6	36.8	37.1	37.3	37.5	37.8
107–109	36.4	36.7	36.9	37.1	37.4	37.6	37.9	38.1	38.4
110–112	37.0	37.2	37.5	37.7	38.0	38.2	38.5	38.7	38.9
113–115	37.5	37.8	38.0	38.2	38.5	38.7	39.0	39.2	39.5
116–118	38.0	38.3	38.5	38.8	39.0	39.3	39.5	39.7	40.0
119–121	38.5	38.7	39.0	39.2	39.5	39.7	40.0	40.2	40.5
122–124	39.0	39.2	39.4	39.7	39.9	40.2	40.4	40.7	40.9
125–127	39.4	39.6	39.9	40.1	40.4	40.6	40.9	41.1	41.4
128–130	39.8	40.0	40.3	40.5	40.8	41.0	41.3	41.5	41.8

*Percent fat calculated by the formula by Siri. Percent fat = [(4.95/BD) – 4.5] × 100, where BD = body density.

A - 23
S - 40
L - 20
83

H - 48
W - 41
0.854

Chart 3 Percent Fat Estimates for Sum of Triceps, Abdominal, and Calf Skinfolds

Men		Women	
Sum of Skinfolds	Percent Fat	Sum of Skinfolds	Percent Fat
8–10	3.2	23–25	16.8
11–13	4.1	26–28	17.7
14–46	5.0	29–31	18.5
17–19	6.0	32–34	19.4
20–22	6.0	35–37	20.2
23–25	7.8	38–40	21.0
26–28	8.7	41–43	21.9
29–31	9.7	44–46	22.7
32–34	10.6	47–49	23.5
35–37	11.5	50–52	24.4
38–40	12.5	53–55	25.2
41–43	13.4	56–58	26.1
44–46	14.3	59–61	26.9
47–49	15.2	62–64	27.7
50–52	16.2	65–67	28.6
53–55	17.1	68–70	29.4
56–58	18.0	71–73	30.2
59–61	18.9	74–76	31.1
62–64	19.9	77–79	31.9
65–67	20.8	80–82	32.7
68–70	21.7	83–85	33.6
71–73	22.6	86–88	34.4
74–76	23.6	89–91	35.5
77–79	24.5	92–94	36.1
80–82	25.4	95–97	36.9
83–85	26.4	98–100	37.8
86–88	27.3	101–103	38.6
89–91	28.2	104–106	39.4
92–94	29.1	107–109	40.3
95–97	30.1	110–112	41.1
98–100	31.0	113–115	42.0
101–103	31.9	116–118	42.8
104–106	32.8	119–121	43.6
107–109	33.8	122–124	44.5
110–112	34.7	125–127	45.3
113–115	35.6	128–130	46.1
116–118	36.6	131–133	47.0
119–121	37.5	134–136	47.8
122–124	38.4	137–139	48.7
125–127	39.3	140–142	49.5

Chart 4 Standards for Body Fatness (Percent Body Fat)

Classification	Males	Females
Essential fat	No less than 5%	No less than 10%
Borderline	5%–9%	10%–16%
High performance	5%–15%	10%–23%
Good fitness (healthy)	10%–20%	17%–28%
Marginal	21%–25%	29%–35%
Overfat	25%+	35%+

Calculating Fatness from Skinfolds (Fitnessgram Method)

1. Sum the three skinfolds (triceps, abdominal, and calf) for both men and women. Use horizontal abdominal measure.
2. Use the skinfold sum and your age to determine your percent fat using Chart 3. Locate your sum of skinfold in the left column and your age at the top of the chart. Your estimated body fat percentage is located where the values intersect.
3. Use the Standards for Body Fatness (Chart 4) to determine your fatness rating.

Calculating Fatness from Self-Measured Skinfolds

1. Use either the Jackson-Pollock or Fitnessgram method but make the measures on yourself rather than have a partner do the measures. When doing the tricep measure use the self-measurement technique for both men and women. (See page 290.)
2. Calculate fatness using the methods described previously.
3. Use Chart 4 to determine ratings.

Height-Weight Measurements

1. *Height*—Measure your height in inches or centimeters. Take the measurement without shoes, but add 2.5 centimeters or 1 inch to measurements, as the charts include heel height.
2. *Weight*—Measure your weight in pounds or kilograms without clothes. Add 3 pounds or 1.4 kilograms because the charts include weight of clothes. If weight must be taken with clothes on, wear indoor clothing that weigh 3 pounds or 1.4 kilograms.
3. Determine your frame size using the elbow breadth. The measurement is most accurate when done with a broad-based sliding caliper. However, it can be done using a skinfold caliper or can be estimated with a metric ruler. The right arm is measured when it is elevated with the elbow bent at 90 degrees and the upper arm horizontal. The back of the hand should face the person making the measurement. Using the caliper, measure the distance between the epicondyles of the humerus (inside and outside bony points of the elbow). Measure to the nearest millimeter (1/10 of a centimeter). If a caliper is not available, place the thumb and the index finger of the left hand on the epicondyles of the humerus and measure the distance between the fingers with a metric ruler. Use your height and elbow breadth in centimeters to determine your frame size (Chart 5), you need not repeat this procedure each time you use a height-weight chart.

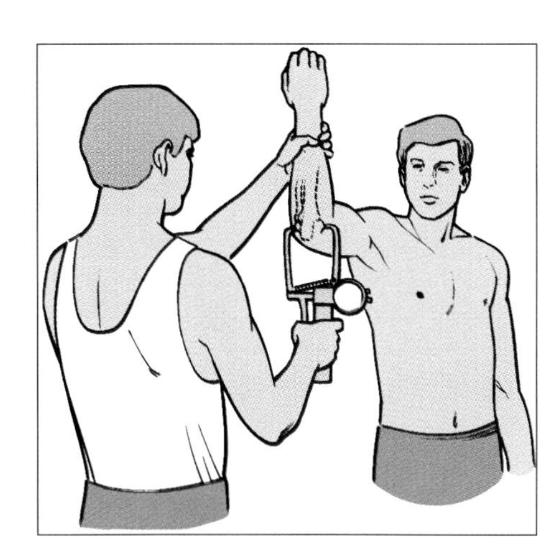

4. Use Chart 6 to determine your healthy weight range. The new healthy weight range charts do not account for frame size. However, you may want to consider frame size when determining a personal weight within the health weight range. People with a larger frame size typically can carry more weight within the range than those with a smaller frame size.

Chart 5 Frame Size Determined from Elbow Breadth (mm)

	Elbow Breadth (mm).		
Height	Small Frame	Medium Frame	Large Frame
Males			
5′2″ or less	<64	64–72	>72
5′3″–5″6 1/2″	<67	67–74	>74
5′7″–5′10 1/2″	<69	69–76	>76
5′11″–6′2 1/2″	<71	71–78	>78
6′3″ or less	<74	74–81	>81
Females			
4′10 1/2″ or less	<56	56–64	>64
4′11″–5′2 1/2″	<58	58–65	>65
5′3″–5′6 1/2″	<59	59–66	>66
5′7″–5′10 1/2″	<61	61–68	>69
5′11″ or less	<62	62–69	>69

Courtesy of the Metropolitan Life Insurance Company.

Height is given including 1-inch heels.

Chart 6 Healthy Weight Ranges for Adult Women and Men

Women			Men		
Feet	Height Inches	Pounds	Feet	Height Inches	Pounds
4	10	91–119	5	9	129–169
4	11	94–124	5	10	132–174
5	0	97–128	5	11	136–179
5	1	101–132	6	0	140–184
5	2	104–137	6	1	144–189
5	3	107–141	6	2	148–195
5	4	111–146	6	3	152–200
5	5	114–150	6	4	156–205
5	6	118–155	6	5	160–211
5	7	121–160	6	6	164–216
5	8	125–164			

SOURCE: Data from 1995 Dietary Guidelines U.S. Department of Agriculture and Department of Health and Human Services.

Chart 7 Body Mass Index

Height	100	105	110	115	120	125	130	135	140	145	150	155	160	165	170	175	180	185	190	195	200	205	210	215	220	225	230	235	240	245	250
5'0"	20	21	21	22	23	24	25	26	27	28	29	30	31	32	33	34	35	36	37	38	39	40	41	42	43	44	45	46	47	48	49
5'1"	19	20	21	22	23	24	25	26	26	27	28	29	30	31	32	33	34	35	36	37	38	39	40	41	42	43	43	44	45	46	47
5'2"	18	19	20	21	22	23	24	25	26	27	27	28	29	30	31	32	33	34	35	36	37	37	38	39	40	41	42	43	44	45	46
5'3"	18	19	19	20	21	22	23	24	25	26	27	27	28	29	30	31	32	33	34	35	35	36	37	38	39	40	41	42	43	43	44
5'4"	17	18	19	20	21	21	22	23	24	25	26	27	27	28	29	30	31	32	33	33	34	35	36	37	38	39	39	40	41	42	43
5'5"	17	17	18	19	20	21	22	22	23	24	25	26	27	27	28	29	30	31	32	32	33	34	35	36	37	37	38	39	40	41	42
5'6"	16	17	18	19	19	20	21	22	23	23	24	25	26	27	27	28	29	30	31	31	32	33	34	35	36	36	37	38	39	40	40
5'7"	16	16	17	18	19	20	20	21	22	23	23	24	25	26	27	27	28	29	30	31	31	32	33	34	34	35	36	37	38	38	39
5'8"	15	16	17	17	18	19	20	21	21	22	23	24	24	25	26	27	27	28	29	30	30	31	32	33	33	34	35	36	36	37	38
5'9"	15	16	16	17	18	18	19	20	21	21	22	23	24	24	25	26	27	27	28	29	30	30	31	32	32	33	34	35	35	36	37
5'10"	14	15	16	17	17	18	19	19	20	21	22	22	23	24	24	25	26	27	27	28	29	29	30	31	32	32	33	34	34	35	36
5'11"	14	15	15	16	17	17	18	19	20	20	21	22	22	23	24	24	25	26	26	27	28	29	29	30	31	31	32	33	33	34	35
6'0"	14	14	15	16	16	17	18	18	19	20	20	21	22	22	23	24	24	25	26	26	27	28	28	29	30	31	31	32	33	33	34
6'1"	13	14	15	15	16	16	17	18	18	19	20	20	21	22	22	23	24	24	25	26	26	27	28	28	29	30	30	31	32	32	33
6'2"	13	13	14	15	15	16	17	17	18	19	19	20	21	21	22	22	23	24	24	25	26	26	27	28	28	29	30	30	31	31	32
6'3"	12	13	14	14	15	16	16	17	17	18	19	19	20	21	21	22	22	23	24	24	25	26	26	27	27	28	29	29	30	31	31
6'4"	12	13	13	14	15	15	16	16	17	18	18	19	19	20	21	21	22	23	23	24	24	25	26	26	27	27	28	29	29	30	30

Weight

Low | Good fitness zone | Marginal | Obese

Body Mass Index (BMI)

Use the steps listed below or use Chart 7 to calculate your BMI.

1. Divide your weight in pounds by 2.2 to determine your weight in kilograms.
2. Multiply your height in inches by 0.0254 to determine your height in meters.
3. Square your height in meters (multiply your height in meters by your height in meters).
4. Divide the value you obtain in step 3 (square of height in meters) into the value you obtain in step 1 (weight in kilograms).
5. If you use these steps to determine your BMI, use the Rating Scale for Body Mass Index (Chart 8) to obtain a rating for your BMI.

Chart 8 Rating Scale for Body Mass Index

Classification	BMI
Obese (high risk)	Over 30
Marginal	25–30
Good fitness zone	17–24.9
Low	Less than 17

NOTE: An excessively low BMI is not desirable. Low BMI values can be indicative of eating disorders and other health problems. The government rating for marginal is "overweight."

Determining the Waist-to-Hip Circumference Ratio

The waist-to-hip circumference ratio is recommended as the best available index for determining risk and disease associated with fat and weight distribution. Disease and death risk are associated with abdominal and upper body fatness. When a person has both high fatness and a high waist-to-hip ratio, additional risks exist. The following steps should be taken in making measurements and calculating the waist-to-hip ratio.

1. Both measurements should be done with a nonelastic tape. Make the measurements while standing with the feet together and the arms at the sides, elevated only high enough to allow the measurements. Be sure that the tape is horizontal and around the entire circumference. Record scores to the nearest millimeter or 1/16th of an inch. Use the same units of measure for both circumferences (millimeters or 1/16th of an inch). The tape should be pulled snugly but not to the point of causing an indentation in the skin.
2. *Waist measurement*—Measure at the natural waist (smallest waist circumference). If there is no natural waist, the measurement should be made at the level of the umbilicus. Measure at the end of a normal inspiration.
3. *Hip measurement*—Measure at the maximum circumference of the buttocks. It is recommended that you wear thin-layered clothing (such as a swimming suit or underwear) that won't add significantly to the measurement.
4. Divide the hip measurement into the waist measurement or use the waist-to-hip nomogram (Chart 9) to determine your waist-to-hip ratio.
5. Use the Waist-to-Hip Ratio Rating Scale (Chart 10) to determine your rating for the waist-to-hip ratio.

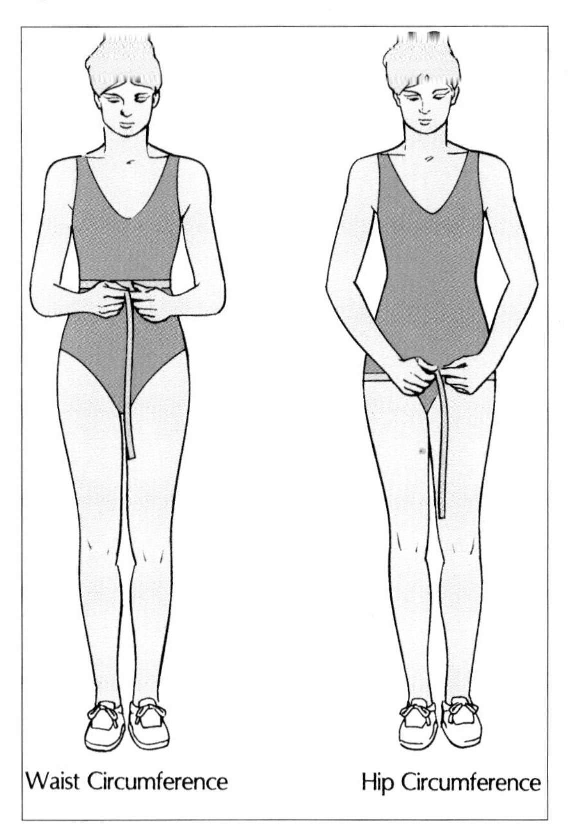

Note: Using a partner or a mirror will aid you in keeping the tape horizontal.

Chart 9 Waist-to-Hip Ratio Nomogram

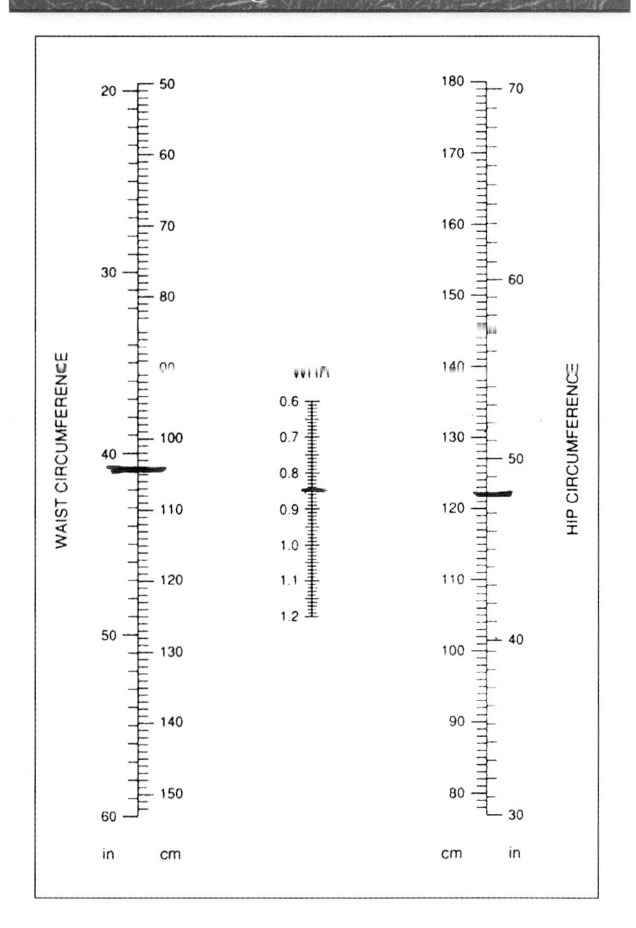

Chart 10 Waist-to-Hip Ratio Rating Scale

Classification	Men	Women
High risk	>1.0	>0.85
Moderately high risk	0.90–1.0	0.80–0.85
Lower risk	<0.90	<0.80

Lab 15B: Evaluating Body Composition: Height/Weight and Circumference Measures

Name	Section	Date

Purpose: To assess body composition using a variety of procedures, to learn the strengths and weaknesses of each technique, and to use the results to establish personal standards for evaluating body composition.

General Procedures: Follow the specific procedures for the three different self-assessment techniques. If possible, work with a partner you trust to help with measurements that you have difficulty making on yourself. If you are just learning a measurement technique, it is important to practice the skills of making the measurement. If you do measurements over time, use the same instrument (if possible) each time you measure. If your measurements vary widely, take more than one set until you get more consistent results. If possible, have an expert make measurements on you using the two procedures.

Height and Weight Measurements

Procedures:

1. Read the directions for height and weight measurements in the lab resource materials.
2. Determine your healthy weight range using Chart 6 in the lab resource materials. You may want to use your elbow breadth (Chart 5). People with smaller frame sizes should typically weigh less than those with a larger frame size within the healthy weight range. You may need the assistance of a partner to make the elbow breadth measurement.
3. Record your scores in the Results section.

Results:

Weight ☐ Healthy weight range ☐

Height ☐

Make a check by the statements that are true about your measurements.

☐ You are confident in the accuracy of the scale you used.

☐ You are confident that the height technique is accurate.

The more checks you have, the more likely your measurements are accurate.
If you are a very active person with a high amount of muscle, use this method with caution.

The Body Mass Index

Procedures:

1. Use the height and weight measures from Part 1 above.
2. Determine your BMI score by using Chart 7 or the directions in the lab resource materials. Determine your rating using Chart 8.
3. Record your scores and rating in the Results section.

Results:

Body mass index ☐ Rating ☐

If you are a very active person with a high amount of muscle, use this method with caution.

Waist-to-Hip Ratio

Procedures:

1. Measure your waist and hip circumferences using the procedures in the lab resource materials.
2. Divide your hip circumference into your waist circumference or use Chart 9 in the lab resource materials to calculate your waist-to-hip ratio.
3. Determine your rating using Chart 10 in the lab resource materials.
4. Record your scores in the Results section.

Results:

Waist circumference ☐

Hip circumference ☐

Waist-to-hip ratio ☐ Rating ☐

Make a check by the statements that are true about your measurements.

☐ You are confident in the accuracy of the waist and hip measurement.

Make a check by the statements that are true about you.

☐ I am a male 5′9″ or less and have a waist girth of 34 or more.

☐ I am a male 5′10″ to 6′4″ and have a waist girth of 36 or more.

☐ I am a male 6′5″ or more and have a waist girth of 38 or more.

☐ I am a female 5′2″ or less and have a waist girth of 29 or more.

☐ I am a female 5′3″ to 5′10″ and have a waist girth of 31 or more.

☐ I am a female 5′11″ or more and have a waist girth of 33 or more.

If you checked one of the boxes above, the waist-to-hip ratio is especially relevant for you.

Conclusions and Implications:

In the space provided below, discuss your results for the three height, weight, and circumference procedures. Note any discrepancies in the measurements. Indicate the strengths and weaknesses of the various methods. Which of the measures do you think provided you with the most useful information? If you also did the skinfold measures (Lab 15A), discuss your body composition based on all of the information you have collected (skinfolds and height, weight, and circumference measures).

Lab 15C: Determining Your Daily Energy Expenditure

Name　　　Section　　　Date

Purpose: To learn how many calories you expend in a day.

Procedures:

1. Estimate your basal metabolism using step 1 in the Results section. First determine the number of minutes you sleep.
2. Monitor your activity expenditure for one day using Chart 1. Record the number of 5-, 15-, and 30-minute blocks of time that you perform each of the different types of physical activities (e.g., if an activity lasted 20 minutes, you would use one 15-minute block and one 5-minute block). Be sure to distinguish between moderate (Mod) or vigorous (Vig) intensity in your logging. If you perform an activity that is not listed, specify the activity on the line labeled "Other" and estimate if it is moderate or vigorous. You may want to keep copies of Chart 1 for future use. One extra copy is provided.
3. Sum the total number of minutes of moderate and vigorous activity. Determine your calories expended during moderate and vigorous activity using steps 2 and 3.
4. Determine your nonactive minutes using step 4. This is all time that is not spent sleeping or being active.
5. Determine your calories expended in nonactive minutes using step 5.
6. Determine your calories expended in a day using step 6.

Results:

Daily Caloric Expenditure Estimates

Step 1:

Basal calories = .0076 × ______ (Body wt (lbs)) × ______ (Minutes of sleep) = ______ (Basal calories) (A)

Step 2:

Calories (moderate activity) = .036 × ______ (Body wt (lbs)) × ______ (Minutes of moderate activity) = ______ (Calories in moderate activity) (B)

Step 3:

Calories (vigorous activity) = .053 × ______ (Body wt (lbs)) × ______ (Minutes of vigorous activity) = ______ (Calories in vigorous activity) (C)

Step 4:

Minutes (nonactive) = 1,440 min. − ______ (Minutes of sleep) − ______ (Minutes of moderate activity) − ______ (Minutes of vigorous activity) = ______ (Nonactive minutes)

Step 5:

Calories (rest and light activity) = .011 × ______ (Body wt (lbs)) × ______ (Nonactive minutes) = ______ (Calories in other activities) (D)

Step 6:

Calories expended (per day) = ______ (A) + ______ (B) + ______ (C) + ______ (D) = ______ (**Daily calories**)

Answer these questions about your daily calorie expenditure estimate.

Yes	No	
☐	☐	Were the activities you performed similar to what you normally perform each day?
☐	☐	Do you think your daily estimated calorie expenditure is an accurate estimate?
☐	☐	Do you think you expend the correct amount of calories in a typical day to maintain the body composition (body fat level) that is desirable for you?

Conclusions and Interpretations: In several paragraphs, discuss your daily calorie expenditure. Comment on your answers to the questions listed above. In addition, comment on whether you think you should modify your daily calorie expenditure for any reason.

Chart 1 Daily Activity Log

Day of Monitoring:

Physical Activity Category		5 Minutes	15 Minutes	30 Minutes	Minutes
Lifestyle Activity		1 2 3 4 5 6	1 2 3 4 5 6	1 2 3	
Dancing (general)	Mod				
Gardening	Mod				
Home repair/maintenance	Mod				
Occupation	Mod				
Walking/hiking	Mod				
Other:	Mod				
Aerobic Activity		1 2 3 4 5 6	1 2 3 4 5 6	1 2 3	
Aerobic dance (low impact)	Mod				
	Vig				
Aerobic eq. (rowing, stair, ski)	Mod				
	Vig				
Bicycling	Mod				
	Vig				
Running	Mod				
	Vig				
Skating (roller/ice)	Mod				
	Vig				
Swimming (laps)	Mod				
	Vig				
Other:	Mod				
	Vig				
Sport/Recreation Activity		1 2 3 4 5 6	1 2 3 4 5 6	1 2 3	
Basketball	Mod				
	Vig				
Bowling/billiards	Mod				
Golf	Mod				
Martial arts (judo, karate)	Mod				
	Vig				
Racquetball/tennis	Mod				
	Vig				
Soccer/hockey	Mod				
	Vig				
Softball/baseball	Mod				
Volleyball	Mod				
	Vig				
Other:	Mod				
Flexibility Activity		1 2 3 4 5 6	1 2 3 4 5 6	1 2 3	
Stretching	Mod				
Other:	Mod				
Strengthening Activity		1 2 3 4 5 6	1 2 3 4 5 6	1 2 3	
Calisthenics (push-ups/sit-ups)	Mod				
Resistance Exercise	Mod				
Other:	Mod				
				Minutes of moderate activity	
				Minutes of vigorous activity	
				Total minutes of activity	

Chart 2 Daily Activity Log

Day of Monitoring:

Physical Activity Category		5 Minutes	15 Minutes	30 Minutes	Minutes
Lifestyle Activity		1 2 3 4 5 6	1 2 3 4 5 6	1 2 3	
Dancing (general)	Mod				
Gardening	Mod				
Home repair/maintenance	Mod				
Occupation	Mod				
Walking/hiking	Mod				
Other:	Mod				
Aerobic Activity		1 2 3 4 5 6	1 2 3 4 5 6	1 2 3	
Aerobic dance (low impact)	Mod				
	Vig				
Aerobic eq. (rowing, stair, ski)	Mod				
	Vig				
Bicycling	Mod				
	Vig				
Running	Mod				
	Vig				
Skating (roller/ice)	Mod				
	Vig				
Swimming (laps)	Mod				
	Vig				
Other:	Mod				
	Vig				
Sport/Recreation Activity		1 2 3 4 5 6	1 2 3 4 5 6	1 2 3	
Basketball	Mod				
	Vig				
Bowling/billiards	Mod				
Golf	Mod				
Martial arts (judo, karate)	Mod				
	Vig				
Racquetball/tennis	Mod				
	Vig				
Soccer/hockey	Mod				
	Vig				
Softball/baseball	Mod				
Volleyball	Mod				
	Vig				
Other:	Mod				
Flexibility Activity		1 2 3 4 5 6	1 2 3 4 5 6	1 2 3	
Stretching	Mod				
Other:	Mod				
Strengthening Activity		1 2 3 4 5 6	1 2 3 4 5 6	1 2 3	
Calisthenics (push-ups/sit-ups)	Mod				
Resistance Exercise	Mod				
Other:	Mod				
				Minutes of moderate activity	
				Minutes of vigorous activity	
				Total minutes of activity	

Concept 16

Nutrition

The amount and kinds of food you eat affect your health and wellness.

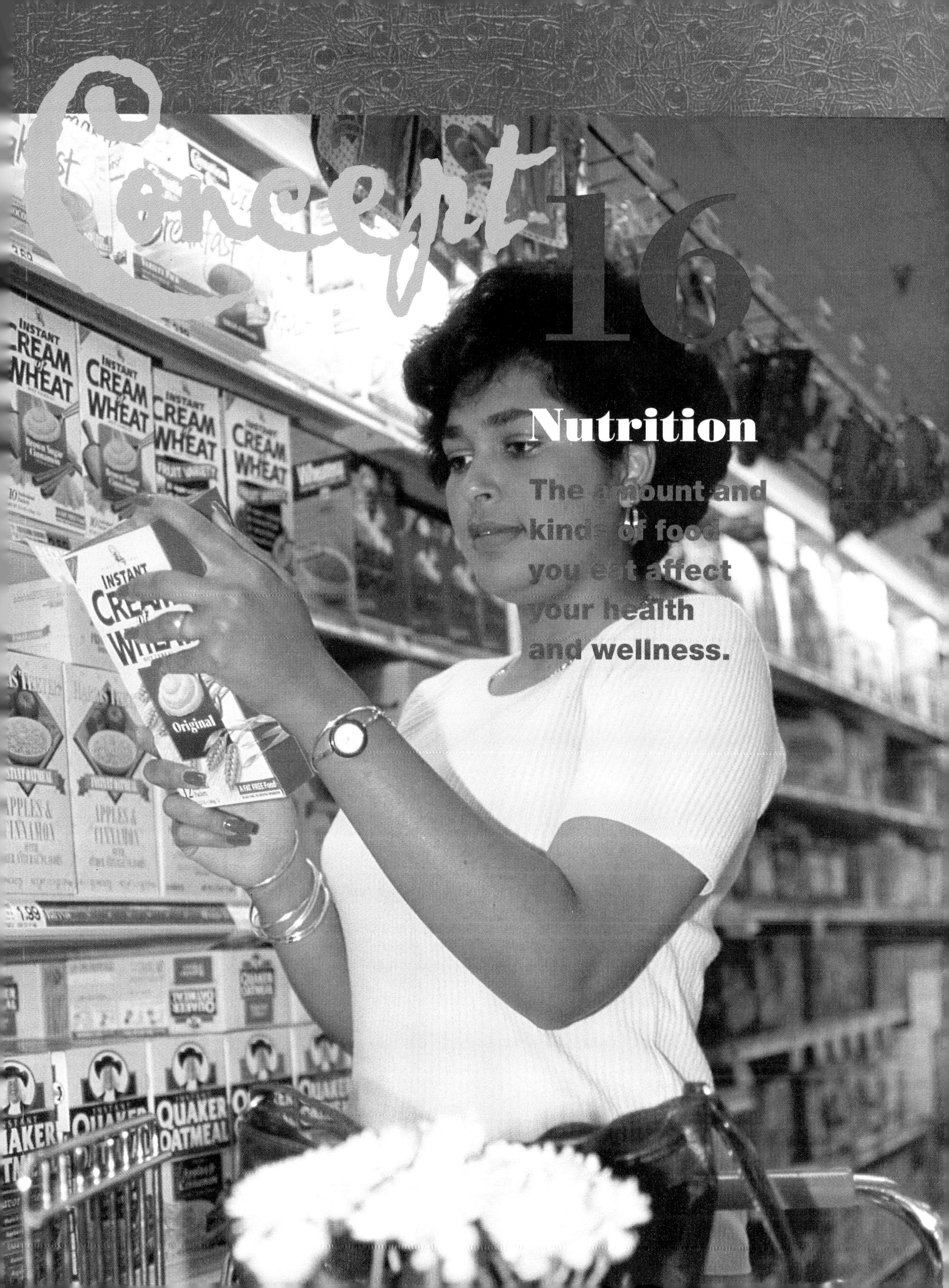

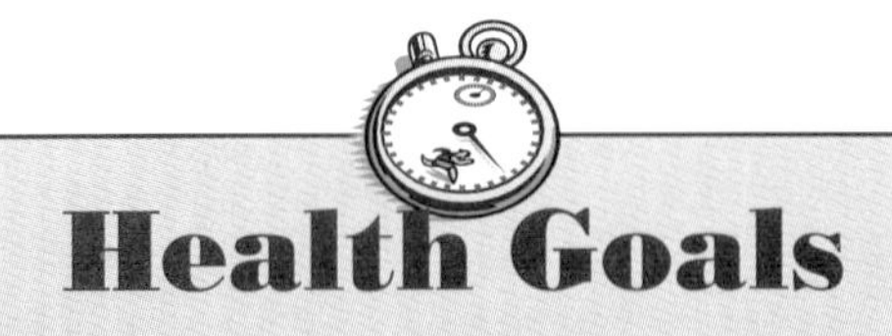

for year 2010

Promote health and reduce chronic disease associated with dietary factors and weight.

Increase proportion of people who eat healthy snacks.

Increase proportion of people who eat no more than 30 percent of calories as fat.

Increase proportion of people who eat no more than 10 percent of calories as saturated fat.

Increase proportion of people who eat at least five servings of vegetables and fruits daily.

Increase proportion of people who eat at least six servings of grain products daily.

Increase proportion of people who meet dietary recommendation for calcium.

Reduce proportion of people who consume excess sodium.

Reduce incidence of iron deficiency and anemia (especially children and women).

Increase proportion of worksites that offer nutrition and/or weight management classes.

Introduction

The importance of good nutrition for optimal health is well established. Most people believe that nutrition is important but still find it difficult to maintain a healthy diet. One reason is that foods are usually developed, marketed, and advertised for convenience and taste rather than for health or nutritional quality. Another reason is that many individuals have misconceptions about what constitutes a healthy diet. Some of these misconceptions are propagated by so called "experts" with less than impressive credentials and those with commercial interests. Others are created by the confusing, and often contradictory, news reports about new nutrition research. In spite of the fact that nutrition is an advanced science, there are still many unanswered questions.

In this concept some basic nutrition guidelines are presented to inform the reader and dispel various nutrition myths. A special section is presented on nutrition and physical performance to assist those interested in sports and high-level performance. If you are interested in learning more about nutrition than is covered here you are encouraged to seek the advice of a registered dietitian or to study reliable books, journals, or government documents (see Suggested Readings and Web Review).

The Facts about Basic Nutrition and Health

The amount and kinds of food you eat affect your health and well-being.

There are about 45 to 50 nutrients in food that are believed to be essential for the body's growth, maintenance, and repair. These are classified into six categories: carbohydrates (and fiber), fats, proteins, vitamins, minerals, and water. The first three provide energy, which is measured in calories. Specific dietary recommendations for each of the six nutrients are presented later in this concept.

www.mhhe.com/phys_fit/webreview16 Click 01

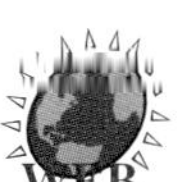

Recommended Daily Allowances (RDA) values published by the Food and Nutrition Board of the National Academy of Sciences have served as the standard for nutritional adequacy for the past two decades. Recently the Academy, in partnership with Health Canada, has recognized the need for additional nutrition standards resulting in the establishment of four types of values all classified under the heading of **Dietary Reference Intakes** (DRI). RDA values are established when adequate scientific information is available for most foods (Recommended Nutrient Intake—RNI values—in Canada). They are based on **Estimated Average Requirements** (EAR) values when they are available. **Adequate Intake** (AI) is an alternative term used to describe the amount of a nutrient people should consume when scientific data is not adequate to establish RDA values. **Tolerable Upper Intake Level** (UL) is a new type of dietary reference. To date UL values have been established for only a few nutrients. The goal is to establish UL values for all, or at least most nutrients, in the next few years. The guidelines will make it clear that while too little of a nutrient can be harmful to health, so can too much. For now, RDA values are the most relevant reference term, though UL values will become more meaningful when they are established for most nutrients. In many ways the RDAs are threshold values similar to the threshold of training values for physical activity. The target zone for healthy eating would range from the RDA values to the UL values.

The quantity of nutrients recommended varies with age and other considerations; for example, young children need

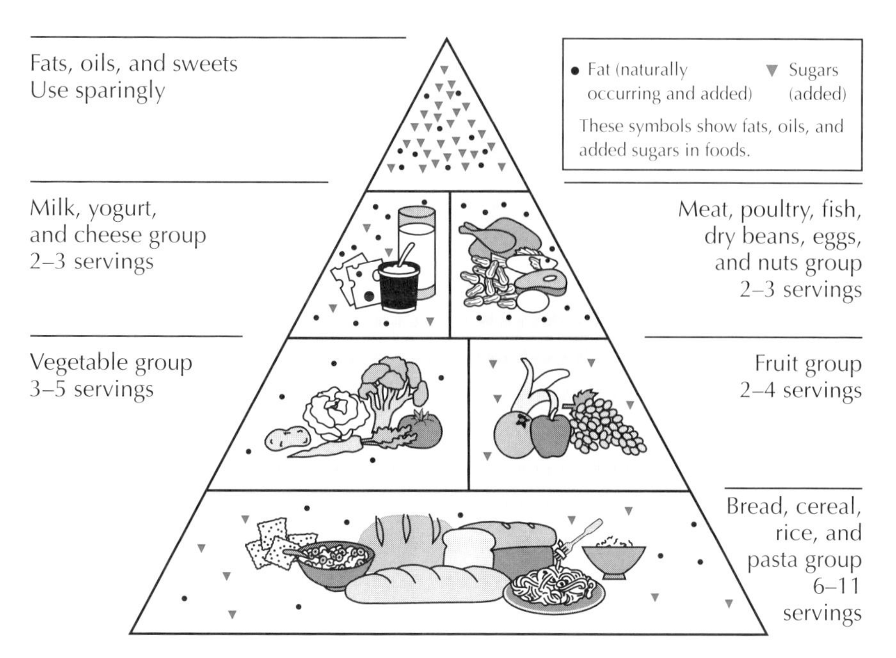

Figure 1
The food guide pyramid.
SOURCE: Data from the U.S. Department of Agriculture.

more calcium than adults and pregnant women or postmenopausal women need more calcium than other women. Accordingly dietary reference intakes, including RDAs, have been established for several age/gender groups. In this book, the values used are those that are appropriate for most adult men and women.

Some foods contain some of all six classes of nutrients (e.g., whole wheat bread) whereas others contain only one (e.g., sugar). No food is a "complete" food because none contains all of the specific essential nutrients.

> Eating the recommended servings of food from the food guide pyramid will provide key nutrients and enable a person to meet dietary recommendations.

The food guide pyramid (Figure 1) was designed to guide people in the selection of nutritious food. Selecting the appropriate number of servings from each portion of the pyramid will assure inclusion of necessary nutrients in the diet. A greater number of servings is recommended from the foods near the base of the pyramid (complex carbohydrates) with fewer servings from the upper levels. Foods from the lower level of the pyramid are "nutritionally dense," meaning that they have more nutrients per calorie than low-density foods. For example, a 200-calorie piece of Boston cream pie (from tip of pyramid) has very few vitamins and minerals and is high in fat and refined carbohydrates. On the other hand, 200 calories of tuna has very little fat; 100 percent of the RDA for protein, niacin, and vitamin B_{12}; and substantial B_6 and phosphorus. Eating nutritionally dense food is particularly important for someone on a low-

Recommended Daily Allowance (RDA) The minimum amount of a specific nutrient that should be included in the daily diet to meet the health needs of nearly all people in a specific age/gender group.

Dietary Reference Intakes (DRI) A generic term used to describe four types of values used to describe appropriate amounts of nutrients in the diet (AI, EAR, RDA, and UL).

Estimated Average Requirement (EAR) A term that described the amount of a nutrient that meets the needs of at least 50 percent of the people in a specific age/gender group.

Adequate Intakes (AI) A term used instead of recommended dietary allowance (RDA) when sufficient data are not available to establish RDA values for a specific nutrient.

Tolerable Upper Intake Level (UL) A term used to describe the maximum level of a daily nutrient that will not pose a risk of adverse health effects for most people.

Food Groups

Bread, cereal, rice, and pasta		
1 slice of bread	1 ounce of ready-to-eat cereal	1/2 cup of cooked cereal, rice or pasta

Vegetable		
1 cup of raw leafy vegetables	1/2 cup of other vegetables, cooked or chopped raw	3/4 cup of vegetable juice

Fruit		
1 medium apple, banana, orange	1/2 cup of chopped, cooked, or canned fruit	3/4 cup of fruit juice

Milk, yogurt, and cheese		
1 cup of milk or yogurt	1-1/2 ounces of natural cheese	2 ounces of process cheese

Meat, poultry, fish, dry beans, eggs, and nuts	
2–3 ounces of cooked lean meat, poultry, or fish	1/2 cup of cooked dry beans, 1 egg, or 2 tablespoons of peanut butter count as 1 ounce of lean meat

Figure 2
What counts as a serving?
SOURCE: Data from the U.S. Department of Agriculture.

Aim for fitness...

- Aim for a healthy weight.
- Be physically active each day.

Build a healthy base...

- Let the Pyramid guide your food choices.
- Choose a variety of grains daily, especially whole grains.
- Choose a variety of fruits and vegetables daily.
- Keep food safe to eat.

Choose sensibly...

- Choose a diet that is low in saturated fat and cholesterol and moderate in total fat.
- Choose beverages and foods to moderate your intake of sugars.
- Choose and prepare foods with less salt.
- If you drink alcoholic beverages, do so in moderation.

Figure 3
Dietary guidelines for Americans: The ABC's
SOURCE: U.S. Department of Agriculture, U.S. Department of Health and Human Services, Washington, DC, 2000.

calorie diet because it is especially hard to get all the essential nutrients when you do not eat very much food.

There are other models used to describe methods for helping people eat healthy nutritious diets. For example, the American Heart Association has adapted the pyramid to aid in selection of foods for heart disease prevention, a pyramid for older adults is now available, and in Canada the Food Guide is used to help people choose nutritious foods (see Appendix E).

Counting food servings is important to assuring that adequate choices are made from the pyramid.

Figure 2 provides you with examples of what constitutes a serving for each food group. Use this information to help you see if you have made the appropriate number of choices from the pyramid. National health goals for nutrition specifically target fruits, vegetables, and grains.

Though many people in western society do not eat adequate portions of nutritionally dense foods even when they are readily available, there is evidence that the diets of Americans have improved in recent years. Over the past two to three decades, the percentage of calories from fat has decreased and the intake of fruits (up 19 percent), vegetables (up 22 percent), and grains (up 47 percent) has increased. Still the number of servings of fruit now averages 1.5 per day, an amount lower than the dietary recommendation of two servings per day. It is encouraging that vegetable intake (3.6 per day) is above the recommended amount of three servings per day. Discouraging is the fact that nearly half of the vegetable intake is from potatoes, and half of the potato intake is from French fries.

New dietary guidelines are available to help you plan for sound nutrition.

Federal law requires the publication of national dietary guidelines every five years. The most recent guidelines were published in 2000 (see Figure 3). These guidelines provide the basis

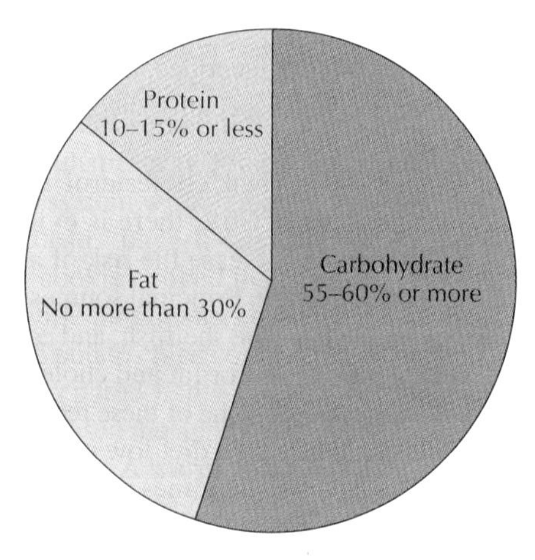

Figure 4
Recommended dietary intake.

for federal nutrition policy and nutrition education activities. They are also intended to provide advice to Americans about making healthy food choices. The current guidelines include more specific recommendations about maintaining a healthy weight and being physically active every day. The revised guidelines also differ from previous guidelines in making more specific suggestions about food selection. They recommend that consumers use the food pyramid to guide their food choices (as opposed to just eating a variety of foods) and also specifically recommend eating a variety of fruits and vegetables *daily.*

> The number of calories needed per day depends upon the body's metabolic rate (MR), which, in turn, depends upon such factors as age, sex, size, muscle mass, glandular function, emotional state, climate, and exercise.

www.mhhe.com/phys_fit/webreview16 Click 02

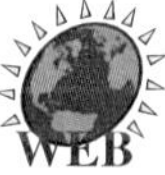

Your **basal metabolic rate (BMR)** is the basis for your caloric needs. The higher the BMR, the more calories you burn at rest. Your **metabolic rate (MR)** is a combination of your BMR and calories expended in normal daily activities. The MR is usually higher in males, young people, large people, lean and muscular people, and in nervous people; in cold and hot weather; and during exercise.

A moderately active college-age woman needs about 2,000 calories per day, whereas a moderately active man of the same age needs about 2,800 calories. A female athlete in training might burn 2,600 to 4,500 calories; a male athlete in training might expend 3,500 to 6,000. If your weight remains at the optimum, the caloric content of your diet is correct. If weight varies from optimal, the caloric content of the diet may need to be altered.

The three primary sources of calories in the diet are fat, protein, and carbohydrates. The typical adult consumes too much fat and too little carbohydrate, especially complex carbohydrates. Health goals want Americans to reduce the amount of dietary fat and increase the amount of complex carbohydrates in the diet (see Figure 4). Currently, only 33 percent of people aged 2 and above meet the goal of eating no more than 30 percent of the diet as fat, and 35 percent consume more than 10 percent saturated fat. For fruits and vegetables, the proportion of the population eating adequate servings is 40 percent and for grains 52 percent.

> Eating well can reduce risk of various health problems and increase quality of life.

As will be more clearly described in the sections that follow, the risk of many diseases is reduced by proper nutrition. Among the conditions especially affected by eating patterns are heart disease, stroke, diabetes, colon cancer, high blood pressure, and osteoporosis. Proper nutrition can also enhance the quality of life by improving the ability to carry out work and leisure-time activities without fatigue.

Dietary Recommendations for Fat: The Facts

> Excess fat in the diet, particularly saturated fat, is associated with an increased risk of disease and is inversely related to optimal health.

www.mhhe.com/phys_fit/webreview16 Click 03

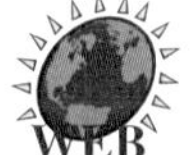

Humans need some fat in their diet because fats are carriers of vitamins A, D, E, and K. They are a source of essential linoleic acid, make food taste better, and provide a concentrated form of calories, which serve as an important source of energy during moderate to

Metabolic Rate (MR) The rate at which the body produces heat that is measured in calories; an indication of the body's activities, including exercise and normal body functions.

Basal Metabolic Rate (BMR) Metabolic rate at complete rest or sleep.

Krauss R. M. et al. "AHA Dietary Guidelines Revision 2000: A Statement for Health-Care Professionals from the Nutrition Committee of the American Heart Association." *Circulation*. 102(2000): 2284–99.

Honein. M. A. et al. "Impact of Folic Acid Fortification of the U.S. Food Supply on the Occurrence of Neural Tube Defects." *Journal of the American Medical Association*. 285(23)(2001): 3022.

Ludwig, D.S. et al. "Dietary Fiber, Weight Gain, and Cardiovascular Disease Risk Factors in Young Adults." *Journal of the American Medical Association*. 282(1999):1539–1546.

Manore, M. M., and Thompson, J. A. *Sport Nutrition for Health and Performance*. Champaign, IL: Human Kinetics, 2000.

Manore, M. M., Barr, S. I., and Butterfield, G. E. "Position of the American Dietetic Association: Nutrition and Athletic Performance." *Journal of the American Dietetic Association*, 5(1)(2001): 1543–1556.

Manore, M. M. "Vitamins and Minerals. Part I: How Much Do You Need?" *ACSM's Health and Fitness Journal*. 5(1)(2001): 33–36.

Manore, M. M. "Vitamins and Minerals. Part II: Who Needs Supplements?"*ACSM's Health and Fitness Journal*. 5(3)(2001): 33–36.

Manore, M. M. "Vitamins and Minerals. Part III: Can You Get Too Much?" *ACSM's Health and Fitness Journal*. 5(5)2001: 26–28.

People. "Diet Riot." *People*, 12 June 2000, 104–110.

Questioning 40/30/30: A Guide to Understanding Sports Nutrition Advice. A booklet published jointly by the American College of Sport Medicine, the American Dietetics Association, the Women's Sports Foundation and the Cooper Institute for Aerobics Research, 1997.

Thompson, S. R., Weber, M. M., and Brown, L. B. "The Relationship Between Health and Fitness Magazine Readings and Eating-Disordered Weight-Loss Methods Among High School Girls." *American Journal of Health Education*. 32(3)(2001): 133–138.

U.S. Department of Agriculture and U.S. Department of Health and Human Services. *Report of the Dietary Guidelines Advisory Committee*. Washington, D.C.: U.S. Department of Agriculture and U.S. Department of Health and Human Services, 2000.

U.S. Department of Health and Human Services, *Healthy People 2010*. 2nd ed. With *Understanding and Improving Health* and *Objectives for Improving Health*, 2 vols. Washington, DC: U.S. Government Printing Office, November 2000, Chapter 19, "Nutrition and Overweight."

Van Loan, M. D. "Do You Restrict Your Food Intake? The Implications of Food Restriction on Bone Health." *ACSM's Health and Fitness Journal*. 5(1)(2001): 11–14.

Wardlaw, G.M. *Contemporary Nutrition*. 5th ed. St. Louis: McGraw-Hill, 2002.

Williams, M. H. *Nutrition for Health, Fitness, and Sports*. 6th ed. St. Louis: McGraw-Hill, 2002.

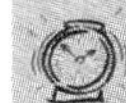

Physical Fitness News Update

Despite good intentions, many Americans have diets that do not satisfy general nutrition guidelines. For example, a recent national survey estimated that only 23 percent of Americans eat five or more servings of fruits and vegetables a day. As research on behavior change progresses, it is becoming more evident that our environment plays a critical role in our ability to maintain change. In an effort to improve our diet, there have been a number of proposals that may help modify America's eating patterns.

Nutritional Media Campaign

Some health advocates suggest that frequent, hard-hitting media campaigns are needed to change Americans' eating patterns. The U.S. government currently spends one million dollars a year to promote the "*5 a day*" fruit and vegetable campaign. In contrast, the largest fast-food companies spend over a billion dollars a year and the soft drink industry more than 500 million a year. With a bigger budget, a targeted media campaign may be able to promote better awareness about nutrition.

Taxes on Junk Food

Arguing that the prevalence of junk food in our society is a root cause of our poor eating patterns, some health advocates have proposed taxes on junk food. It is estimated that a one cent tax on soft drinks would raise an estimated $1.5 billion a year. This money could go to help with current medical expenditures or to be targeted to educational efforts to improve diets.

Subsidies for Fruits and Vegetables

Another environmental factor that influences diets is the high cost of healthy foods. To address this issue, some have proposed government subsidies to lower the costs of produce. If apples were ten cents instead of fifty to seventy-five cents, it is likely that more people would eat them.

Lab 16B: Selecting Nutritious Foods

Name	Section	Date

Purpose: To learn to select a nutritious diet, to determine the nutritive value of favorite foods, and to compare a nutritious foods values to a favorite foods values.

Procedure:

1. Select a breakfast, lunch, and dinner from the foods list in Appendix D. Include between-meal snacks with the nearest meal. If you cannot find foods you would normally choose, select those most similar to choices you might make.
2. Select a breakfast, lunch, and dinner from foods you feel would make the most nutritious meals. Include between-meal snacks with nearest meal.
3. Record your "favorite foods" and "nutritious foods" on the log on the back of this sheet. Record the calories for proteins, carbohydrates, and fats for each of the foods you choose.
4. Total each column for the "favorite" and the "nutritious" meal.
5. Determine the percentages of your total calories that are protein, carbohydrate, and fat by dividing each column total by the total number of calories consumed.
6. Answer the questions in the Conclusions and Implications section.

Results: Record your results below. Calculate percent of calories from each source by dividing total calories into calories from each food source (protein, fat, or carbohydrate).

	Favorite Foods		Nutritious Foods	
Source	Calories	% of Total Calories	Calories	% of Total Calories
Protein				
Fat				
Carbohydrates				
Total		100%		100%

Conclusion and Implications: In several sentences, discuss differences you found between your nutritious diet and your favorite diet. Discuss the quality of your nutritious diet as well as other things you learned from doing this lab.

"Favorite" versus "Nutritious" Food Choices for Three Daily Meals

Breakfast Favorite	*Food Choices*				*Breakfast Nutritious*	*Food Choices*			
Food No.	***Cal.***	***Pro. Cal.***	***Car. Cal.***	***Fat Cal.***	***Food No.***	***Cal.***	***Pro. Cal.***	***Car. Cal.***	***Fat Cal.***
Totals					***Totals***				

Lunch Favorite	*Food Choices*				*Lunch Nutritious*	*Food Choices*			
Food No.	***Cal.***	***Pro. Cal.***	***Car. Cal.***	***Fat Cal.***	***Food No.***	***Cal.***	***Pro. Cal.***	***Car. Cal.***	***Fat Cal.***
Totals					***Totals***				

Dinner Favorite	*Food Choices*				*Dinner Nutritious*	*Food Choices*			
Food No.	***Cal.***	***Pro. Cal.***	***Car. Cal.***	***Fat Cal.***	***Food No.***	***Cal.***	***Pro. Cal.***	***Car. Cal.***	***Fat Cal.***
Totals					***Totals***				
Daily Totals (Calories)					***Daily Totals (Calories)***				
Daily % of Total Calories					***Daily % of Total Calories***				

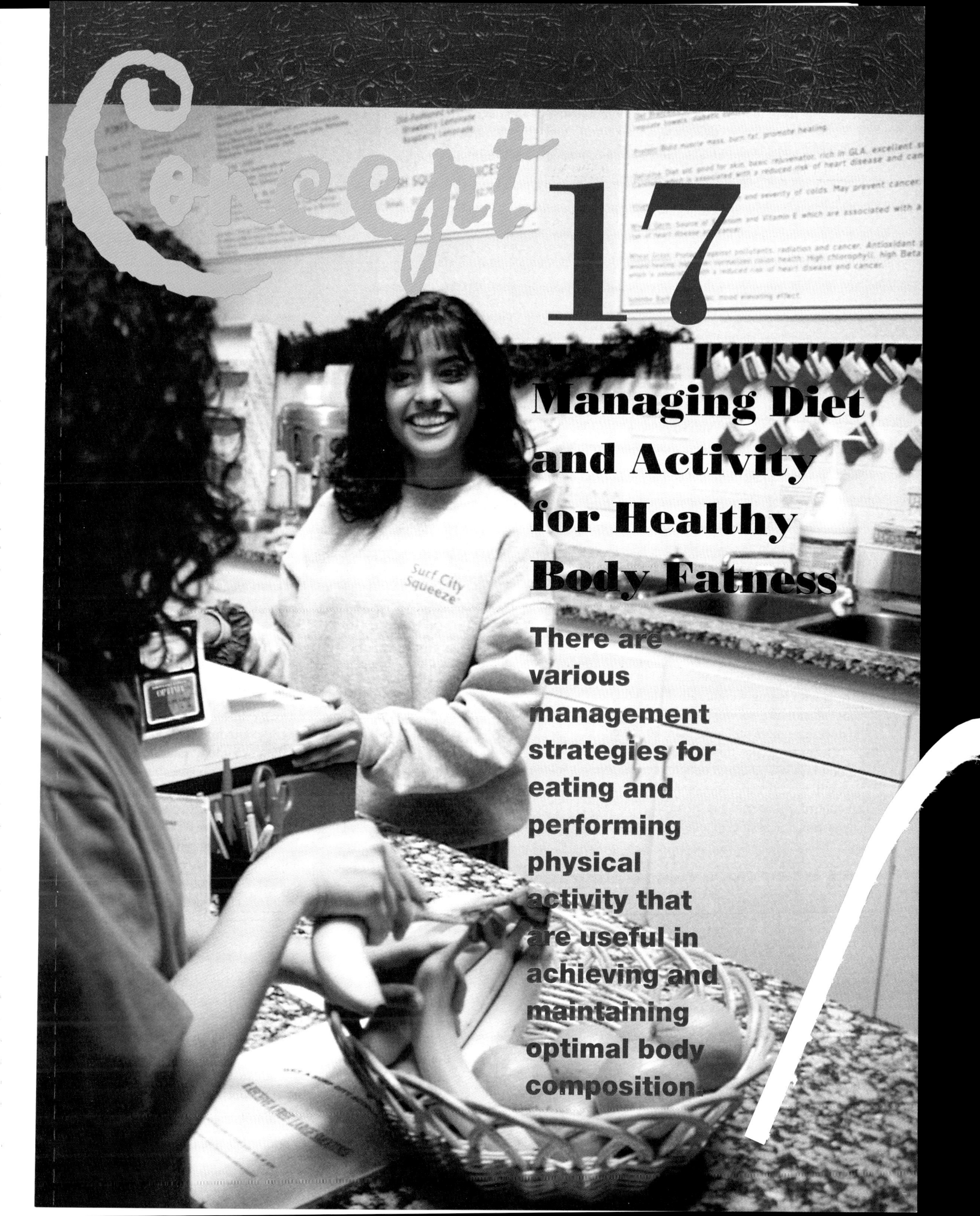

Concept 17

Managing Diet and Activity for Healthy Body Fatness

There are various management strategies for eating and performing physical activity that are useful in achieving and maintaining optimal body composition.

Suggested Readings

American Dietetics Association. "Weight Management: Position of the American Dietetics Association." *Journal of the American Dietetics Association.* 97(1997):71–74.

Anderson, R. E. "Exercise, Active Lifestyle, and Obesity: Making an Exercise Prescription Work." *The Physician and Sports Medicine.* 27(10) (1999):41–50.

Clark, K. "Replacing Fat: Have We Managed a Miracle?" *ACSM's Health and Fitness Journal.* 3(2)(1999):22–26.

Coleman, E. "AHA Dietary Guidelines." *Sports Medicine Digest.* 22(2000): 133.

Krauss R. M. et al. "AHA Dietary Guidelines Revision 2000: A Statement for Health-Care Professionals from the Nutrition Committee of the American Heart Association." *Circulation.* 102(2000): 2284–99.

Manore, M. M., and Thompson, J. A. *Sport Nutrition for Health and Performance.* Champaign, IL: Human Kinetics, 2000.

Manore, M. M., Barr, S. I., and Butterfield, G. E. "Position of the American Dietetic Association: Nutrition and Athletic Performance." *Journal of the American Dietetic Association,* 5(1)(2001): 1543–1556.

People. "Diet Riot." *People.* 12 June 2000, 104–110.

Questioning 40/30/30: A Guide to Understanding Sports Nutrition Advice. A 22-page booklet published jointly by the American College of Sports Medicine, the American Dietetics Association, the Women's Sports Foundation, and the Cooper Institute for Aerobics Research, 1997.

Tate, D.F., Wing, R.R., and Winett, R.A. "Using Internet Technology to Deliver a Behavioral Weight Loss Program." *Journal of the American Medical Association.* 285(9)(2001): 1172–1177.

U.S. Department of Health and Human Services. *Healthy People 2010.* 2nd ed. With *Understanding and Improving Health* and *Objectives for Improving Health.* 2 vols. Washington, DC: U.S. Government Printing Office, November 2000, Chapter 19, "Nutrition and Overweight."

Van Loan, M. D. "Do You Restrict Your Food Intake? The Implications of Food Restriction on Bone Health." *ACSM's Health and Fitness Journal.* 5(1)(2001): 11–14.

Williams, M. *Nutrition for Health, Fitness and Sports.* 6th ed. St. Louis:McGraw-Hill, 2002.

Wardlaw, G. M. *Contemporary Nutrition,* 5th ed. St. Louis: McGraw-Hill, 2002.

Wilmore, J. H. "Exercise, Obesity and Weight Control." In Corbin, C. B., and Pangrazi, R. P. (ed.). *Towards a Better Understanding of Physical Fitness and Activity,* Scottsdale, AZ: Holcomb-Hathaway, 1999, Chapter 16.

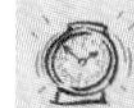

Physical Fitness News Update

Influence of Environmental Factors on Energy Balance

Considerable attention has been devoted to better understanding the causes and consequences of the obesity epidemic our society is currently facing. We have been able to combat most any infectious disease, but the problem of obesity that is posing a current threat is one that is dependent on our lifestyles. A consensus conference was recently held to discuss the latest research on obesity prevention. At this meeting, Dr. Jim Hill presented a model that describes how environmental factors influence the energy balance equation. The essence of the model is that we are continually confronted with environments that make it easy to consume large quantities of energy-dense food. We also live in an environment in which most physical tasks are no longer necessary and people have little time or interest in physically active recreation. To minimize the risks of gaining weight, it is important to modify both dietary behaviors and activity behaviors.

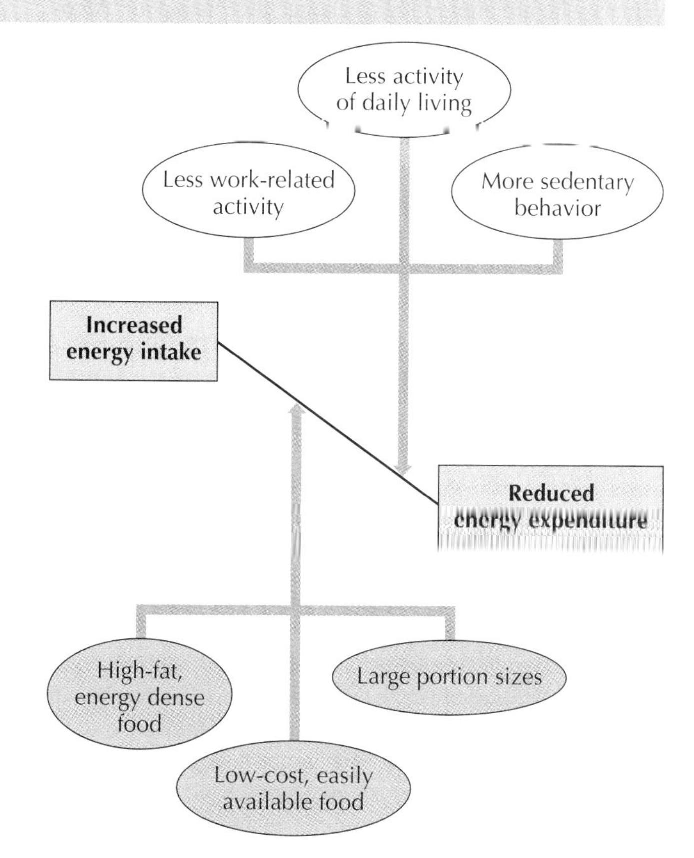

Source: Model adapted from Hill et al., 1999.

Lab 17A: Selecting Strategies for Managing Eating

Name | Section | Date

Purpose: To help you select strategies for managing eating to control body fatness.

Procedures:

1. Read the strategies listed in Chart 1.
2. Make a check in the box beside five to ten of the strategies that you think will be most useful to you.
3. Answer the questions in the Conclusions and Implications section.

Chart 1 Strategies for Managing Eating to Control Body Fatness

✓	Check 5 to 10 strategies that you might use in the future.
	Shopping Strategies
	Shop from a list.
	Shop with a friend.
	Shop on a full stomach.
	Check food labels.
	Consider foods that take some time to prepare.
	Methods of Eating
	When you eat, do nothing but eat. Don't watch television or read.
	Eat slowly.
	Do not eat food you do not want.
	Follow an eating schedule.
	Do your eating in designated areas such as kitchen or dining room only.
	Leave the table after eating.
	Avoid second servings.
	Limit servings of condiments.
	Limit servings of nonbasics such as dessert, breads, and soft drinks.
	Eat several meals of equal size rather than one big meal and two small ones.
	Eating in the Work Environment
	Take your own food to work.
	Avoid snack machines.
	If you eat out, plan your meal ahead of time.
	Do not eat while working.
	Avoid sharing foods from coworkers including birthday cakes, etc.
	Have activity breaks during the day.
	Have water available to substitute for soft drinks.
	Have low-calorie snacks to substitute for office snacks.

✓	Check 5 to 10 strategies that you might use in the future.
	Eating on Special Occasions
	Practice ways to refuse food.
	Avoid tempting situations.
	Eat before you go out.
	Don't stand near food sources.
	If you feel the urge to eat, find someone to talk to.
	Strategies for Eating Out
	Limit deep-fat fried foods.
	Ask for information about food content.
	Limit use of condiments.
	Choose low-fat foods (e.g., skim milk, low-fat yogurt).
	Choose chicken, fish, or lean meat.
	Order á la carte.
	If you eat desserts, avoid those with sauces or toppings.
	Eating at Home
	Keep busy at times when you are at risk of overeating.
	Store food out of sight.
	Avoid serving food to others between meals.
	If you snack, choose snacks with complex carbohydrates such as carrot sticks or apple slices.
	Freeze leftovers to avoid temptation of eating them between meals.

Conclusions and Implications:

1. In several sentences, discuss your need to use strategies for effective eating. Do you need to use them? Why or why not?

2. In several sentences, discuss the effectiveness of the strategies contained in Chart 1. Do you think they can be effective for people who have a problem controlling their body fatness?

Lab 17B: Keeping Records for Fat Control

Name **Section** **Date**

Purpose: To allow you to keep records of calories taken in and calories expended to help you maintain a healthy level of body fat.

Procedures:

1. Establish a calorie intake goal for one day.
2. Determine the calories you consumed in one day using information from the dietary records you kept previously (Lab 16A Nutrition). If you did not perform that lab, perform it to provide information for this activity.
3. Record your daily calories consumed in the Results section.
4. Determine the calories you expended in one day using information from the calorie expenditure records you kept previously (Lab 15B Body Composition). If you did not perform that lab, perform it to provide information for this activity.
5. Record your daily calories expended in the Results section.
6. Determine your daily calorie imbalance by subtracting your calories consumed from calories expended.
7. Provide the additional information requested in the Results section.
8. Answer the questions in the Conclusions and Implications section.

Results:

Subtract calories expended from those consumed for the day to determine your calorie imbalance.

Daily calories actually consumed		Daily calories actually expended		Calorie imbalance
	–		=	+
				–

Divide the calories imbalance into 3,500 calories to determine how many days it would take your daily calorie imbalance to cause a gain or loss of one pound.

3,500 / [ ] Calorie imbalance = [ ] Days to gain or lose one pound of fat.

Conclusions and Implications:

1. In several sentences, discuss the calorie imbalance (or lack of one) that existed for the one day described in this lab. Are the daily intake and expenditure values recorded for this lab typical of a normal day for you? If not, what do you think would be more typical? Would you like to continue a plan of eating and activity that would result in a calorie intake/expenditure similar to what you experienced in this lab?

Section VI

Stress Management

Concept 18

Stress and Health

Mental and physical health are affected by an individual's ability to avoid or adapt to stress.

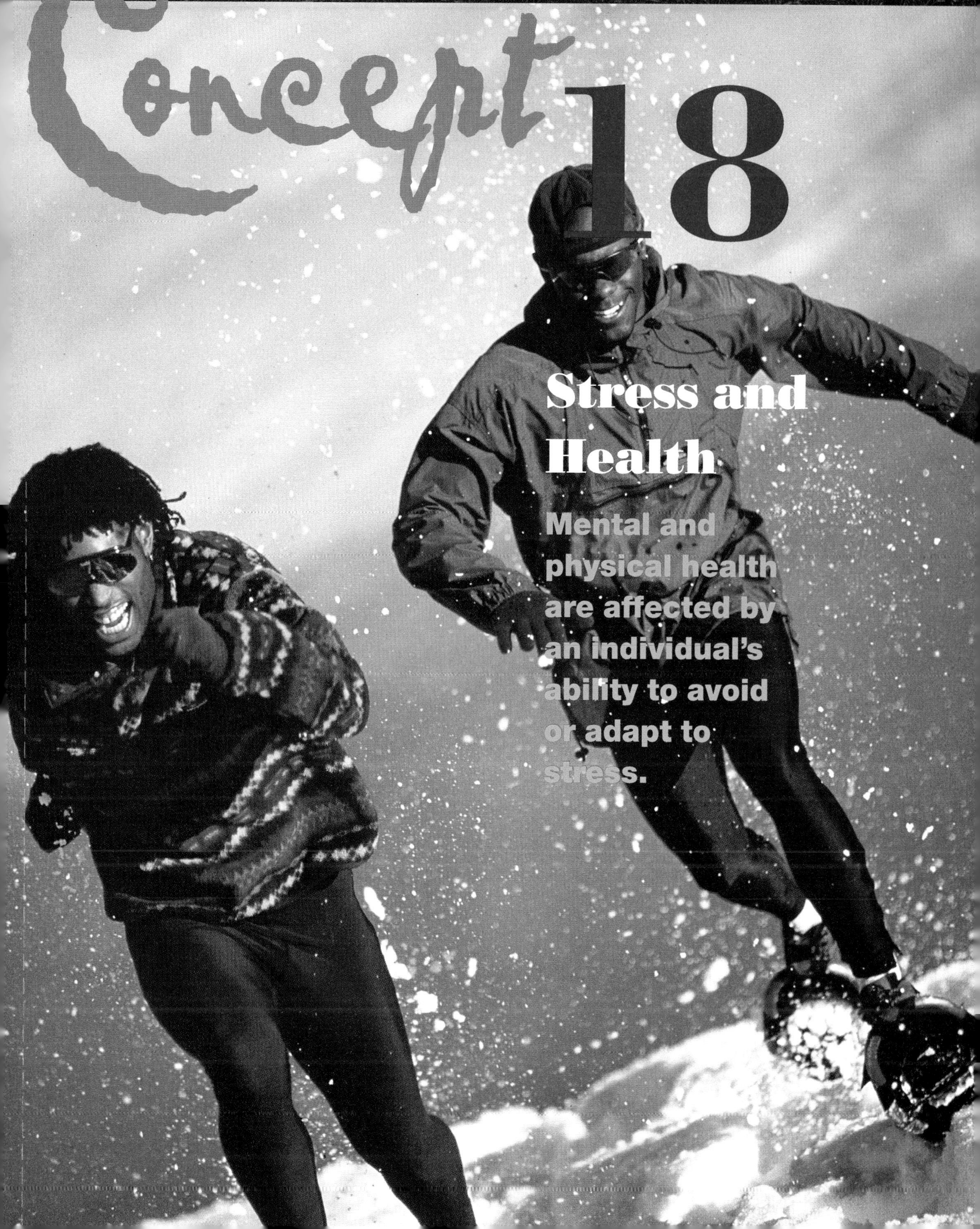

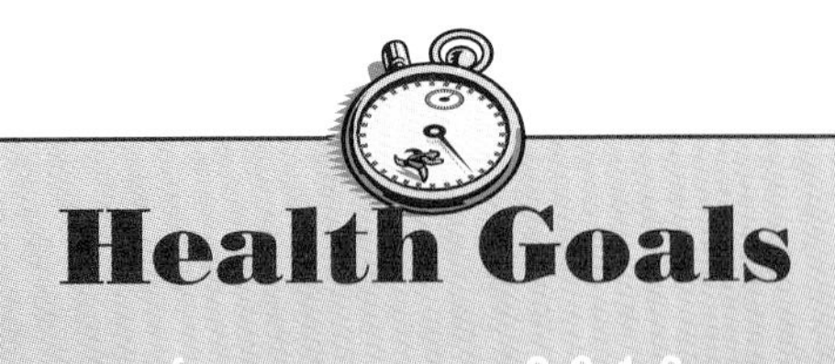

Improve mental health and ensure access to appropriate, quality mental health services.

Increase mental health treatment, including treatment for depression and anxiety disorders.

Increase mental health screening and assessment.

Reduce suicide and suicide attempts, especially among young people.

Increase availability of worksite stress reduction programs.

Introduction

Stress has been linked to between 50 and 70 percent of all illnesses. Some mental and physical conditions that can be psychosomatic (or stress-caused) include high blood pressure and heart disease; psychiatric disorders, such as depression and schizophrenia; indigestion; colitis; poor posture; headaches; insomnia; diarrhea; constipation; increased blood-clotting time; increased cholesterol concentration; diuresis; edema; and low back pain. Other serious diseases, such as cancer, can be influenced by a person's state of mind. In many cases, there is considerable time between a major stressor and the onset of a disease, so we do not always associate the two. Because of this, it is likely that the effect of stress on our body's function is underestimated.

Stress affects nearly everyone to some degree. In fact, approximately 67 percent of adults indicate that they feel "great stress" at least one day a week. Because stress is such a common problem in our society, stress management is viewed as a priority lifestyle similar to physical activity and a healthy diet. This concept will review the cause and consequence of stress. The following concept will provide practical guidelines on how to manage stress more effectively.

The Facts about Stress and Tension

Stress is a normal part of life.

All living creatures are in a continual state of **stress** (some more, some less). It is so pervasive that the body has a built-in mechanism that helps it respond and adapt to stress. When the body experiences a significant **stressor,** it triggers an emotional response that, in turn, evokes the autonomic nervous system to activate the "fight-or-flight" response. This adaptive and protective mechanism stimulates the adrenal glands to secrete hormones (epinephrine and cortisol) that prepare the body for what is perceived as a threat or assault on the whole organism. Almost all body systems are alerted to a heightened state of readiness as a result of this hormonal response. In some instances, this alarm reaction of the body may be essential to survival, but when evoked inappropriately or excessively, it may be more harmful than the effects of the original stressor. For example, a fight-or-flight response may cause a coronary spasm that could lead to a heart attack.

Too little stress is undesirable.

Stress is not always harmful. In fact, a lack of stress, sometimes called "rust out," can lead to boredom, apathy, and less than optimal health. Moderate stress may enhance behavioral adaptation and is necessary for maturation and health. It stimulates psychological growth. It has been said that "freedom from stress is death" and "stress is the spice of life."

Individuals tend to adapt best to moderate stress.

According to Hans Selye, the father of modern stress theory, the physiological and emotional effects of stress are adaptive responses that assist the body in adjusting to the stress. You would expect mild stress to produce mild **adaptations,** and strong stress to produce strong adaptive responses, but this is not so. High levels of threat tend to evoke ineffective, disorganized behavior that impairs the ability to function effectively. Figure 1 shows this relationship between stress and adaptive responses. The amount of stress that you can adapt to comfortably is what Selye called **eustress** and would, in a sense, be the target zone for stress (see Figure 2). The excessive level of stress that compromises our function and well-being is known as **distress.**

Individuals react and adapt differently to stressors.

What one person finds stressful may not be stressful to another person. Stress mobilizes some to greater efficiency, while it confuses and disorganizes others. For example, sky diving or riding a roller coaster would be thrilling for some people, but for others it would be a very stressful and unpleasant experience. An individual's response to stress depends upon the intensity of the threat, the type of situation in which it occurs, and such personal variables as cultural background, tolerance levels, past experience, cognitive style, and personality.

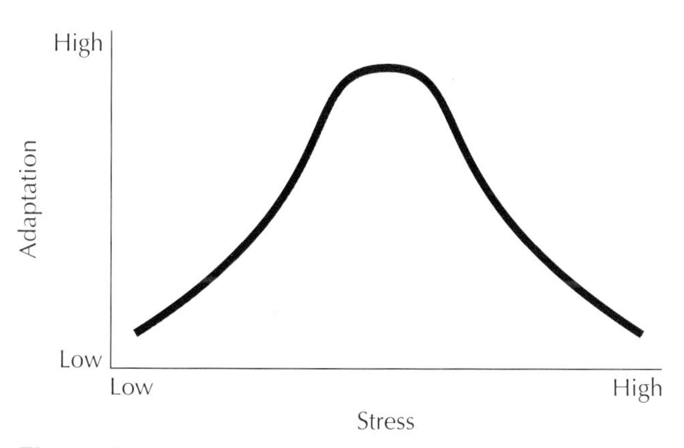

Figure 1
Stress and adaptive responses.

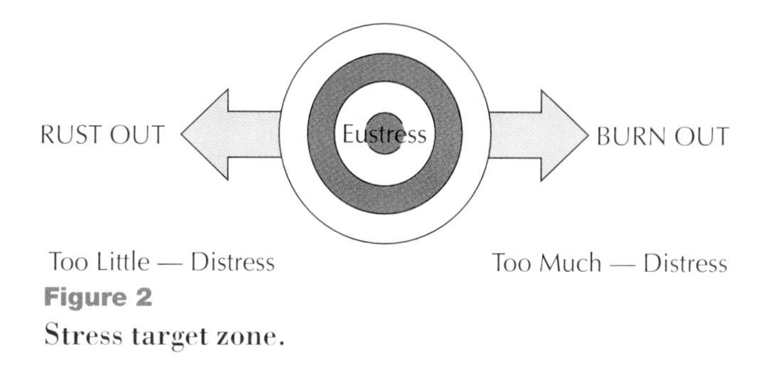

Figure 2
Stress target zone.

Many contemporary health psychologists acknowledge the complexity of the stress response and view stress as an interactive process. From this perspective, the nature of the stressor is not as important as the way a person appraises stress and what coping strategies are used to deal with stress. Two people can experience the same stressor but may respond very differently depending on how they appraise it and/or cope with it. These issues will be explored in more detail in this and the following concept.

The Facts about Sources of Stress

Stress can come from a variety of sources.

There are many kinds of stressors. Environmental stressors include heat, noise, overcrowding, climate, and terrain. Physiological stressors may be such things as drugs, caffeine, tobacco, injury, infection or disease, and physical effort.

Emotional stressors are the most frequent and important stressors affecting humans. Some people refer to these as "psychosocial" stressors. These include life-changing events, such as a change in work hours or line of work, family illnesses, problems with superiors, deaths of relatives or friends, and increased responsibilities. In school, pressures such as grades, term papers, and oral presentations may induce stress. A recent national study of daily experiences indicates that more than 60 percent of all stressful experiences fall in 13 areas. These areas are listed in Table 1.

Table 1 Leading Sources of Stress

Source	%
1. Arguments or tense moments	8.6
2. Disagreements on issues at work	7.8
3. Concern over physical health of others	7.0
4. Work overload and demands	6.7
5. Worry about other's problems or well-being	6.4
6. Financial issues	4.6
7. Disciplining children	3.5
8. Disagreement over family issues	3.1
9. Being late or missing appointments	3.1
10. Differences of opinions on values	2.7
11. Home overload and demands	2.7
12. Household and car repairs	2.6
13. Tension over household chores	2.6

SOURCE: National Study of Daily Experiences, with permission of David Almeida.

Financial problems are a significant source of stress for college students.

Today, the average age of college students is estimated to be in the upper 20s. This is because many people go back to

Stress The nonspecific response (generalized adaptation) of the body to any demand made upon it in order to maintain physiological equilibrium. This positive or negative response results from emotions that are accompanied by biochemical and physiological changes directed at adaptation.

Stressor Anything that places a greater than routine demand on the body or evokes a stress reaction.

Adaptation The body's efforts to restore normalcy.

Eustress Positive stress, or stress that is mentally or physically stimulating.

Distress Negative stress, or stress that contributes to health problems.

school while working or change careers later in life. No matter what your age, financial problems are stressful (see Table 1). However, students who are not self-sufficient or who have to work as well as attend school, are especially likely to experience stress associated with money. Students are often given access to credit cards even though they may have little experience managing money. To avoid financial problems and their associated stresses, all people would be advised to adhere to the following guidelines:

- Prepare a budget and stick to it. A budget should include an itemized list of planned expenditures. The amount budgeted for all expenses should be less than total income.
- Avoid using credit or credit cards. Credit allows you to buy things you cannot afford but it also reduces your buying power by 5 to 25 percent. Saving to buy the things you want and need allows you to get more for your money.
- Communicate with significant others about spending. Lack of communication is associated with many money problems.

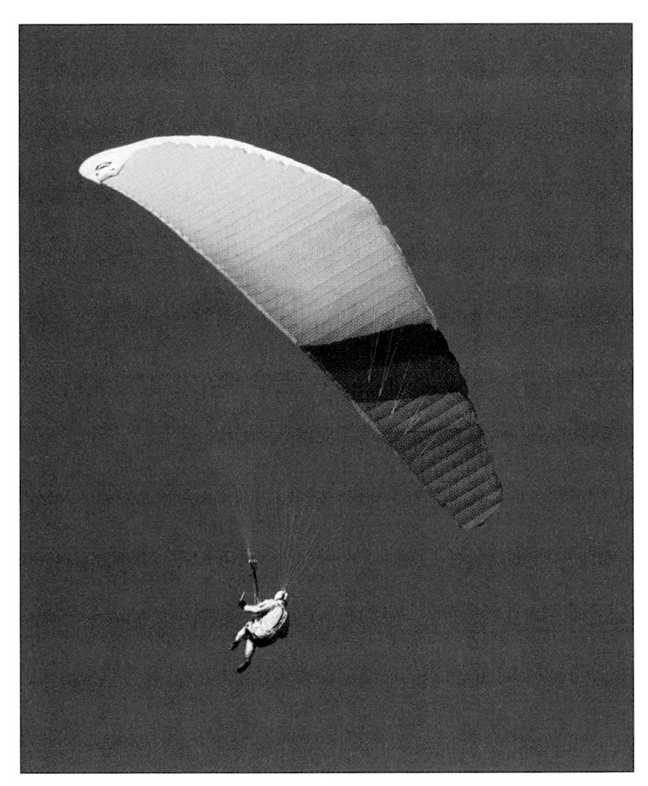

One person's stress is another's pleasure.

Stressors vary in severity.

Because stressors vary in magnitude and duration, many experts categorize them by severity. Major stressors are those that create major emotional turmoil or require tremendous amounts of adjustment. This category includes personal crises (major health problems or death in family, divorce/separation, financial problems, legal problems, etc.), job/school-related pressures or major age-related transitions (college, marriage, career, retirement). Minor stressors are generally viewed as shorter term or less severe. This category includes events or problems such as traffic hassles, peer/work relations, time pressures, or family squabbles, just to name a few. Major stressors can alter our daily patterns of stress and impair our ability to handle the minor stressors or hassles of life. Conversely, minor stressors can accumulate and create more significant problems. It is important to be aware of both types of stressors.

The nature and magnitude of stressors change during the life span.

Depending on your perspective, some periods in life may be more stressful than others, but each phase provides its own challenges and experiences. Some argue that adolescence represents the most stressful time of life. There are drastic changes in a person's body and numerous psychosocial challenges that must be overcome. College provides additional mental challenges as well as financial pressures and the pressures of living independently. During the early adult years, there are tremendous pressures and responsibilities to juggle career and family obligations. Late adulthood presents still other new challenges such as coping with declining functioning or illness. While the nature of the stressor changes, the presence of stress remains consistent. Learning to manage stress can make it easier to handle the changing stresses in life.

Stress can be self-induced and pleasurable, or unpleasurable.

www.mhhe.com/phys_fit/webreview18 Click 01

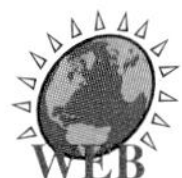

While many people blame external sources for their stress, much of our stress is self-induced. For example, athletes deliberately place themselves in stressful, competitive situations, lawyers and surgeons attempt the challenge of difficult cases or operations, and pregnant women willingly accept the psychological and physiological stress of bearing children. For some, stress can be addictive. Many **Type A personalities** seek out stressful situations and seemingly thrive on the pressure. Self-induced stress may also be an unpleasant but necessary interlude that cannot be avoided. For example, the risk of falling is necessary in learning to ride a bicycle.

At one time, all people with Type A personalities were thought to be at special risk of health problems, especially heart diseases. More recent studies indicate that many Type A personalities adapt to stress well, while others do not. Those who do not express their anger and have hostility associated with stressful situations are more likely to be at risk. A recent study showed that anger and hostility are as much factors for women as men. In addition to the physical health risks, recent research suggests that individuals who are high in hostility are likely to have poor social support and greater susceptibility to chronic depression.

Negative, ambiguous, and uncontrollable events are usually the most stressful.

While stress can come from both positive and negative events, negative ones generally cause more distress. This is because negative stressors usually have harsher consequences and little benefit. Positive stressors on the other hand usually have enough benefit to make them worthwhile. So, while the stress of getting ready for a wedding may be tremendous, it is not as bad as the negative stress associated with losing a job.

Ambiguous stressors are harder to accept than problems that are more clearly defined. In most cases, if the cause of a stressor or problem can be identified, then active measures can be taken to improve the situation. For example, if you are stressed about a project at work or school, you can employ specific strategies to help you complete the task on time. Stress brought on by a relationship with friends or coworkers, on the other hand, may be harder to understand. In some cases, it may not be possible to determine the primary source or cause of the problem. These situations are more problematic because there are fewer clear-cut solutions.

Another factor that makes events stressful is a lack of control. Stress brought on by illness, accidents, or natural disasters fit into this category. Because little can be done to change the situation, these events leave us feeling powerless. If the stressor is something that can be dealt with more directly, then efforts at minimizing the stress are likely to be effective. This helps us to feel more in control.

Jobs and schoolwork are common sources of stress for college students.

www.mhhe.com/phys_fit/webreview18 Click 02

For college students, schoolwork can be a full-time job and those who have to work outside of school must handle the stresses of both "jobs." Although the college years are often thought of as a break from the stresses of the "real world," college life has its own unique stressors. Obvious sources of stress include exams, public speaking requirements, and becoming comfortable with talking to professors. Students are often living independent of family for the first time and at the same time negotiating new relationships—with roommates, dating partners, etc. Young people entering college are also faced with a less structured environment and simultaneously with the need to control their own schedules. Though there are a number of advantages to this environment, students are faced with a greater need to manage their time effectively. Chapter 19 will introduce a number of ways to effectively cope with the unique stresses of the college environment.

The Facts about the Appraisal of Stress

Your appraisal of a stressful situation influences its severity.

Stressors by themselves generally do not cause problems unless they are perceived or appraised as stressful. Appraisal usually involves a consideration of the consequences of the situation and an evaluation of the resources that are available to help you cope with the situation. Stressors that have major consequences and little hope of resolution pose the greatest threat. By trying to maintain an optimistic view of stressful situations, you can minimize the effect of stress on your lifestyle. A recent study found a strong correlation between a person's outlook (optimistic vs. pessimistic) and the severity of pain related to gastrointestinal disorders. There is even evidence that individuals who are more optimistic will live longer on average.

Certain personality characteristics have been found to be associated with the ability to deal with stressful situations.

www.mhhe.com/phys_fit/webreview18 Click 03

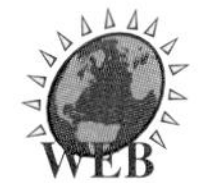

While all people are exposed to stress, some people handle it better than others. Much of the difference lies in how people appraise a stressful situation. Certain characteristics (collectively referred to as **hardiness**) have been found to influence a person's reaction

Type A Personality A personality type characterized by impatience, ambition, and aggression; Type A personalities may be more prone to the effects of stress but may also be more able to cope with stress.

Hardiness A collection of personality traits thought to make a person more resistant to stress.

to stressful situations. Individuals possessing hardiness have been found to appraise and respond to stress in a more favorable ways than people without it. Research in a college population indicates that individuals who are high in hardiness are at reduced risk for illness, due to the way they perceive stress and the coping mechanisms they use in response to stressful situations (see Figure 3). The dimensions of hardiness are:

Commitment: The stressors of everyday life can be overwhelming to many people. While stress cannot be avoided, a sense of commitment to your life and your aspirations can make stress more tolerable. Hardy individuals possess a strong sense of commitment and are willing to put up with adversity to keep pushing toward their desired goals.

Challenge: Many people experience considerable stress from the high-pressure demands of school and work. Much of the stress is caused by concern about being able to meet these new demands and the fear associated with failure. Hardy individuals see new responsibilities and situations as challenges rather than stressors. With this perspective, new situations become opportunities for growth rather than chances for failure.

Control: As previously mentioned, situations tend to be more stressful when they are out of our control. Rather than easily giving up when situations seem out of control, hardy individuals find ways to assume control over their problems. Being proactive rather than reactive is an effective strategy to combating stress. It is important to acknowledge that many stressors may be out of your control. In these situations, it is important to just "go with the flow." Depending on the degree of control that is available, some coping strategies may be more effective than others. Specific recommendations are provided in the next concept.

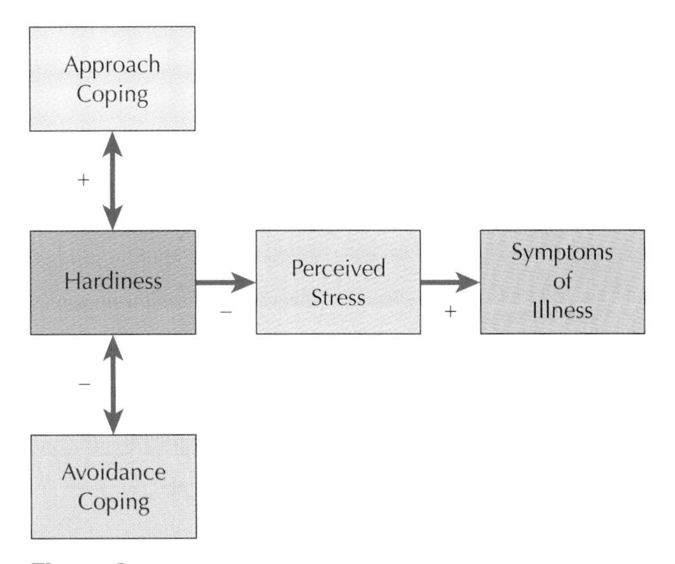

Figure 3
Hardiness and Illness.
Adapted from Soderstrom, M.

The Facts about Responses to Stress

Responses to stressors can be short- or long-lived.

Some stress persists only as long as the stressor is present. For example, job-related stress caused by a challenging project would generally subside once that project is completed. Other forms of stress may outlast the experience. For example, getting raped or mugged is an incredibly stressful experience and one that tends to stay with a person long after the crime is over. In some cases, traumatic experiences may lead to Post-Traumatic Stress Disorder (PTSD). Symptoms of PTSD include re-experiencing or "flashbacks" of the traumatic event, avoidance of situations that remind the person of the event, emotional numbing, and increased level of arousal.

Stress can have physical effects on the body.

Many of the commonly observed symptoms of stress are physical in nature. Increases in heart rate and blood pressure and sweaty palms are just some of the many physical changes that are commonly observed following acute stress (see Figure 4). It is important to recognize that these physiological responses to stress are a NORMAL part of the body's response. How one interprets these sensations significantly impacts how one will react emotionally and behaviorally. For example, public speaking is a situation that leads to autonomic arousal for most people. Those who handle these situations well probably recognize that these sensations are normal and may even interpret them as excitement about their upcoming speech. In contrast, those who experience severe and sometimes debilitating anxiety are probably interpreting these same sensations as indicators of fear, panic, and loss of control.

Chronic exposure to stress can lead to other physical symptoms such as headaches, indigestion, and stomach cramps. Muscle tension is another common result of stress. One form of this tension is seen in the unnecessary "bracing" or "splinting" action of muscles—the clinched jaw, hunched shoulders, and white knuckles, or muscles contracting when they are not needed. They may stay contracted for long periods without your being aware of it. This tension can cause muscle spasms and pain that, in turn, becomes an additional stressor.

You can evaluate tension by learning to recognize signs of muscle tension. In Lab 18C, you will have the opportunity to practice evaluating signs of **neuromuscular hypertension.**

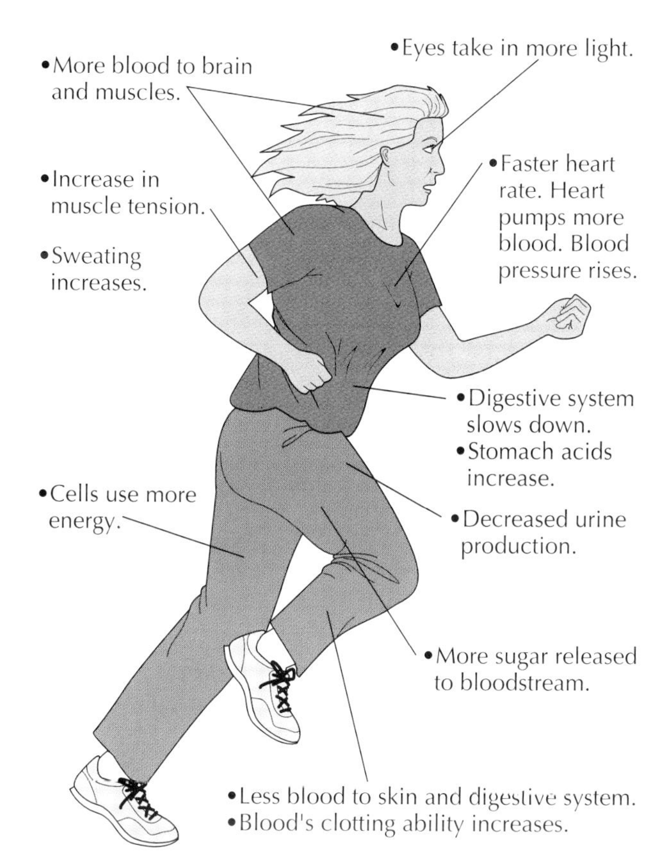

Figure 4
Physical symptoms of stress.

The Facts about Stress and Health

Chronic stress can cause or exacerbate a variety of health problems.

The diathesis-stress model suggests that individuals with a genetic or biological predisposition for a particular illness will express that illness when environmental stresses are sufficient. Someone with a family history of depression is likely to develop depression when under significant stress. Thus, stress is viewed as an important cause of or contributor to many health problems. It has been linked to chronic health maladies that plague individuals on a daily basis such as headaches, indigestion, insomnia, and the common cold. It has also been linked to major health problems such as depression and coronary heart disease. In fact, a recent study indicated that "out-of-control stress" was the leading preventable source of increased health care cost in the workforce; roughly equivalent to the costs of health problems related to smoking.

Fatigue is often a sympton of chronic stress. It can result from lack of sleep, emotional strain, pain, disease, or a combination of these factors. Fatigue can be classified as either **physiological fatigue** or **psychological fatigue,** but both can result in a state of exhaustion or **chronic fatigue syndrome.**

Neuromuscular Hypertension Unnecessary or exaggerated muscle contractions; excess tension beyond that needed to perform a given task; also called hypertonus.

Anxiety A state of apprehension with a compulsion to do something; excessive anxiety is a tension disorder with physiological characteristics.

Psychological Fatigue A feeling of fatigue usually caused by such things as lack of exercise, boredom, or mental stress that results in a lack of energy and depression; also referred to as "subjective" or "false" fatigue.

Physiological Fatigue A deterioration in the capacity of the neuromuscular system as the result of physical overwork and strain; also referred to as "true" fatigue.

Chronic Fatigue Syndrome A clinical condition characterized by a pronounced fatigue or debilitating tiredness.

Stress can have mental and emotional effects on the body.

The challenges caused by psychosocial stress may lead to a variety of mental and emotional effects. In the short-term, stress can impair concentration and attention span. **Anxiety** is an emotional response to stress that is characterized by apprehension. Because the response usually involves expending a lot of nervous energy, anxiety can lead to fatigue and muscular tension. Unresolved personal stressors can also lead to depression.

Stress can lead to changes in behavior.

Stress can cause people to adopt nervous habits like biting their nails. It can also cause normally calm people to become irritable and short-tempered. Other behavioral responses to stress include altered eating and sleeping patterns, smoking, and use of alcohol and other drugs.

Excessive stress reduces the effectiveness of the immune system.

Research on the immune system indicates that stress compromises the function of your body's immune system. With an inefficient immune system, it is more difficult to fight off bacterial infections and to recover from medical treatments. An altered immune function also increases a person's susceptibility to allergens. Therefore allergies and asthma attacks may be more severe under periods of high stress. Other autoimmune disorders such as rheumatoid arthritis are also worsened by stress.

Depression is associated with excessive negative stress.

People who are excessively stressed are more likely to be depressed than people who have optimal amounts of stress in their lives. Health care costs for depressed people are 70 percent higher than for those who are not, and costs for people reporting high levels of stress are 50 percent higher than their less-stressed colleagues. Recent research has shown that drugs commonly prescribed to reduce depression can be effective in many cases but that they often do not get to the source of the life stressors that cause depression and often have side effects that are not positive.

Stress can indirectly influence health.

Chronic levels of stress put a tremendous burden on a person's lifestyle. Many people find it difficult to maintain a healthy lifestyle during periods of high stress. Smoking, drinking, drugs, and unhealthy foods are some of the common vices or escapes that people resort to during periods of stress.

In addition to increased tendencies for negative behaviors, stress can result in a reduced tendency toward positive behaviors such as regular physical activity and sufficient sleep. The combination of more negative behaviors and less positive behaviors can lead to additional health problems.

Strategies for Action: The Facts

Self-assessments of stressors in your life can be useful in managing stress.

In Lab 18A you will have the opportunity to evaluate your stress levels using the Life Experience Survey. In Lab 18B you will assess your hardiness, a characteristic associated with effectively coping with stress. If you find that you are high in stress, you can use the techniques described in the next concept to help reduce your stress levels.

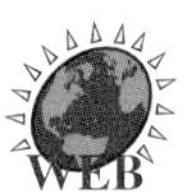

Web Review

Web review materials for Concept 18 are available at *www.mhhe.com/phys_fit/webreview18 Click 04.*

American Institute of Stress
www.stress.org

American Psychological Association
www.apa.org

National Center for Post Traumatic Stress Disorder
www.ncptsd.org

National Institute for Occupational Safety and Health
www.cdc.gov/niosh/stresshp.html

National Institute of Mental Health
www.nimh.nih.gov

Suggested Readings

Benson, H. "Mind-Body Pioneer." *USA Today*, 1 June 2001.

Babyak, M. et al. "Exercise Treatment for Major Depression: Maintenance of Therapeutic Benefit at 10 Months." *Psychosomatic Medicine*. (62)(5) (2000): 633–638.

Burns, D. D. *The Feeling Good Handbook*. New York: Plume, 1999.

Corbin, D. E. (ed.). *Perspectives: Stress Management*. Boulder, CO: Coursewise Publishing Co., 1999.

Fredrickson, B. "Cultivating Positive Emotions to Optimize Health and Well-Being." *Prevention and Treatment*. 3(2000) a web journal (http://journals/prevention/vol3/pre0030001a.html)

Girdano, D., and Everly, G. *Controlling Stress and Tension*. 6th ed. Needham, MA: Allyn and Bacon, Inc., 2000.

Greenberg, J. S. *Comprehensive Stress Management*. 7th ed. St. Louis: McGraw-Hill, 2002.

Hudd, S. et al. "Stress at College: Effects on Health Habits, Health Status, and Self-Esteem." *College Student Journal*. (34)(2)(2000): 217–227.

Landers, D. "The Influence of Exercise on Mental Health." In Corbin, C. B., and Pangrazi, R. P. (ed.). *Towards a Better Understanding of Physical Fitness and Activity*. Scottsdale, AZ: Holcomb-Hathaway, 1999, Chapter 16.

Seligman, M. E. *Learned Optimism: How to Change Your Mind and Your Life*. New York: Pocket Books, 1998.

Shelton, R. C. et al. "Effectiveness of St. John's Wort in Major Depression." *Journal of the American Medical Association* (285)(15)(2001): 1978–1986.

U.S. Department of Health and Human Services. *Healthy People 2010*. 2nd ed. With *Understanding and Improving Health* and *Objectives for Improving Health*. 2 vols. Washington, DC: U.S. Government Printing Office, November 2000, Chapter 18, "Mental Health and Mental Disorders."

Lab 18B: Evaluating Your Hardiness

Name	Section	Date

Purpose: To evaluate your level of hardiness and to help you identify the ways in which you appraise and respond to stressful situations.

Procedure:

1. Complete the Hardiness Questionnaire. Make an X over the circle that best describes what is true for you personally.
2. Summarize your score using the scoring chart.
3. Evaluate your score using the Hardiness Rating Chart and record your ratings.
4. Interpret the results by answering the questions, and discussing the conclusions and implications in the space provided.

Hardiness Questionnaire

Questions	Not True	Rarely True	Sometimes True	Often True	Score
1. I look forward to school and work on most days.	1	2	3	4	
2. Having too many choices in life makes me nervous.	4	3	2	1	
3. I know where my life is going and look forward to the future.	1	2	3	4	
4. I prefer to not get too involved in relationships.	4	3	2	1	
Commitment Score Sum 1–4					
5. My efforts at school and work will pay off in the long run.	1	2	3	4	
6. You just have to trust your life to fate to be successful.	4	3	2	1	
7. I believe that I can make a difference in the world.	1	2	3	4	
8. Being successful in life takes more luck and good breaks than effort.	4	3	2	1	
Control Score Sum 5–8					
9. I would be willing to work for less money if I could do something really challenging and interesting.	1	2	3	4	
10. I often get frustrated when my daily plans and schedule get altered.	4	3	2	1	
11. Experiencing new situations in life is important to me.	1	2	3	4	
12. I don't mind being bored.	4	3	2	1	
Challenge Score Sum 9–12					

Results:

Commitment score		Commitment rating	
Control score		Control rating	
Challenge score		Challenge rating	
(Sum the three scores)			
Hardiness score		Hardiness rating	

Hardiness Rating Chart:

Rating	Individual Hardiness Scale Scores	Total Hardiness Scores
High hardiness	14–16	40–48
Moderate hardiness	10–13	30–39
Low hardiness	Less than 10	Less than 30

Conclusions and Implications:

1. In several sentences, discuss your three hardiness scores. Commitment scores reflect a dedication toward personal goals and life in general. Control scores reflect a belief that events in your life are within your control. Challenge scores reflect an ability to see stressful situations as opportunities for growth. Do you think these scores have implications for you? Are there changes you can make?

2. In several sentences, discuss your total hardiness score. This collection of traits has been referred to as the "stress-resistant personality" since hardy individuals have been found to respond better to stressful situations. Do you think your score is accurate for you? Do you think the score has implications for you?

Concept 19

Stress Management, Relaxation, and Time Management

While stress cannot be avoided, proper stress management techniques can help to reduce the impact of stress in your life.

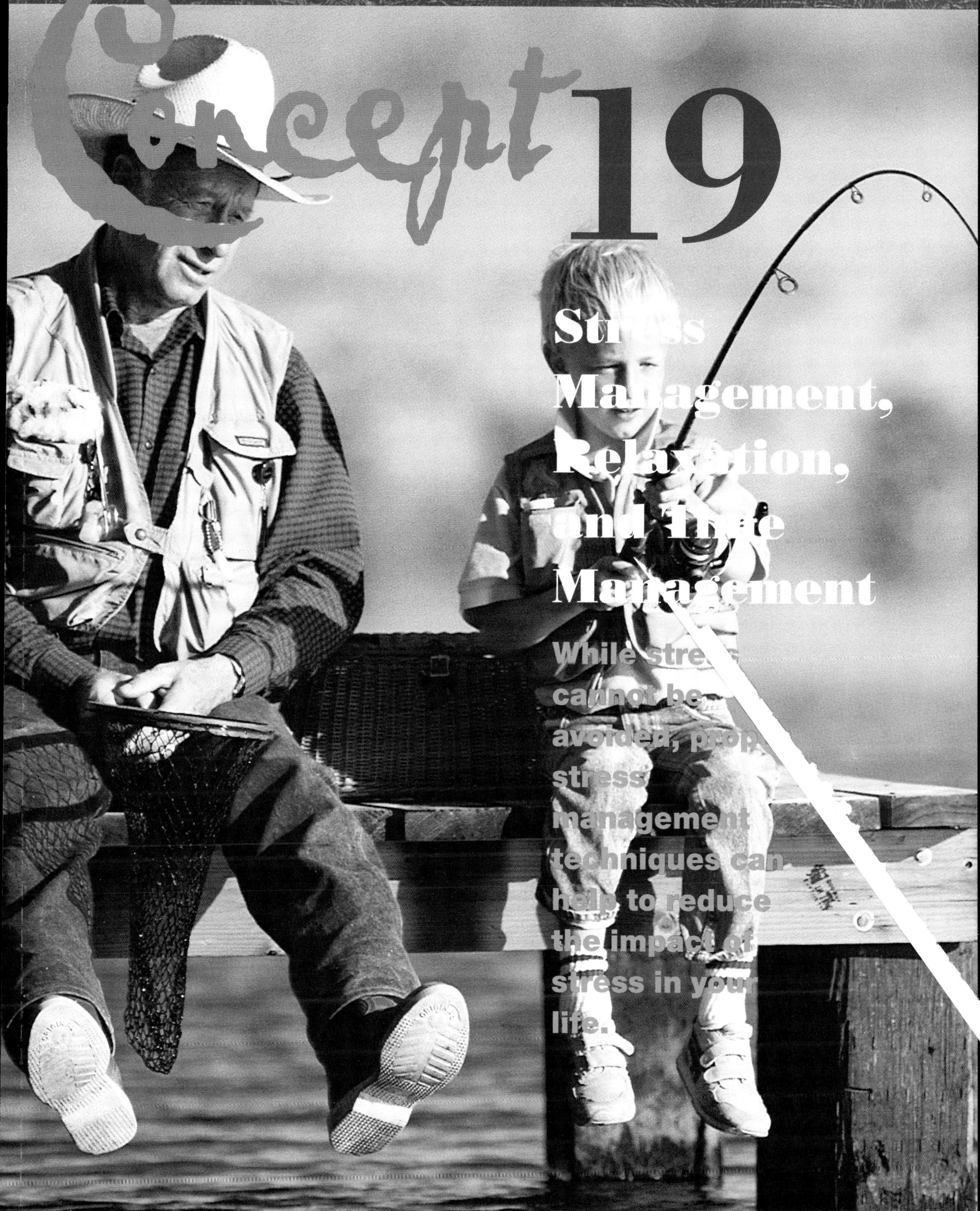

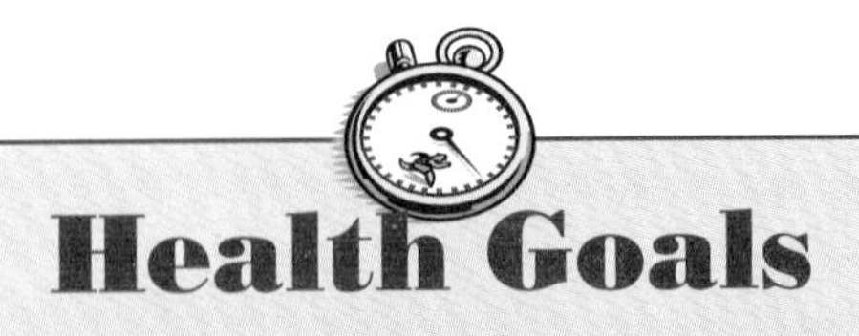

Improve mental health and ensure access to appropriate, quality mental health services.

Increase mental health treatment, including treatment for depression and anxiety disorders.

Increase mental health screening and assessment.

Reduce suicide and suicide attempts, especially among young people.

Increase availability of worksite stress reduction programs.

Introduction

When stress gets the best of you, it is important to find ways to cope with stress. **Problem-focused coping strategies** (problem solving, social support) are recommended when the stressful situations are largely within your control. **Emotion-focused coping strategies** (music, relaxation exercises, exercise) are recommended when the stress is largely out of your control or when you just want some immediate relief from the stress at hand. Most stressors will require both types of strategies. Drugs, alcohol, and food are not good choices for reducing stress since these can lead to more problems than they are intended to solve. This concept will review several approaches for effective stress management.

The Facts about Coping with Stress

Unresolved stress poses the greatest physical and emotional danger.

While some stressors are short lived, many stressors persist over a long period of time. The ability to adapt, or cope with these stressors, largely determines their ultimate effect. If effective coping strategies are used, the effects of a stressful situation can be more tolerable. In many cases, by "staying positive" reasonable solutions or compromises can be found for many problems. On the other hand, if ineffective coping strategies are used, many problems can actually become worse. This can lead to even more stress and more severe outcomes. While stress cannot be avoided, stress can be managed. Effective stress management is a skill that can contribute to both health and quality of life.

Coping strategies can be classified as "problem-focused" or "emotion-focused" depending on the nature of their influence.

Individuals deal with stress in a variety of ways; however, the methods of **coping** can generally be classified as problem-focused, emotion-focused, or avoidant. Problem-focused coping strategies are aimed at changing the source of the stress. Emotion-focused coping strategies, on the other hand, attempt to regulate the emotions resulting from stress. While either of these types of strategies may be effective in various circumstances, avoidant coping strategies, like ignoring or escaping the problem, are likely to be ineffective for almost everyone.

A key in stress management is to select coping strategies that are appropriate for the type of stress that you are experiencing. If you are confronting a situation that is largely out of your control, then problem-focused efforts to change the situation are unlikely to be effective. For these situations, it is more effective to use emotion-focused coping strategies that help to minimize the effects of the stress. On the other hand, if you are experiencing stress from issues or events that you can control, then more problem-focused efforts are likely to improve the situation.

Coping with most stress requires a variety of thoughts and actions.

Stress forces our bodies to work under less than optimal conditions; yet, this is the time when we need to function at our best. Effective coping may require some efforts to regulate the emotional aspects of the stress and other efforts directed toward solving the problem. For example, if you are experiencing stress over grades in school, you have to accept your current grades and also take active steps to improve them. It does no good to worry about events that are behind you. Instead, it is important to look ahead for ways to solve the problems at hand.

Table 1 Strategies for Stress Management

Category	Description
Problem-focused Strategies	**Strategies that directly seek to solve or minimize the stressful situation.**
• Accepting	• Realizing that the problem was brought on by you and committing yourself to not let it happen again.
• Re-appraising	• Viewing experience as a learning or growth opportunity.
• Praying	• Looking for spiritual guidance to overcome the problem.
• Problem solving	• Making a plan of action to solve the problem and following the necessary steps to make the situation better.
• Controlling	• Trying to make yourself feel better or looking for ways to get past the situation.
• Seeking active social support	• Getting help or advice from others who can provide specific assistance for your situation.
Emotion-focused Strategies	**Strategies that minimize the emotional and physical effects of the situation.**
• Confronting	• Expressing anger over a situation, or challenging authorities to try to change the situation.
• Relaxing	• Using relaxation techniques to reduce the symptoms of stress.
• Exercising	• Using physical activity to reduce the symptoms of stress.
• Seeking passive social support	• Talking with someone about what you are experiencing or accepting sympathy and understanding.
Avoidant Coping Strategies	**Strategies that attempt to distract the individual from the problem.**
• Ignoring	• Refusing to think about the situation or trying to pretend there was no problem.
• Escaping	• Looking for ways to feel better or to stop thinking about the problem, including eating or using nicotine, alcohol, or other drugs.

Coping with this situation may therefore require both problem- and emotion-focused strategies. Emotion-focused strategies are needed to stop worrying about your current situation, and problem-focused strategies are needed to remove the source of the stress.

Physical Activity and Stress Management: The Facts

Regular activity and a healthy diet can help you adapt to stressful situations.

An individual's capacity to adapt is not a static function, but fluctuates with energy, drive, and courage. The better your overall health, the better you can withstand the rigors of tension without becoming susceptible to illness or other disorders. Physical activity is especially important because it conditions your body to function effectively under challenging physiological conditions.

Physical activity can provide relief from stress and aid in muscle tension release.

Physical activity has been found to be effective at relieving stress, particularly white-collar job stress. Studies show that regular exercise decreases the likelihood of stress disorders and reduces the intensity of the stress response. It also shortens the time of recovery from an emotional trauma. Its effect tends to be short term, so one must continue to exercise regularly for it to have a continuing effect. Aerobic exercise is believed to be especially effective in reducing anxiety and relieving stress (though a wide

Coping A person's constantly changing cognitive and psychological efforts to manage stressful situations. Coping strategies can be either active or passive.

Problem-focused Coping Strategies A method of adapting to stress that is based on changing the source or cause of stress.

Emotion-focused Coping Strategies A method of adapting to stress that is based on regulating the emotions that cause stress.

Avoidant Coping Strategies Seeking immediate, temporary relief from stress through distraction or self-indulgence.

variety of other activities are also good). Whatever your choice of exercise, it is likely to be more effective as an antidote to stress if it is something you find enjoyable.

> Stretching exercises and rhythmical exercises especially aid in relaxation.

People who work long hours at a desk can release tension by getting up frequently and stretching, by taking a brisk walk down the hall, or by performing "office exercises."

Exercising to music or to a rhythmic beat has been found to be relaxing and even "hypnotic." Some exercises designed specifically for relaxation are illustrated in Table 2.

> Various mechanisms have been proposed to explain the stress reductions following physical activity.

www.mhhe.com/phys_fit/webreview19 Click 01

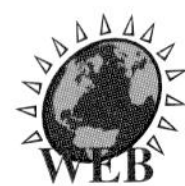

Numerous studies have examined the anxiety-reducing effects of physical activity. Because physical activity leads to a variety of changes in the mind and body, it has proven difficult to identify the mechanisms through which it exerts its effect. Some of the leading theories are described here:

- *Distraction* (***time-out hypothesis***): Physical activity provides a break from the demands of normal life. This change in focus may allow the brain to process or reinterpret stressful scenarios or to relax. This theory would suggest that participating in other focused activities (e.g., playing the piano) may have similar beneficial effects on stress.
- *Increased endorphins* (***endorphin hypothesis***): The evidence is equivocal but some research has suggested that exercise causes the release of natural painkilling chemicals known as endorphins that may be related to the affective changes in mood.
- *Neurotransmitter hypothesis:* Regular physical activity reduces the levels of catecholamines (epinephrine and norepinephrine) and cortisol, hormones involved in the stress response. Thus, regular bouts of activity can reduce the end result of stress. Some evidence indicates that physical activity also influences levels of other neurotransmitters, such as dopamine, that are associated with relaxation.
- *Self-esteem hypothesis:* For many people, the completion of a task like exercise boosts confidence and a sense of self-mastery. These perceptions can boost self-esteem and help people feel better about themselves and their situation.
- *Thermogenic hypothesis:* During exercise, the body's core temperature increases as a result of the increased muscular activity. There is some evidence that these elevations may produce therapeutic benefits. Many people report that a sauna or warm shower can promote relaxation—possibly by the same mechanism.

The Facts about Conscious Relaxation Techniques

> Conscious relaxation techniques can be an effective way to combat stress.

Conscious relaxation techniques reduce stress and tension by directly altering the symptoms. When you are stressed, heart rate, blood pressure, and muscle tension all increase to help your body deal with the challenge. Conscious relaxation techniques act to reduce these normal effects and bring the body back to a more relaxed state. Most techniques employ the "three Rs" of relaxation to help the body relax: (1) reduce mental activity, (2) recognize tension, and (3) reduce respiration. Because these techniques do not change the nature or impact of a stressor, they are considered to be a passive or emotion-focused coping strategy.

> There are a variety of conscious relaxation techniques.

Six examples of these techniques are described here:

- *"The Quick Fix"*—To get relief from a stressful situation during the day, take a timeout for 5 or 10 minutes by finding a quiet place away from the situation with as

Time-Out Hypothesis A possible mechanism for the beneficial effects of exercise on stress.

Endorphins Hormones released by the body during periods of stress or exertion that are thought to suppress pain and promote relaxation.

Table 2
Relaxation Exercises

1. Neck Stretch

Roll the head slowly in a half-circle from 9:00 to 8:00 to 7, 6, 5, 4, and 3, then reverse from 3 to 9. Close your eyes and feel the stretch. Do *not* make a full circle by tipping the head back. Repeat several times.

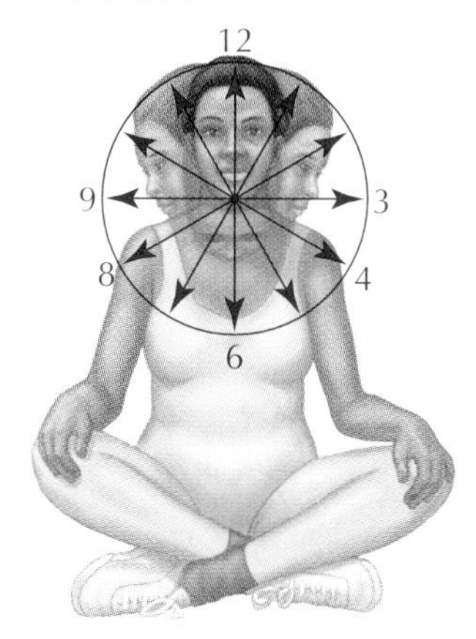

2. Shoulder Lift

Hunch the shoulders as high as possible (contract) and then let them drop (relax). Repeat several times. Inhale on the lift; exhale on the drop.

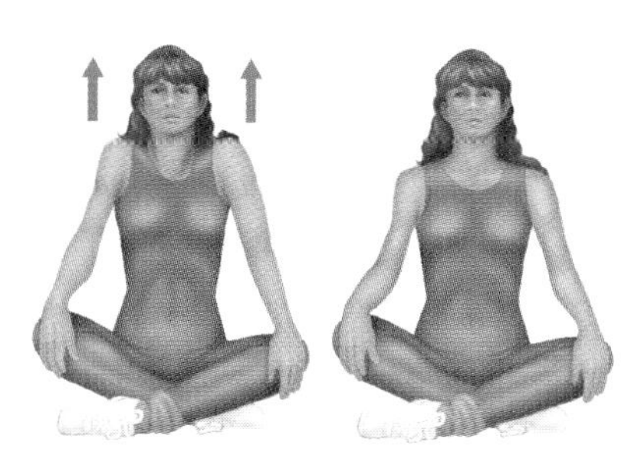

3. Trunk Stretch and Drop

Stand and reach as high as possible; tiptoe and stretch every muscle, then collapse completely, letting knees flex and trunk, head, and arms dangle. Repeat two or three times. Inhale on the stretch and exhale on the collapse.

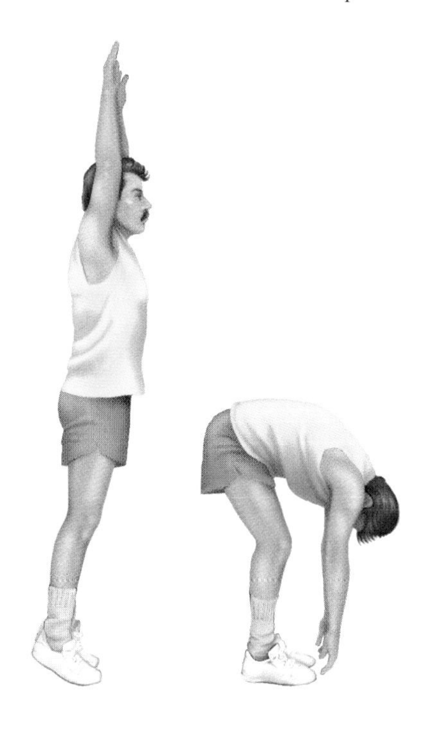

4. Trunk Swings

Following the trunk stretch and drop (see illustration 3), remain in the "drop" position and with a minimum of muscular effort, set the trunk swinging from side to side by shifting the weight from one foot to the other, letting the heels come off the floor alternately. Keep the entire body (especially the neck) limp.

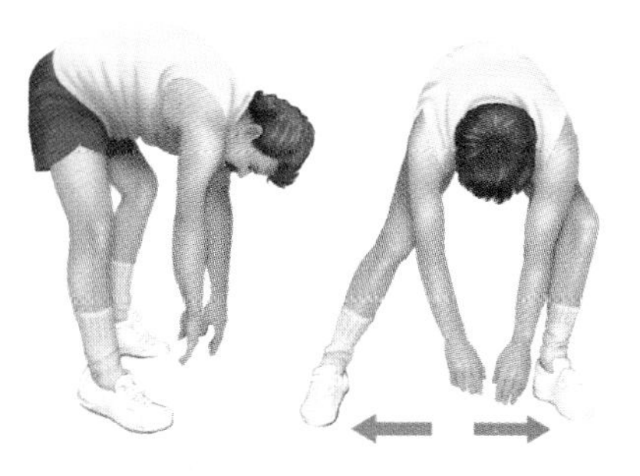

5. Tension Contrast

With arms extended overhead, lie on your side. Tense the body as stiff as a board, then let go and relax, letting the body fall either forward or backward in whatever direction it loses balance. Continue letting go for a few seconds after falling and allow yourself to feel like you are still sinking. Repeat on the other side.

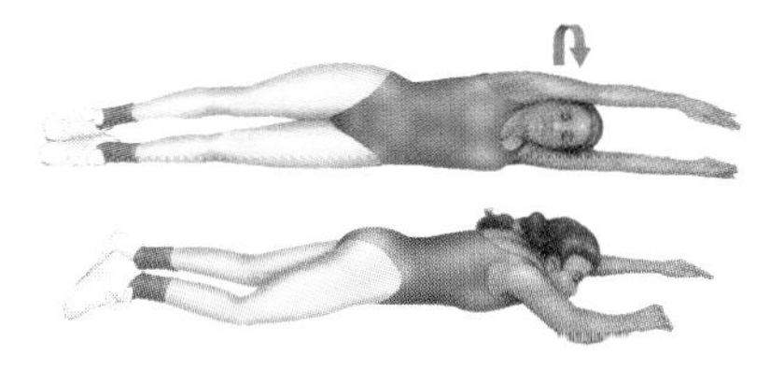

few distractions as possible. Sit, loosen your clothes, take off your shoes, and close your eyes. Then follow these steps: (1) Inhale deeply for about 4 seconds; then exhale, letting the air out slowly for about 8 seconds (twice as long as the inhalation). Do this several times. (2) Mentally visualize a pleasant image, such as a peaceful lake or stream; continue to relax and breathe deeply. (3) When your time is up, breathe deeply and stretch luxuriously; go back to your work refreshed and with a changed attitude. You may need to do this several times a day.

- *Jacobson's Progressive Relaxation Method*—You must be able to recognize how a tense muscle feels before you can voluntarily release the tension. In this technique, contract the muscles strongly, then relax. Each of the large muscles is relaxed first, and later the small ones. The contractions are gradually reduced in intensity until no movement is visible. Always, the emphasis is placed on detecting the feeling of tension as the first step in "letting go," or "going negative." Jacobson, a pioneer in muscle relaxation research, emphasized the importance of relaxing eye and speech muscles, because he believed these muscles trigger reactions of the total organism more than other muscles. A sample contract-relax exercise routine for relaxation is presented in Lab 19B.
- *Autogenic (Self-generated) Relaxation Training*—Several times daily, sit or lie in a quiet room with eyes closed. Block out distracting thoughts by passively concentrating on preselected words or phrases. This technique has been used to focus on heaviness of limbs, warmth of limbs, heart rate regulation, respiratory rate and depth regulation, and coolness in the forehead. It evokes changes opposite to those produced by stress. Research has shown that people who are skilled in this technique can decrease oxygen consumption, change the electrical activity of the brain, slow the metabolism, decrease blood lactate, lower body temperature, and slow the heart rate.
- *Biofeedback–Autogenic Relaxation Training*—Biofeedback training utilizes machines that monitor certain physiological processes of the body and provide visual or auditory evidence of what is happening to normally unconscious bodily functions. When combined with autogenic training, subjects have learned to relax and reduce the electrical activity in their muscles, lower blood pressure, decrease heart rate, change their brain waves, and decrease headaches, asthma attacks, and stomach acid secretion. Biofeedback is helpful in treating phobias, stage fright, drug abuse, sexual dysfunction, stuttering, and other psychological problems.
- *Imagery*—Thinking autogenic phrases, you can visualize such feelings as "sinking into a mattress or pillow," or you can think of being a "limp, loose-jointed puppet with no one to hold the strings." You can imagine being a "half-filled sack of flour resting on an uneven surface" or pretend to be "a sack of granulated salt left out in the rain, melting away." Some people seem to respond better to the concept of "floating" than to feeling "heavy." It also includes visualizing pleasant, relaxing scenes as mentioned in the description of "The Quick Fix." You attempt to place yourself in the scene and experience all of the sounds, colors, and scents. Whatever the image you wish to conjure,

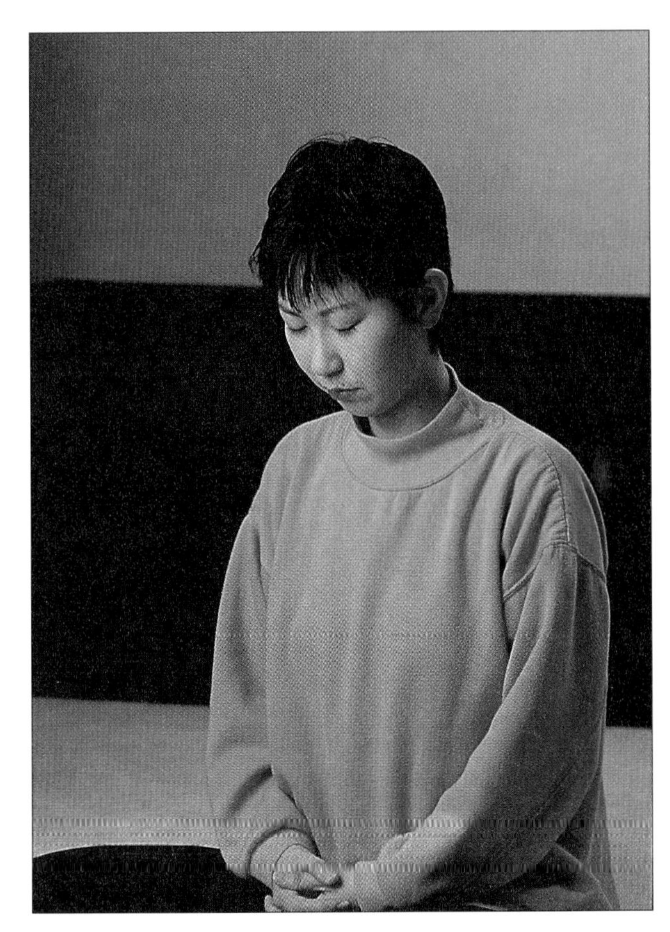

Prayer and meditation can reduce physical symptoms of stress and can help you cope.

imagery can help take your mind off anxieties and distractions and, at the same time, release unwanted tension in the muscles using the principle of "mind over matter."

- *Prayer*—Recent studies have shown that prayer can decrease blood pressure for many people and can be a source of internal comfort. It can have other calming effects that are associated with reduced distress. It can also provide confidence to function more effectively, thereby reducing stresses associated with ineffectiveness at work or in other situations.

Some Facts about Muscle Tension and Sleep

> There are a variety of techniques that can reduce muscle tension.

One of the symptoms of stress is muscle tension. Muscle tension can lead to pain, which in turn can negatively influence quality of life, especially for older adults. Various procedures typically used by physical therapists (e.g., ultrasound, heat, cold, and massage) can be helpful in relieving muscle tension. Care should be taken to ensure that these procedures are used properly, typically by experts. Recently, the National Institutes of Health concluded that acupuncture has value in relieving muscle tension and associated pain. Again, it is important that the person administering the treatment has appropriate credentials. Most of the treatments described here are for the relief of already existing muscle tension. They are passive techniques that may give relief to symptoms but may do little to eliminate the cause of the problem.

> Stress can impair sleep and lack of sleep can be a source of stress.

One of the effects of negative stress is insomnia or inability to sleep. Business pressures, worries about college exams, concerns for loved ones who are ill, and other stressors can cause insomnia. On the other hand, lack of sleep is a stressor itself. Using the coping strategies described in this concept can help people who have insomnia. A common myth is that older people need less sleep than younger people. The amount of sleep you need does not change with age. There are other factors that should also be considered. Some guidelines follow:

- Check with your doctor about medications. Some medicines, such as weight loss pills and decongestants, contain caffeine, ephedrine, or other ingredients that interfere with sleep.

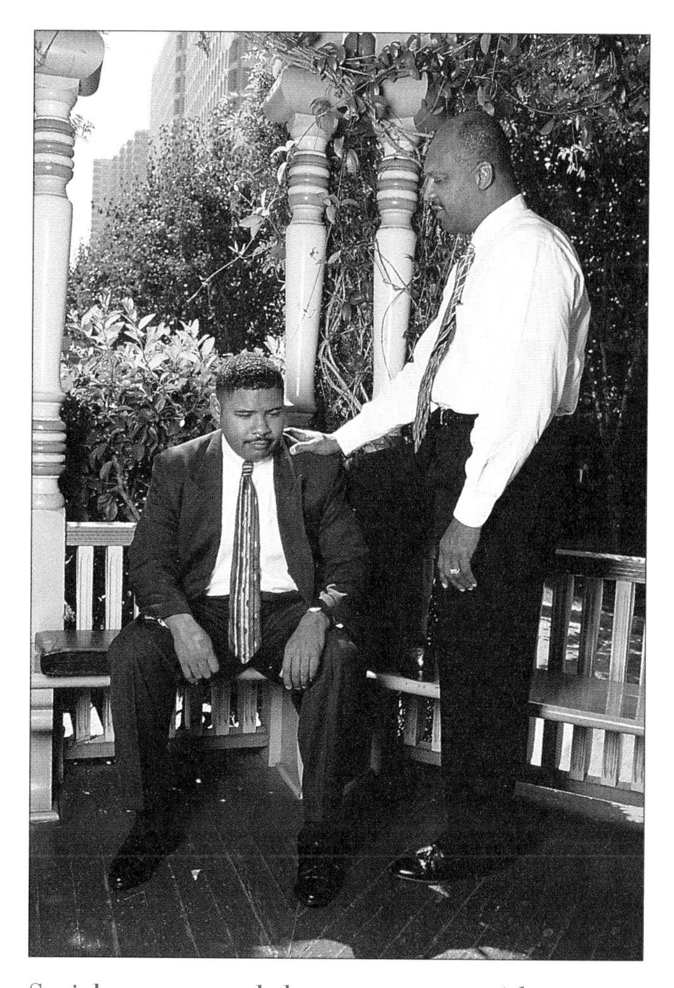

Social support can help a person cope with stress.

- Avoid tobacco use. Nicotine is a stimulant and can interfere with sleep.
- Avoid excess alcohol use. Alcohol may make it easier to get to sleep but may be a reason why you wake up at night and stay awake.
- Exercise late in the day but do not do vigorous activity right before bedtime.
- Sleep in a room that is cooler than normal.
- Avoid hard-to-digest foods late in the day. Fatty and spicy foods should be avoided.
- Avoid large meals late in the day or right before bedtime. A light snack before bedtime should not be a problem for most people.
- Avoid too much liquid before bedtime.
- Avoid naps during the day.
- Go to bed and get up at the same time each day.

Social Support and Stress Management: The Facts

Social support is important for effective stress management.

Social support has been found to play an important role in coping with stress. Social support has been linked to faster recovery from various medical procedures. One study of athletic injuries has shown that people who were the most stressed were injured more often, and those who had the poorest support system were the most likely to be injured. While the mechanism for this effect is not understood, it is clear that social support plays a major role in stress management. Social support can assist in both problem-focused and emotion-focused forms of coping. Friends and family can provide very concrete advice that can help solve a problem, and they can also provide moral support and encouragement.

Social support can come from a variety of sources.

Everyone needs someone to turn to for support when feeling overwhelmed. Support can come from friends, family members, clergy, a teacher, a coach, or a professional counselor. Different sources may provide different forms of support. Even pets have been shown to be a good source of social support with consequent health and quality of life benefits. The goal is to identify and nurture relationships that can provide this type of support. In turn, it is important to look for ways to support and assist others.

There are many types of social support.

Social support can generally be divided into three main components: informational, material, and emotional. Informational (technical support) refers to tips, strategies, or advice that can help a person get through a specific stressful situation. For example, a parent, friend, or coworker may offer insight into how they once resolved similar problems. Material support refers to direct assistance to get a person through a stressful situation. An example would be providing a loan to help pay off a short-term debt.

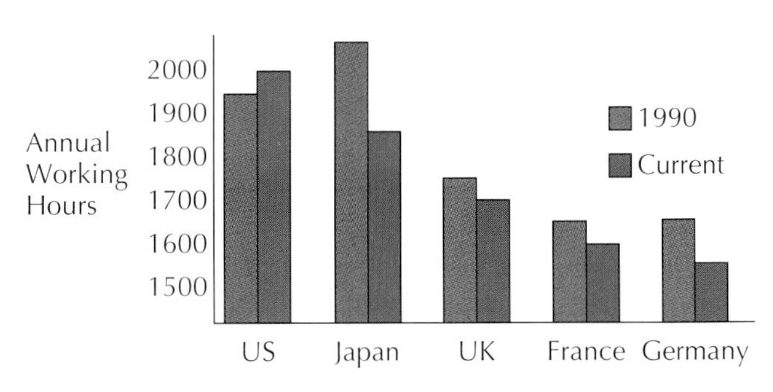

Figure 1
Average annual working hours of five nations.
SOURCE: Organization for Economic Cooperation and Development.

Lastly, emotional support refers to encouragement or sympathy that a person provides to help another cope with a particular challenge.

Obtaining good social support requires close relationships.

Although we live in a social environment, it is often difficult to ask people for help. Sometimes the nature and severity of our problems may not be apparent to others. Other times, friends may not want to offer suggestions or insight because they don't want to appear too pushy. To obtain good support, it is important to develop quality personal relationships with several individuals. Research on the effects of social support clearly indicates that it is the quality of social support, not the quantity, that leads to better health outcomes.

The Facts about Work and Leisure

The amount of time the average person spends at work has increased rather than decreased in the last two decades.

Since 1860, the amount of hours typically spent in work decreased dramatically. The most recent statistics (see Figure 1), however, indicate a trend toward increased work time. A major reason for this recent increase is that more people now hold second jobs than in the past. Also, some jobs of modern society have increasing rather than decreasing time demands. For example, medical doctors and other professionals often work more hours than the 35–44 hours that the majority of people work. Also nearly three times as many married women with children work full time now as compared with 1960.

Experts have referred to young adults as the "overworked Americans" because they work several jobs, maintain dual roles (full-time employment coupled with normal family chores), or they work extended hours in demanding professional jobs. A recent Gallup poll shows that the great majority of adults have "enough time" for work, chores, and sleep but not enough time for friends, self, spouse, and children. When time is at a premium, the factors most likely to be negatively affected are personal health, relationships with children, and marriage or romantic relationships.

It is easy to see that work pressures can be stressful. This suggests a need to manage time effectively and to find activities that are enjoyable during free time.

Unenjoyable work detracts from a person's sense of well-being and quality of life.

Many people enjoy the hours they spend at work more than the hours off the job. It is interesting to note, however, that satisfaction at work has dramatically decreased in the last 50 years. The number of people who enjoy work more than nonwork time was twice as high in 1950 as it was in the 1990s. As indicated in the previous concept, disagreements at work and work overload are the second and fourth leading causes of stress. Nevertheless, work is still important to well-being as indicated by the fact that more than 73 percent of all adults would continue to work even if they had enough money to live without working.

Job satisfaction is important to quality living, but an overcommitment to work can result in decreased well-being. In spite of the fact that most young adults feel that they do not have enough free time, the majority say work is more important than recreation. Few (14 percent) would cut their income to have more leisure time.

All nonwork time is *not* free time.

Among some workers, the demands of "other duties" have increased, allowing fewer hours of truly free time each year. **Committed time** has increased for many people, including traveling to and from work, spending extra time at work-related activities that is unpaid, managing the home and care in addition to work outside the home, and transporting the children.

Free time is very important to the average person.

Most people say that **free time** is important, but surveys indicate that more than half of all adults feel that they get too little of it. Many adults report that they get too little time for **recreation** or to simply relax and "do nothing" (leisure).

Recreation and leisure are important contributors to wellness (quality of life).

www.mhhe.com/phys_fit/webreview19 Click 02

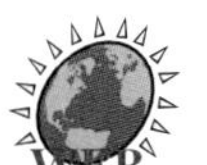

Leisure is time spent "doing things I just want to do" or "doing nothing." Recreation, on the other hand, is often purposeful. Both leisure and recreation can contribute to stress reduction and wellness, though leisure activities are not done specifically to achieve these benefits.

Social Support Any behavior that assists another person in addressing a specific need.

Committed Time Time that is committed to specific activity or purpose.

Free Time Time not committed to work or other duties of the day.

Recreation Recreation literally means creating something anew. In this book, it refers to something that you do for your amusement or for fun to help you divert your attention and to refresh yourself (re-create yourself).

Leisure Time that is free from the demands of work is often called leisure time. Leisure is more than free time; it is also an attitude. Leisure activities need not be means to ends (purposeful) but are ends in themselves.

The value of recreation and leisure in the busy lives of people in Western culture is evidenced by the emphasis public health officials place on availability and accessibility of recreational facilities in the future.

To achieve wellness and stress-reduction benefits, recreation should provide a sense of play.

Play is done of one's own free will. It is most often done for fun or intrinsic rather than extrinsic reasons. Activities performed for material things such as trophies and medals can be considered recreational as long as the principal reason for doing the activity is a sense of fun and playfulness. If the activity is done primarily for extrinsic reasons, it may not provide wellness benefits and is probably not true recreation. For example, playing golf to impress the boss is an extrinsic reason that may increase life stress rather than decrease it.

There are many meaningful types of recreation.

www.mhhe.com/phys_fit/webreview19 Click 03

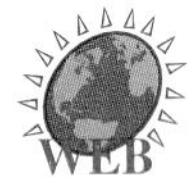

Many recreational activities involve moderate to vigorous physical activity. If fitness is the goal, these activities should be chosen. Involvement in nonphysical activities also constitutes recreation. For example, reading is a participation activity that can contribute significantly to other wellness dimensions, such as emotional/mental and spiritual. Passive involvement (spectating) is a third type of participation.

Passive participation has been criticized by some people who feel that active participation is an important ingredient of meaningful recreation. Experts are quick to point out that spectating can be very refreshing and meaningful. For example, watching a good play at the theater qualifies as meaningful recreation and could be true leisure. Likewise, active participation in community theater can be meaningful recreation. To achieve the wellness benefits of recreation, liberal participation and meaningful passive involvement (spectating) are encouraged. Involvement as a spectator does not preclude active participation. However, since free time available for recreation is often limited, excessive spectating can result in decreased active participation. Recent statistics indicate that much of the increase in recreational spending over the past five years is associated with physical activities as evidenced by dramatic increases in money spent for golfing, fitness and sports club memberships, and bowling.

Television viewing has its limitations but is not without its advantages as a recreational activity.

Television is a free-time activity that deserves special mention. Evidence presented elsewhere in this book shows that people who spend a great deal of time watching television tend to be fatter and less physically active than people who spend less time watching television. On the other hand, 58 percent of adults feel that watching television is a "good" use of free time. Nevertheless, as many as four in 10 people feel that they watch too much television. According to a recent Gallup poll, television is still the favorite way to spend an evening for most Americans, and more people feel that television is good rather than bad for society. Like other activities, it can qualify as leisure and recreation, and for many people can be useful in stress reduction.

The Facts about Time Management

Effective time management is essential to adapting to the stresses of modern living.

Many people in our culture lead stress-filled lives and see the need for lifestyle changes but fail to carry out their plans for various reasons. Most often mentioned is the lack of time. "I would like to exercise, but I don't have the time." "My two jobs don't allow me as much time as I would like to spend with my family." "I know I need to relax and enjoy myself, but I just can't find the time." You may never find time to do all of the things you want to do, but you can learn to manage time more effectively to help you cope with the stresses of daily living. In Lab 19E you will get the opportunity to practice the time-management skills outlined in the section that follows.

There are some steps that can be followed to help you manage your time effectively.

Step 1—Establish Priorities

Analyze what you value in life. Most Americans indicate that they want to reduce time spent in work-related activities and spend more time in recreation, at leisure, and with family or friends. Make a list of your priorities. Are these priorities currently being met? Are there activities for which you would like to have more time? Are there people with whom you would like to spend more time?

Step 2—Monitor Your Current Time Use

What we say we value does not always provide the basis for the way we spend our time. Keep a daily log of actual time expenditures to help you see how you could save time to devote to activities you value.

Step 3—Analyze Your Current Time Use

Each day has only 24 hours, and time available for daily activities is fixed. To have more time for priorities, schedules must be modified. Analysis of daily logs can help you determine how you spend your time. Ask yourself these questions:

- *In what activities can I spend less time?* Be honest. It's easy to say you'll spend less time on work, but can you really do it? Sometimes committed time other than work can be the problem. For example, some joggers spend so much time running that they have less time to spend with family.
- *What can I do to reduce time spent in these activities?* Maybe you can "kill two birds with one stone." For example, recreational time could be used to build fitness. Recreational time could also be family time (e.g., jog with the family). The key is finding activities that truly fulfill priorities for everyone involved. Finding work or recreational activities closer to home may save time.

Step 4—Make a Schedule

Writing a daily schedule can help you use time more effectively. This will allow you to enjoy life as a result of meeting priorities and spending time doing the things that enrich life for you and others important to you. A schedule should not be a rigid plan; it should be flexible enough to allow spontaneous activities.

If you cannot adhere to your time schedule, it should be modified. Your plan may not be realistic, and trying to adhere to it could cause you stress. In that case, the schedule is a problem rather than a solution to a problem.

Committed time can also be free time. It is possible to make a commitment to reserve time for activities that are important to you. Taking the time to "re-create" yourself or to enjoy family and friends is important. Sometimes the only way to "find the time" is to plan for it. Charts for helping you manage time effectively are provided in Lab 19E accompanying this concept.

Strategies for Action: Steps for Stress Management

There are some steps that you can follow to effectively manage stress.

Because everyone responds differently to stressful situations, stress management is a highly individual process. What works for one person may not work for you. The following facts provide steps to manage stress.

The first step in managing stress is to recognize the causes and to be aware of the symptoms.

You need to recognize the situations in your life that are the stressors. Try to identify the things that make you feel "stressed-out." Everything from minor irritations, such as traffic jams, to major life changes, such as births, deaths, or job loss, can be stressors. Or a stress overload of just too many demands on your time can make you feel that you are no longer in control. You may feel so overwhelmed that you become depressed.

Make yourself aware of how your body feels when you are under stress. Are your muscles beginning to tighten? Are you gritting your teeth, gripping the steering wheel tightly, drumming your fingers, tapping your foot, or hunching your shoulders? Can you feel your heart beating faster, your breathing rate becoming faster and more shallow? Are you perspiring, shaking, or getting a headache? By being aware of your most common stressors you will have a better chance of avoiding them or learning how to cope with them. In Lab 19A you will have the opportunity to evaluate muscle tension.

Play Play is something one does of his/her own free will. The play experience is fun, intrinsically rewarding, and a self-absorbing means of self-expression. It is characterized by a sense of freedom or escape from life's normal rules.

The second step is to use some type of relaxation technique or coping strategy for relief of stress.

www.mhhe.com/phys_fit/webreview19 Click 04

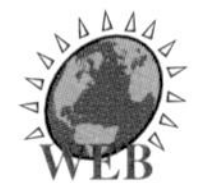

When you are aware of what stress does to your body, you can do something to relieve those symptoms immediately as well as on a regular and more long-term basis. While there is no magical cure for stress or tension, there are a variety of therapeutic approaches that may be effective in helping you cope with stress. These approaches can slow your heart and respiration, relax tense muscles, clear your mind, and help you relax mentally and emotionally. Perhaps most importantly, these techniques can improve your outlook and help you better cope with the stressful situation. In Lab 19B you will perform a progressive relaxation program. Performing Lab 19B only once will not prepare you to use relaxation techniques effectively. Remember, learning to relax is a skill that must be practiced.

Some treatments are less desirable than others because they act only as "crutches" or "fire extinguishers" and do not get at the root of the problem. Hypnosis may lead to fantasy and dependency. Alcoholic beverages, tranquilizers, and painkillers may give temporary relief and may be prescribed by a physician as part of the treatment, but they do not resolve the problem and may even mask symptoms or cause further problems such as addiction. Drugs do not provide a long-term solution to chronic stress or tension. Contrary to vitamin and mineral advertisements, there are no proven benefits to supplementing the diet with vitamin C or so-called "stress" vitamin formulations. Several different passive relaxation techniques were described earlier, such as massage, heat, deep breathing, and music.

Of course, using coping strategies and finding social support as described earlier in the concept are critical to successful stress management. In Lab 19C you will assess some of your current coping strategies. In Lab 19D you will assess your current support system to help you determine ways in which you can improve it.

The third step is to seek solutions for avoiding or controlling the stress in your life.

While some stressors are unavoidable, much of the stress that we face on a daily basis is self-inflicted and may be somewhat preventable. By taking active control over your lifestyle, you can reduce your risks of experiencing additional stress. Seeking balance and moderation in your lifestyle are good guides toward minimizing stress. Give some priority to proper rest, recreational activities, and diversion in order to prevent burnout. Diversion can be a temporary change from one activity to another (e.g., change from studying to mowing the lawn) or a change of scenery.

Depending on your situation and personality, reducing future exposure to stress may require additional changes in your work habits or interaction style. For example, if you are a person who responds to stress by working harder, then better time management may be an important way to prevent additional stress. If you are a person who can't say no, then assertiveness training may be beneficial. You may even need a change of job or a vacation.

The fourth step is to be as fit and healthy as possible.

The more fit and healthy you are, the better able you are to cope with stress. Selye suggested that physical fitness serves as an inoculation against stress; others have called it a "buffer." A healthy diet and proper rest also are important in managing stress. Leading a healthy lifestyle can help you cope with current stressors and can also help you avoid additional stress in the future.

The fifth step is to change your way of thinking.

Research suggests that it is possible to reduce stress by "changing the way you think." At one time or another, virtually all people have "distorted thinking" that can create unnecessary stress. Distorted thinking is also referred to as "negative or automatic thinking." To alleviate stress, it can be useful to recognize some of the common types of distorted thinking. If you can learn to recognize distorted thinking, you can change the way you think and in many cases reduce your stress levels. Some common types of distorted thinking are listed in Table 3.

If you have ever used any of the ten types of distorted thinking described in Table 3, you may find it useful to consider different methods of "untwisting" your thinking. Using the strategies for untwisting your thinking (see Table 4) can be useful in changing negative thinking to positive thinking.

If you really want to change your way of thinking to avoid stress, you may have to practice the guidelines outlined in Table 4. To do this, you can think of a recent situation that caused stress. It can be useful to describe the situation on paper, then try to see if you used distorted thinking in the situation (see Table 3). If so, write down which types of distorted thinking you used. Finally, determine if any of the

Table 3 Checklist of Cognitive Distortion

Type of Cognitive Distortion	Description
1. All or None Thinking	You look at things in absolute, black-and-white categories.
2. Overgeneralization	You view a negative event as a never-ending pattern of defeat.
3. Mental Filter	You dwell on the negatives and ignore the positives.
4. Discounting the Positives	You insist that your accomplishments and positive qualities don't count.
5. Jumping to Conclusions	(A) Mind reading–You assume that others are reacting negatively to you when there is no definite evidence of this; (B) Fortune telling—You arbitrarily predict that things will turn out badly.
6. Magnification or Minimization	You blow things out of proportion or shrink their importance inappropriately.
7. Emotional Reasoning	You reason from how you *feel:* "I feel like an idiot, so I must be one." Or "I don't *feel* like doing this, so I'll put it off."
8. "Should Statements"	You criticize yourself or other people with "shoulds" or "shouldn'ts." "Musts," "oughts," and "have tos" are similar offenders.
9. Labeling	You identify with your shortcomings. Instead of saying, "I made a mistake" you tell yourself "I am a jerk," or "a fool," or a "loser."
10. Personalization and Blame	You blame yourself for something that you weren't entirely responsible for, or you blame other people and overlook ways that your own attitudes and behaviors might contribute to the problem.

From David D. Burns, *The Feeling Good Handbook,* New York: Plume Books, 1999, used by permission.

Table 4 Ten Ways to Untwist Your Thinking

The 10 Ways	Description
1. Identify the Distortion	Write down your negative thoughts so you can see which of the 10 cognitive distortions you're involved in. This will make it easier to think about the problem in a more positive and realistic way.
2. Examine the Evidence	Instead of assuming that your negative thought is true, if you feel that you never do anything right, you could list several things that you have done successfully.
3. The Double-Standard Method	Instead of putting yourself down in a harsh, condemning way, talk to yourself in the same compassionate way you would talk to a friend with a similar problem.
4. The Experimental Technique	Do an experiment to test the validity of your negative thought. For example, if during an episode of panic, you become terrified that you're about to die of a heart attack, you could jog or run up and down several flights of stairs. This will prove that your heart is healthy and strong.
5. Thinking in Shades of Gray	Although this method might sound drab, the defects can be illuminating. Instead of thinking about your problems in all-or-none extremes, evaluate things on a range from 0 to 100. When things don't work out as well as you hoped, think about the experience as a partial success rather than a complete failure. See what you can learn from the situation.
6. The Survey Method	Ask people questions to find out if your thoughts and attitudes are realistic. For example, if you believe that public speaking anxiety is abnormal and shameful, ask several friends if they ever felt nervous before they gave a talk.
7. Define Terms	When you label yourself "inferior" or "a fool" or "a loser," ask, "What is the definition of 'a fool'? You will feel better when you see that there is no such thing as "a fool" or "a loser."
8. The Semantic Method	Simply substitute language that is less colorful or emotionally loaded. This method is helpful for "should statements." Instead of telling yourself "I *shouldn't* have made that mistake," you can say, "It would be better if I hadn't made that mistake."
9. Re-attribution	Instead of automatically assuming that you are "bad" and blaming yourself entirely for a problem, think about the many factors that may have contributed to it. Focus on solving the problem instead of using up all your energy blaming yourself and feeling guilty.
10. Cost-Benefit Analysis	List the advantages and disadvantages of a feeling (like getting angry when your plane is late), a negative thought (like "No matter how hard I try, I always screw up"), or a behavior pattern (like overeating and lying around in bed when you are depressed). You can also use the Cost-Benefit Analysis to modify a self-defeating belief such as, "I must always try to be perfect."

From David D. Burns, *The Feeling Good Handbook,* New York: Plume Books, 1999, used by permission.

guidelines in Table 4 would have been useful. If so, write down the strategy you could have used. When a similar situation arises, you will be prepared to deal with the stressful situation. Repeat this technique, using several situations that have recently caused stress.

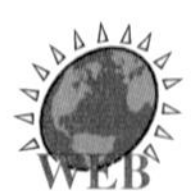

Web Review

Web review materials for Concept 19 are available at *www.mhhe.com/phys_fit/webreview19 Click 05.*

American Institute of Stress
www.stress.org

American Psychological Association
www.apa.org

International Stress Management Association
www.stress-management-isma.org

National Institute of Mental Health
www.nimh.nih.gov

Suggested Readings

Babyak, M. et al. "Exercise Treatment for Major Depression: Maintenance of Therapeutic Benefit at 10 months." *Psychosomatic Medicine.* (62)(5) (2000): 633–638.

Blonna, R. *Coping with Stress in a Changing World.* St. Louis: McGraw-Hill, 1999.

Burns, D. D. *The Feeling Good Handbook.* rev. ed. New York: Plume/Penguin Books, 1999.

Coleman, D., and Gurin, J., eds. *Mind/Body Medicine.* Fairfield, OH: Consumer Reports Books, 1993.

Corbin, D. E. (ed.). *Perspectives: Stress Management.* Boulder, CO: Coursewise Publishing Co., 1999.

Davis, M. et al. *The Relaxation and Stress Reduction Workbook.* 5th ed. Oakland, CA: New Harbinger, 2000.

Girdano, D., and Everly, G. *Controlling Stress and Tension.* 6th ed. Needham Heights, MA: Allyn and Bacon, Inc., 2001.

Greenberg, J. S. *Comprehensive Stress Management.* 7th ed. St.Louis: McGraw-Hill, 2002.

Jacobson, E. *You Must Relax.* New York: McGraw-Hill, 1978.

O'Grady, D. *Taking the Fear Out of Change.* Rainier, WA: Adams Publishing, 1995.

Ortal, M., and Sherman, C. "Exercise Against Depression," *The Physician and Sports Medicine.* 26(10)(1998):55.

Petruzzello, S. et al. "A Meta-Analysis on the Anxiety-Reducing Effects of Acute and Chronic Exercise," *Sports Medicine.* 11(1991):143–182.

Roizen, M. F., and Stephenson, E. A. "Want to Live Longer? Here's Exactly How!" *Prevention,* 1 April 2000.

Rutherford, M. et al. "Pal Power: If Friends Are Gifts We Give Ourselves, It's Good to Be Greedy. Hold On to What You've Got—and Grab Some More." *Time,* 13 November 2000.

Selye, H. *The Stress of Life.* 2nd ed. New York: McGraw-Hill, 1978.

U.S. Department of Health and Human Services, *Healthy People 2010.* 2nd ed. With *Understanding and Improving Health* and *Objectives for Improving Health.* 2 vols. Washington, DC: U.S. Government Printing Office, November 2000, Chapter 18, "Mental Health and Mental Disorders."

Williams, R., and Williams, V. *Anger Kills: 17 Strategies for Controlling Hostility That Can Harm You.* New York: Harper Collins Publishers Inc., 1999.

Physical Fitness News Update

The physical health benefits of exercise have been well established for some time. More recent research suggests that the benefits of exercise extend beyond the physical and into the realm of mental health. Studies have demonstrated that exercise can reduce anxiety, aid in recovery from depression, and assist in efforts to eliminate negative health behaviors such as smoking.

Exercise and Anxiety

There is considerable evidence in nonclinical samples that exercise leads to reductions in anxiety. One recent study found that exercise may also be effective in reducing anxiety among individuals with panic disorder. An aerobic exercise program lead to reductions in panic symptoms relative to a control group. Although exercise was not as effective as medication, it may be a useful addition to other treatment methods for anxiety disorders.

Exercise and Depression

A randomized clinical trial compared antidepressant medication with aerobic exercise, and a combined antidepressant and exercise condition in the treatment of major depressive disorder. Results indicated that the aerobic exercise group faired as well as the other two at the end of treatment. In addition, patients in the exercise only condition were less likely to have a remission to depression at six-month follow-up. It is possible that individuals in the exercise condition felt more responsible for the improvements in their condition and this increase in self-efficacy lead to better long-term outcomes.

Exercise and Health-Risk Behaviors

A recent study tested vigorous exercise as an adjunct to a cognitive-behavioral smoking cessation program for women. The results indicated that women who received the exercise intervention were able to sustain continuous abstinence from smoking for a longer period of time relative to those who did not receive the exercise intervention. Women in the exercise condition also gained less weight during smoking cessation.

Lab 19B: Relaxing Tense Muscles

Name **Section** **Date**

Purpose: To learn how to relax tense muscles.

Procedure:

Part I

1. Lie on your back in a quiet, nondistracting atmosphere while you are learning this relaxation technique. (Later, you will want to be able to use the technique in public, everyday situations, while you are at work, or any time you are under stress.) Get as comfortable as possible. Close your eyes.
2. Do the Contract-Relax Exercise Routine for Relaxation. Contract the muscles to a moderate level of tension (do not use maximum contractions) as you inhale for 5 to 7 seconds. Study where you are feeling the tension. Try to keep the tension isolated to the designated muscle group without allowing it to spill over to other muscles. Use the dominant side of the body first; repeat on the nondominant side.
3. Next, release the tension completely, instantly relaxing the muscles, and exhale. Extend the feeling of relaxation throughout your muscles for 20 to 30 seconds before contracting again. Think of relaxation words like "warm," "calm," "peaceful," and "serene."
4. If time permits, you should practice each muscle group two to five times (until tension is gone) before proceeding to the next group. In a class, you may only have time for one trial. For home practice, do the routine twice a day for 15 minutes.

Contract-Relax Exercise Routine for Relaxation

1. Hand and forearm—Contract your right hand, making a fist; hold 3 counts; relax and keep letting go 6–10 counts. Repeat, then do left fist, then both fists.
2. Biceps—Flex both elbows and contract your biceps; hold 3 counts; relax and continue relaxing 6–10 counts. Repeat.
3. Triceps—Extend both elbows, contract the triceps on the back of the arm. Hold 3 counts; relax 6–10 counts. Repeat.
4. Relax both hands, forearms, and upper arms.
5. Forehead—Raise your eyebrows and wrinkle your forehead; hold 3 counts; relax and continue relaxing 6–10 counts.
6. Cheeks and nose—Make a face; wrinkle your nose and squint; hold 3 counts; relax and continue relaxing 6–10 counts.
7. Jaws—Clench your teeth 3 counts; relax 6–10 counts.
8. Lips and tongue—With teeth apart, press lips together and press tongue to roof of mouth; hold 3 counts; relax 6–10 counts.
9. Neck and throat—Push head backward while tucking chin, pushing against floor or pillow if lying down; if sitting, push against high chairback; hold 3 counts; relax for 6–10 counts.
10. Relax forehead, cheeks, nose, jaws, lips, tongue, neck, and throat. Relax hands, forearms, and upper arms.
11. Shoulder and upper back—Hunch shoulders to ears; hold 3 counts; relax 6–10 counts.
12. Relax lips, tongue, neck, throat, shoulders, and upper back.
13. Abdomen—Suck in abdomen; hold 3 counts; relax 6–10 counts.
14. Lower back—Contract and arch the back; hold 3 counts; relax 6–10 counts.
15. Thighs and buttocks—Squeeze your buttocks together and push your heels into the floor (if lying down) or against a chair rung (if sitting); hold 3 counts; relax 6–10 counts.
16. Relax shoulders and upper back, abdomen, lower back, thighs, and buttocks.
17. Calves—Pull instep and toes toward shins; hold 3 counts; relax 6–10 counts.
18. Toes—Curl toes; hold 3 counts; relax 6–10 counts.
19. Relax every muscle in your body.

**Note:* Eventually, you should progress to a combination of muscle groups and gradually eliminate the "contract" phase of the program. Refer to Jacobson (1978) or Greenberg (1996).

Part II Perform each of the relaxation exercises that follow (see page 365 for pictures).

1. **Neck Stretch**—Roll the head slowly in a half-circle from 9:00 to 8:00 to 7, 6, 5, 4, and 3, then reverse from 3 to 9. Close your eyes and feel the stretch. Do *not* make a full circle by tipping the head back. Repeat several times.
2. **Shoulder Lift**—Hunch the shoulders as high as possible (contract) and then let them drop (relax). Repeat several times. Inhale on the lift; exhale on the drop.
3. **Trunk Stretch and Drop**—Stand and reach as high as possible; tiptoe and stretch every muscle, then collapse completely, letting knees flex and trunk, head, and arms dangle. Repeat two or three times. Inhale on the stretch and exhale on the collapse.
4. **Trunk Swings**—Following the trunk stretch and drop, remain in the "drop" position and with a minimum of muscular effort, set the trunk swinging from side to side by shifting the weight from one foot to the other, letting the heels come off the floor alternately. Keep the entire body (especially the neck) limp.
5. **Tension Contrast**—With arms extended overhead, lie on your side. Tense the body as stiff as a board, then let go and relax, letting the body fall either forward or backward in whatever direction it loses balance. Continue letting go for a few seconds after falling and allow yourself to feel like you are still sinking. Repeat on the other side.

Results:

Yes No Did you find the relaxation exercises effective?

Yes No Do you think you would find them useful as part of your normal daily routine or as a "quick fix" for stress?

Yes No Did you find the contract-relax exercise routine relaxing?

Yes No Do you think you would find it useful as part of your normal daily routine or as a "quick fix" for stress?

Conclusions and Implications:

In several sentences, discuss whether or not you feel that relaxation exercises will be a part of your wellness program.

Lab 19C: Evaluating Coping Strategies

Name | Section | Date

Purpose: To learn how to use appropriate coping strategies that work best for you.

Procedures:

1. Think of five recent stressful experiences that caused you some concern, anxiety, or distress. Describe these situations in Chart 1. Then use Chart 2 to make a rating for changeability, severity, and duration. Assign one number for each category for each situation.
2. In Chart 3 place a check for each coping strategy that you used in coping with each of the five situations you described.
3. Answer the questions in the Conclusions and Implications section.

Results:

Chart 1 Stressful Situations

Think of five different recent stressful situations. Appraise each situation and assign a score (changeable, severity, duration) using the scale in Chart 2.

	Briefly describe the situation.	Changeable	Severity	Duration
1.				
2.				
3.				
4.				
5.				

Chart 2 Appraisal of the Stressful Situations

Use this chart to rate the five situations you described above. Assign a number for changeability, severity, and duration for each situation in Chart 1.

	1.	2.	3.	4.	5.
Was the situation changeable?	Completely within my control	Mostly within my control	Both in and out of my control	Mostly out of my control	Completely outside of my control
What was the severity of the stress?	Very minor	Fairly minor	Moderate	Fairly major	Very major
What was the duration of the stress?	Short-term (weeks)	Moderately short	Moderate (months)	Moderately long	Long (months to year)

Chart 3 Coping Strategies

Directions: Place a check for each coping strategy you used for each of the five situations you described.

Think about your response to the five stressful situations you recently experienced and check the strategies that you used in each situation.	Situation	Situation	Situation	Situation	Situation
Coping Strategy	1	2	3	4	5
1. I apologized or corrected the problem as best I could.					
2. I ignored the problem and hoped that it would go away.					
3. I told myself to forget about it and grew as a person from the experience.					
4. I tried to make myself feel better by eating, drinking, or smoking.					
5. I prayed or sought spiritual meaning from the situation.					
6. I expressed anger to try to change the situation.					
7. I took active steps to make things work out better.					
8. I used music, images, or deep breathing to help me relax.					
9. I tried to keep my feelings to myself and kept moving forward.					
10. I pursued leisure or recreational activity to help me feel better.					
11. I talked to someone who could provide advice or help me with the problem.					
12. I talked to someone about what I was feeling or experiencing.					

Conclusions and Implications:

1. In several sentences, discuss the coping strategies you used. Were they the ones you used the most? The ones you typically use? Were they effective? Would you consider other strategies in the future?

Lab 19D: Evaluating Levels of Social Support

Name	Section	Date

Purpose:
To evaluate your level of social support and to identify ways that you can find additional support.

Procedures:
1. Use Chart 1 to get personal social support scores. Answer each question. Place number of answers in score box. Sum these questions for each score.
2. In the Results section, record your scores and rate your social support (use Chart 2 for ratings).
3. Use Chart 2 to evaluate the quality and nature of your social support network.
4. Answer the questions in the Conclusions and Implications section.

Chart 1 Social Support Questionnaire

The following questions assess various aspects of social support. Base your answer on your actual degree of support, not on the type of support that you would like to have. Place a check in the space that best represents what is true for you.

	Not True	Somewhat True	Very True	
	1	2	3	Score
1. I have close personal ties with my relatives.				
2. I have close relationships with a number of friends.				
3. I have a deep and meaningful relationship with a spouse or close friend.				
Access to social support score:				
4. I have parents and relatives who take the time to listen and understand me.				
5. I have friends or co-workers whom I can confide in and trust when problems come up.				
6. I have a nonjudgmental spouse or close friend who supports me when I need help.				
Degree of social support score:				
7. I feel comfortable asking others for advice or assistance.				
8. I have confidence in my social skills and enjoy opportunities for new social contacts.				
9. I am willing to open up and discuss my personal life with others.				
Getting social support score:				

Scores and Ratings (Use Chart 2 to obtain ratings).

Access to social support score		Rating	
Degree of social support score		Rating	
Getting social support score		Rating	
Total social support score (sum of three scores)		Rating	

Results:

Chart 2 Rating Scale for Social Support

Rating	Item Scores	Total Score
High	8–9	24–27
Moderate	6–7	18–23
Low	Below 6	Below 18

Conclusions and Implications:

1. In several sentences, discuss your overall social support. Do you think your scores and ratings are a true representation of your social support?

2. In several sentences, describe any changes you think you should make to improve your social support system. If you do not think change is necessary, explain why.

Lab 19E: Time Management

Name	Section	Date

Purpose: To help you learn to manage time to meet personal priorities.

Procedure:

1. Follow the four steps outlined in Chart 1 in the Results section.
2. Answer the questions in the Conclusions and Implications section.

Results:

Chart 1 Time Management

Step 1: Establishing Priorities

1. Check circles that reflect your priorities from the list below. Add priorities as necessary.
2. Rate each of the priorities you checked. Use a 1 for highest priority, a 2 for moderate priority, and 3 for low priority.

Check Priorities	*Rating*	*Check Priorities*	*Rating*	*Check Priorities*	*Rating*
◯ more time with family		◯ more time with boy/girlfriend		◯ more time with spouse	
◯ more time for leisure		◯ more time to relax		◯ more time to study	
◯ more time for work success		◯ more time for physical activity		◯ more time to improve myself	
◯ more time for other recreation		◯ other ________		◯ other ________	

Step 2: Monitor Current Time Use

1. On the daily calendar, keep track of daily time expenditure
2. Write in exactly what you did for each time block.

7–9 A.M.	9–11 A.M.	11A.M.–1 P.M.	1–3 P.M.
3–5 P.M.	5–7 P.M.	7–9 P.M.	9–11 P.M.

Chart 1 Time Management *(continued)*

Step 3: Analyze Your Current Time Use

Where can I spend less time? (write below)	Where do I need to spend more time? (write below)

Step 4: Make a Schedule. Write in Your Planned Activities for the Day.

7–9 A.M.	9–11 A.M.	11A.M.–1 P.M.	1–3 P.M.
3–5 P.M.	5–7 P.M.	7–9 P.M.	9–11 P.M.

Conclusions and Implications:

In several sentences, discuss how you might modify your schedule to find more time for important priorities.

Section VII

Making Informed Choices

Concept 20

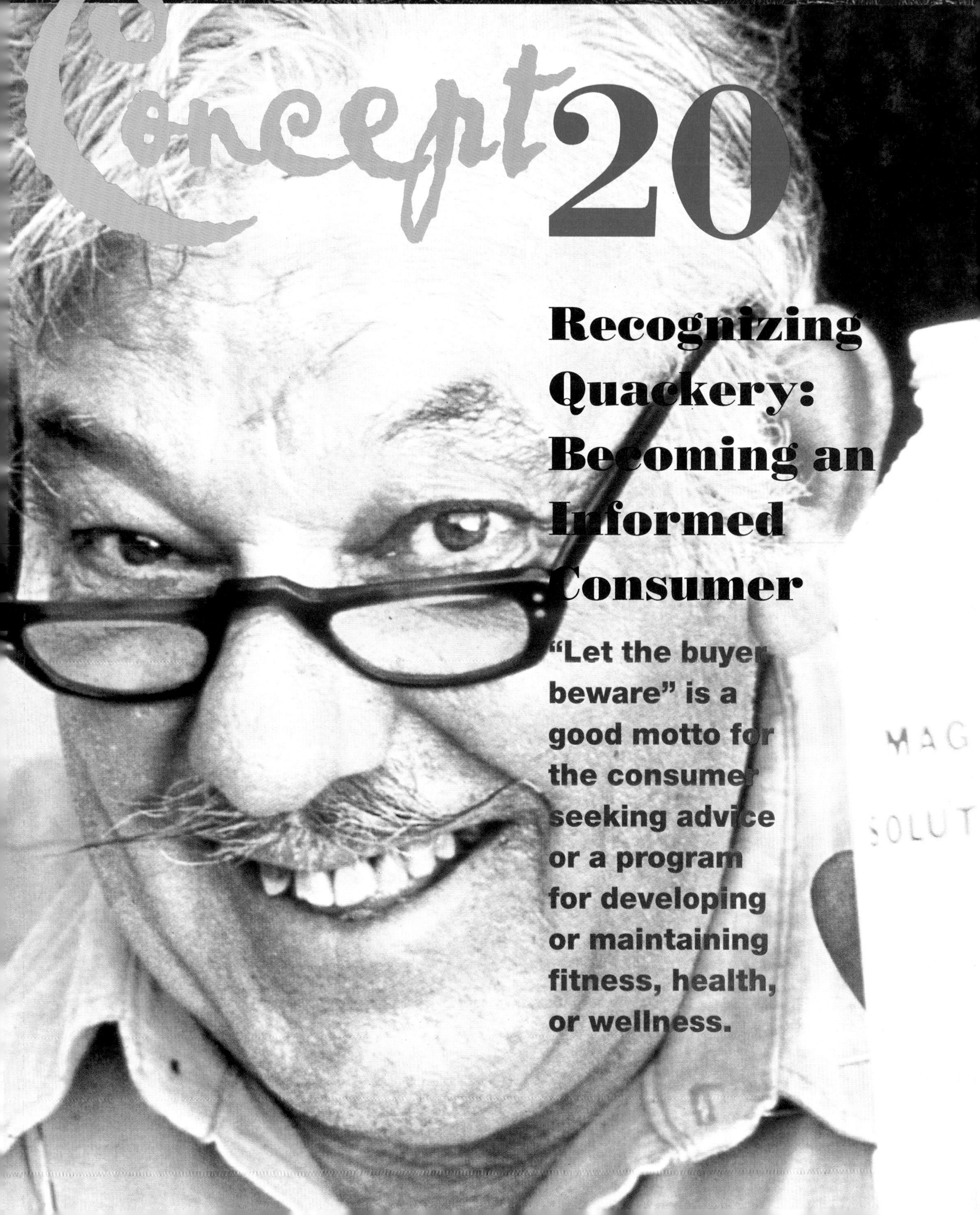

Recognizing Quackery: Becoming an Informed Consumer

"Let the buyer beware" is a good motto for the consumer seeking advice or a program for developing or maintaining fitness, health, or wellness.

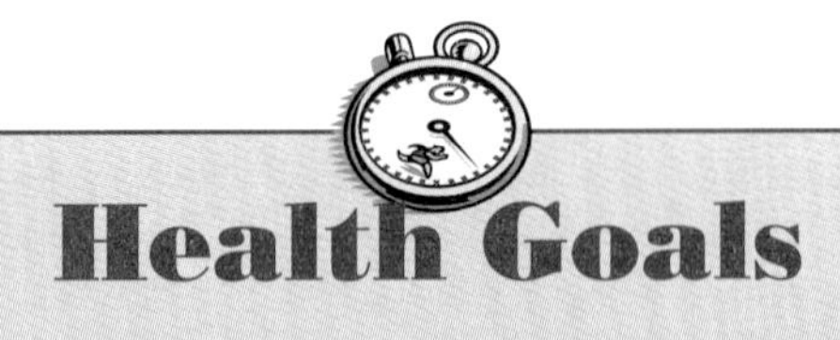

for year 2010

Increase the number of college and university students who receive information on priority health-risk behaviors.

Improve health literacy and increase access to public health information.

Increase health communication activities that include research and evaluation.

Increase adoption and maintenance of appropriate daily physical activity.

Increase proportion of people who meet national dietary guidelines.

Promote healthy and safe communities.

Introduction

People have always searched for the fountain of youth and the easy, quick, and miraculous route to health and happiness. This search has included the area of physical fitness, especially physical activity, nutrition, and weight loss. Because of the popularity of these subjects, the mass media have made it possible to convey as much misinformation as information. All people should seek the truth to protect their health as well as their pocketbooks. This concept discusses some myths and separates fact from fancy.

The Facts about Physical Activity

> Physical activity has many benefits, but it is not a cure all.

Popular books and magazines, television infomercials, and the general media bombard the public with incorrect information about physical activity. The information provided in this book documents the many benefits of physical activity, but it is not a **panacea.** Be suspicious of programs and products that make claims that seem impossible to believe. Consider these general guidelines when making consumer decisions.

- Optimal benefits occur if you select activities from each of the first three levels of the physical activity pyramid.
- Follow the FIT formula for each type of physical activity. Programs that promise complete fitness but do not meet the necessary levels for frequency, intensity, and time, should be strongly questioned.
- Reject programs that promise total fitness in only a few minutes a week, or promise instant benefits.
- Reject programs that promise instant fat loss or promise increases in the size of glands (e.g., breasts).
- Reject programs that promise changes in size of bony structures (e.g., ankles).
- Reject programs that promise "effortless exercise." If it is totally effortless or passive, it is not likely to produce benefits (see section on passive exercise and baths).
- Avoid programs that include dangerous exercises (see Concept 12).
- Be sure that a program provides the benefits that are important to you. Some programs may be beneficial for one reason but not for another. For example, Hatha yoga fails to meet some of the claims made for it. It does not help you lose weight, trim inches, strengthen the glands and organs, or cure health propblems such as the common cold or arthritis. It can be useful, however, in reducing stress, promoting relaxation, and improving flexibility.
- Be wary of claims for exercise machines and health and fitness clubs that make unrealistic promises (see sections on machines/baths and health clubs).
- Be espcially wary of people who make unrealistic promises and stand to gain financially from selling you something.

> Getting rid of cellulite does not require a special exercise, diet, cream or device, as some books and advertisements insist.

Cellulite is ordinary fat with a fancy name. You do not need a special treatment or device to get rid of it. In fact, there is no special "remedy." Fat is fat. To decrease fat, reduce calories and do more physical activity.

> Spot reducing, or losing fat from a specific location on the body, is not possible. It is a fallacy.

When you do physical activity, calories are burned and fat is recruited from all over the body in a genetically determined pattern. You cannot selectively exercise, bump, vibrate, or squeeze the fat from a particular spot. If you were flabby to begin with, local exercise could strengthen the local muscles, causing a change in the contour and the girth of that body part. But exercise affects the muscles, not the fat on that body part. General aerobic exercises are the most effective for burning fat, but you cannot control where the fat comes off.

Surgically sculpting the body with implants and liposuction to acquire physical beauty will not give you physical fitness and may be harmful.

Rather than doing it the hard way, an increasing number of people are having their "love handles" removed surgically and fake calf and pectoral muscles implanted to improve their physique. Liposuction is not a weight loss technique, but rather a contouring procedure. Like any surgery, it is not without risks. There have been fatalities and there is a risk of infection, hematoma, skin slough, and other conditions.

Muscle implants give a muscular appearance, but they do not make you stronger or more fit. The implants are not really muscle tissue, but rather silicon gel or saline such as that used in breast implants, or a hard substitute. Some complications can occur, such as infection and bleeding, but also, some physicians believe the calf implant may put pressure on the calf muscles and cause them to atrophy. A better way to improve physique and fitness is proper exercise.

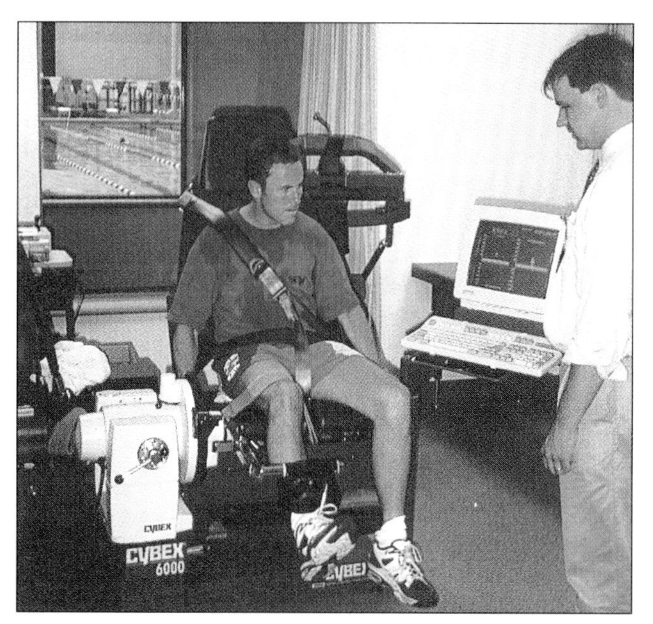

Doing machine exercises can help you recover from injury, but you must provide the movement—not the machine.

The use of hand weights and wrist weights while walking, running, dancing, or bench-stepping can increase the energy cost but requires caution.

There are a variety of devices that have been marketed for increasing the energy expenditure in activities such as walking, running, and other forms of aerobic exercise. Examples include wrist, arm, or ankle weights and small hand held weights. Step benches are another device that can be used to increase energy expenditure for aerobic exercise.

The practice of carrying small weights (not more than 1–3 pounds) while performing aerobic dance, walking, or other aerobic exercise has been found to increase the metabolic cost of the exercise. When the weight is simply carried, the effect is negligible, but when the arms are pumped (bending the elbow and raising the weight to shoulder height and then extending the elbow as the arm swings down), the energy output can increase enough to make a walk comparable to a slow jog. For the person who does not want to walk or jog faster or farther, it could be an effective way of burning more calories or increasing fitness. It may be better to use wrist weights than to carry a weight, since the act of gripping causes an increase in the diastolic blood pressure. Hand weights or wrist weights are more effective than ankle weights because weights that alter your gait pattern can be stressful to the knees. There are hazards to consider in using weights. Coronary patients and people with high blood pressure should be aware that using weights increases both the systolic and diastolic blood pressures. Aerobic dance participants may find it wise to keep the weights below shoulder level if they aggravate the shoulder joint. Anyone with shoulder or elbow joint problems such as arthritis should use weights with caution.

Perhaps a more important consideration is the enjoyment and perception of effort associated with an activity. Walking is a popular activity because it is not especially intense and still offers many health benefits. Though weights can result in more energy expended, if they also make less intense exercise seem too difficult, adding extra weight may result in decreased interest in performing the activity. Be careful not to make simple tasks seem more difficult than they should be. It is better to do less intense activity for a longer period of time rather than trying to make an activity more intense at the expense of regular participation.

If you are a walker you may want to consider using walking poles. Recent evidence suggests that walking poles (similar to canes, one held in each hand) allow faster and potenetially longer walks. Walking poles can also reduce the load on the legs. When you become fatigued, the use of walking poles can result in changes in your walking mechanics. For this reason it is important to be careful to walk with good form, especially when you get tired. For some people arm work is quite fatiguing. If this is true for you, poles may make walking seem more difficult and reduce your enjoyment of the activity.

Panacea A cure all; a remedy for all ills.

The step bench, as used in step-aerobics, was designed to increase the intensity of a work-out without the high impact of some types of aerobic dance. Small weights can also be used in most forms of aerobic dance activities to increase exercise intensity. Some experts suggest that for step-aerobics weights should be limited to intermediate and advanced exercisers because together the bench and the weights provide a double overload. Even for more advanced steppers, it is recommended that weights not exceed 1 to 2 pounds. Up to a point, the aerobic intensity can be increased by adding height to the bench (typically no more than 6–8 inches).

The Facts about Passive Exercise and Passive Devices

> Passive exercise is not effective in weight reduction, spot reduction, increasing strength, or increasing endurance.

WEB

www.mhhe.com/phys_fit/webreview20 Click 01

Passive exercise or devices come in a variety of forms.

- *Rolling machines*—These ineffective wooden or metal rollers, operated by an electric motor, roll up and down the body part to which they are applied. They do not remove, break up, or redistribute fat.
- *Vibrating belts*—These wide canvas or leather belts may be designed for the chin, hips, thighs, or abdomen. Driven by an electric motor, they jerk back and forth, causing loose tissue of the body part to shake. They do not have any beneficial effect on fitness, fat, or figure, and they are potentially harmful if used on the abdomen (especially if used by women during pregnancy, menstruation, or while an IUD is in place). They might also aggravate a back problem.
- *Vibrating tables and pillows*—Some of these quack devices are actually called toning tables. Contrary to advertisements, these passive devices will not improve posture, trim the body, reduce weight, nor will they develop muscle **tonus.** For some people, vibration can help induce relaxation.
- *Continuous Passive Motion (CPM) Tables*—The CPM table is motor driven, but unlike the vibrating table it moves body parts repeatedly through a range of motion. Tables are designed to do such things as passively extend the leg at the hip joint, raise the upper trunk in a sit-up–like motion, or rotate the legs while the client lies relaxed. Many of the same false claims are made for it as for the vibrating table. It also claims to remove cellulite, increase circulation and oxygen flow, and eliminate excess water retention. None of these claims is true, but the table might be justified in claiming to maintain the range of motion in certain body parts for people who cannot move themselves. A similar concept is incorporated in small, portable machines used in hospitals and rehabilitation centers to maintain range of motion in the legs of knee surgery patients, maintain integrity of the cartilage, and decrease the incidence of thrombosis. Certainly the normal, healthy person has nothing to gain from using such a device.
- *Motor-driven cycles and rowing machines*—Like all mechanical devices that do the work for the individual, these motor-driven machines are not effective in a fitness program. They may help increase circulation, and some may even help maintain flexibility, but they are not as effective as active exercise. *Nonmotorized cycles and rowing machines* are very good equipment for use in a fitness program.
- *Massage*—Whether done by a masseur/masseuse or by a mechanical device, massage is passive, requiring no effort on the part of the individual. It can help increase circulation, induce relaxation, prevent or loosen adhesions, retard muscle atrophy, and serve other therapeutic uses when administered in the clinical setting for medical reasons. However, massage has no useful role in a physical fitness program and will not alter your shape. There is no scientific evidence that it can hasten nerve growth, remove subcutaneous fat, or increase athletic performance. Some athletes (e.g., cyclists) find that it aids in recovery from exercise.
- *Electrical muscle stimulators*—Neuromuscular electrical stimulators cause the muscle to contract involuntarily. In the hands of qualified medical personnel, muscle stimulators are valuable therapeutic devices. They can increase muscle strength and endurance selectively and aid in the treatment of edema. They can also help prevent atrophy in a patient who is unable to move, and they may decrease spasticity and contracture, but in a healthy person they do not have the same value as exercise. The multiple muscle group stimulation as done in the so-called "toning" clinics or spas has been proven ineffective for muscle strengthening. These devices can be harmful when used improperly and may induce heart attacks; complicate gastrointestinal, orthopedic, kidney, and other disorders; and aggravate epilepsy, hernias, and varicose veins. They should never be used by the layperson and have no place in a reducing or fitness program.
- *Weighted belts*—Claims have been made that these belts reduce waists, thighs, and hips when worn for several hours under the clothing. In reality, they do none of these things and have been reported to cause actual physical harm. When used in a progressive resistance program, wristlet, anklet, or laced-on weights can help produce an overload and, therefore, develop strength or endurance.
- *Inflated, constricting, or nonporous garments*—These garments include rubberized inflated devices ("sauna belts" and "sauna shorts") and paraphernalia that are airtight plastic or rubberized. Evidence indicates that their girth-reducing claims are *unwarranted.* If exercise is performed while wearing such garments, the exercise,

not the garment, may be beneficial. You cannot squeeze fat out of the pores nor can you melt it!

- *Body wrapping*—Some reducing salons, gyms, or clubs advertise that wrapping the body in bandages soaked in a "magic solution" will cause a permanent reduction in body girth. This so-called treatment is pure quackery. Tight, constricting bands can temporarily indent the skin and squeeze body fluids into other parts of the body, but the skin or body will regain its original size within minutes or hours. The solution is usually similar to epsom salts, which can cause fluid to be drawn from tissue. The fluid is water, not fat, and is quickly replaced. Body wrapping may be dangerous to your health; at least one fatality has been documented.
- *Elastic tights*—These are often worn by athletes such as cyclists for the purpose of decreasing chaffing of the skin. There have been some claims that the tights helped improve venous return and thus recovery from exercise. However, studies have shown that the recovery-response of those who wear tights is no different from those who do not wear them.

Having a good tan is often associated with being fit and looking good, but getting tanned can be risky business.

www.mhhe.com/phys_fit/webreview20 Click 02

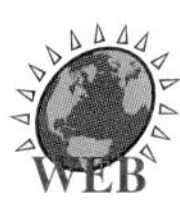

Tanning salons may claim their lamps are safe because they emit only UV-A rays, but these rays can age the skin prematurely and make it look wrinkled and leathery. It may also increase the cancer-producing potential of UV-B rays and cause eye damage. Since there is no warning sign of redness, there is danger of overdosing. Thirty minutes of exposure to UV-A can suppress the immune system. Tanning devices can also aggravate certain skin diseases. The **FDA** advises against the use of any suntan lamp. It is dangerous to use tanning accelerator lotions with the lamps because they can promote burning of the skin. Tanning pills are an even worse choice. They can cause itching, welts, hives, stomach cramps, and diarrhea, and can decrease night vision. Tanning in the sun is also hazardous because it damages the skin, making it age prematurely. It may cause skin cancer. It is best to use products with sun blockers if you must spend long periods in the sun.

The Facts about Baths

Saunas, steam baths, whirlpools, and hot tubs are not effective in weight reduction or in the prevention and cure of colds, arthritis, bursitis, backaches, sprains, or bruises.

Baths do not melt off fat; fat must be metabolized. The heat and humidity from baths may make you perspire, but it is water, not fat, oozing from the pores.

The effect of such baths is largely psychological, although some temporary relief from aches and pains may

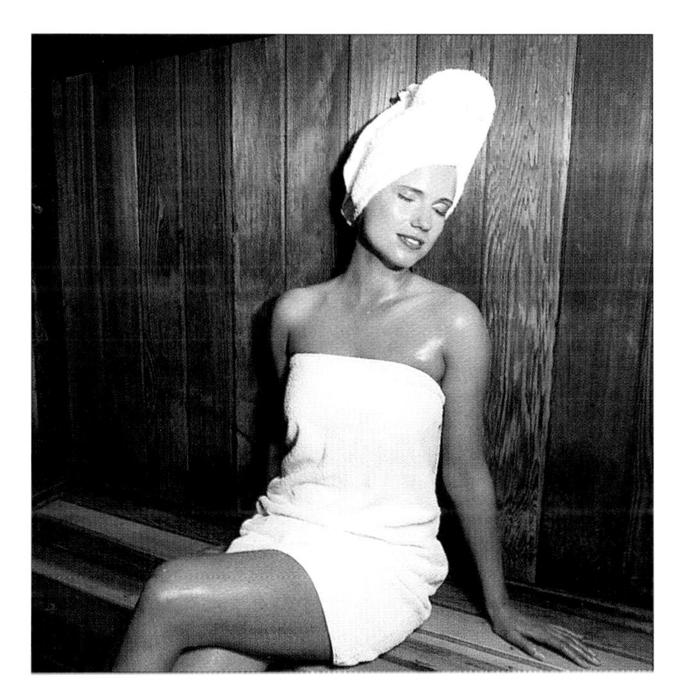

Saunas or other baths may help you relax, but they do not result in fat loss or fitness improvement.

Passive Exercise A type of exercise in which no voluntary muscle contraction occurs; some outside force moves the body part with no effort by the person.

Tonus The most frequently misused and abused term in fitness vocabularies. Tonus is the tension developed in a muscle as a result of passive muscle stretch. Tonus cannot be determined by feeling or inspecting a muscle. It has little or nothing to do with the strength of a muscle.

FDA Abbreviation for the Food and Drug Administration: a federal agency that recommends and enforces government regulations regarding certain foods and drugs.

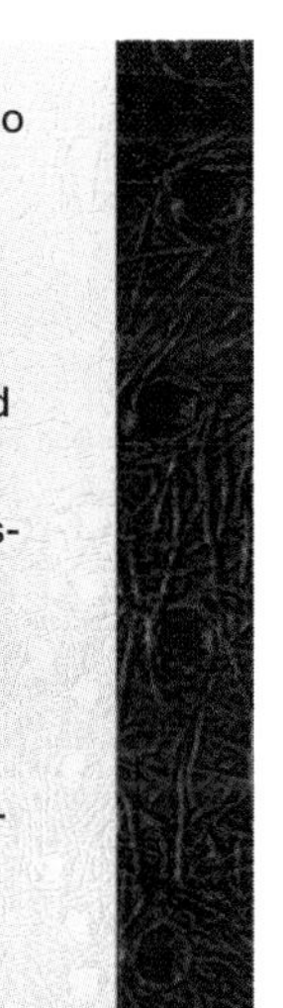

result from the heat. The same relief can be had by sitting in a tub of hot water in your bathroom.

> Various baths are potentially dangerous and should be used and maintained properly.

The following guidelines/precautions should be considered before using a sauna, steam bath, whirlpool, or hot tub:

- Take a soap shower before and after entering the bath.
- Don't wear makeup or skin lotion/oil.
- Wait at least an hour after eating before bathing.
- Cool down after exercise before entering the bath to avoid overheating.
- Drink plenty of water before or during the bath to avoid dehydration.
- Don't wear jewelry.
- Don't sit on a metal stool; do sit on a towel in the steam or sauna bath.
- Don't bathe alone.
- Don't drink alcohol before bathing.
- Get out immediately if you become dizzy; feel hot, chilled, or nauseous; or get a headache.
- Get approval from your physician if you have heart disease, low or high blood pressure, a fever, kidney disease, or diabetes, are obese or pregnant, or are on medications (especially anticoagulants, stimulants, hypnotics, narcotics, or tranquilizers).
- Prolonged use can be hazardous for the elderly or for children.
- Don't exercise in a sauna or steam bath.
- Skin infections can be spread in a bath; make certain it is cleaned regularly and that the hot tub or whirlpool has proper pH and chlorination.
- Follow these recommendations on temperature and duration of stay:

  Sauna: should not exceed 190°F (88°C) and duration should not exceed 10 to 15 minutes.

  Steam bath: should not exceed 120°F (49°C) and duration should not exceed 6 to 12 minutes.

  Whirlpool/hot tub: should not exceed 100°F (37°C) and duration should not exceed 5 to 10 minutes.

The Facts about Quacks

> You can usually tell the difference between an expert and a quack because a quack does not use scientific methods.

A good example of this fact is seen in a study that attempted to obtain documentation for products claiming to enhance athletic performance. It was found that there was no published scientific evidence to support the promotional claims of 42 percent of the products. Thirty-two percent had some scientific documentation but were marketed in a misleading manner, and 21 percent were without any human clinical trials.

Some of the ways to identify quacks, frauds, and rip-offs are to look for these clues:

- They do not use the scientific method of controlled experimentation that can be verified by other scientists.
- To a large extent, they use testimonials and anecdotes to support their claims rather than scientific methods. There is no such thing as a valid testimonial. Anecdotal evidence is no evidence at all.
- They advise you to buy something you would not otherwise have bought.
- They have something to sell.
- They claim everyone can benefit from the product or service they are selling. There is no such thing as a simple, quick, easy, painless remedy/tonic or other concoction that is good for many ailments or useful for conditions for which medical science has not yet found a remedy.
- They promise "quick," "miraculous" results. There is no such thing as a perfect no-risk treatment.
- The claims for benefits are broad, covering a wide variety of conditions.
- They may offer a money-back guarantee. A guarantee is only as good as the company.
- They may claim the treatment or product is approved by the FDA. *Note:* Federal law does not permit the mention of the FDA in any way that suggests marketing approval.
- They may claim the support of experts, but the experts are not identified.
- The ingredients or materials in the product may not be identified.
- They may claim there is a conspiracy against them by "bureaucrats," "organized medicine," the FDA, the **AMA,** and other experts and governmental bodies. Never believe a doctor who claims the medical community is persecuting him/her or that the government is suppressing a wonderful discovery.
- Their credentials may be irrelevant to the area in which they claim expertise.
- They use scare tactics, such as "if you don't do this, you will die of a heart attack."
- They may appear to be a sympathetic friend who wants to share with you a "new discovery."
- They may quote from a scientific journal or other legitimate source, but they misquote or quote out of context to mislead you; or they may mix a little bit of truth with a lot of fiction.
- They may cite research or quote from individuals or institutions that have questionable reputations for scientific truth.
- They may claim it is a "new discovery" (usually it is said to have originated in Europe). There is never a great medical breakthrough that debuts in an obscure

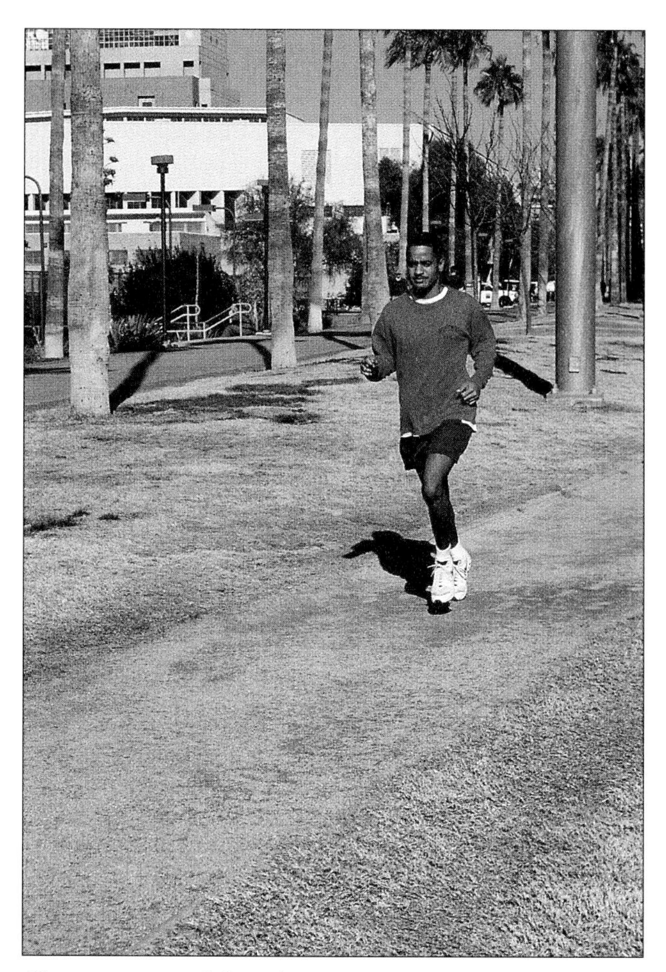

Changing your lifestyle, rather than "quick solutions" is the key to health, fitness, and wellness.

magazine or tabloid. There are no secret cures or magic formulae that have not been recognized by the scientific community, a picture on the cover of *Time* magazine, nomination for a Nobel prize, etc.

- The product or organization named is often similar to that of a famous person or creditable institution (e.g., the Mayo diet had no connection with the Mayo Clinic).
- They often sell products through the mail, which does not allow you to examine the product personally. There are no miracle products available only by mail order or from a single source.

There are some common-sense precautions one can take to avoid being a victim of a rip-off.

The following suggestions can help protect you:

- Read the ad carefully, especially the small print.
- Do not send cash; use a check, money order, or credit card so you'll have a receipt.
- Do not order from a company with only a P.O. box, unless you know the company.
- Do not let high-pressure sales tactics make you rush into a decision.
- Do not order from a company requiring use of an 800 telephone number and a credit card (they may be trying to avoid federal statutes).
- When in doubt, check out the company through your Better Business Bureau (BBB).
- If you have a complaint, write to the company first, but keep a copy of all receipts, checks, and correspondence.
- If that fails, write to the Direct Marketing Association. You may also report to the BBB, postmaster (if it was a mail order), state attorney general, and/or the Federal Trade Commission (FTC).

The Facts about Equipment

The consumer who plans to purchase exercise equipment should keep in mind certain guidelines to get the most for the money.

The following suggestions will help you select equipment:

- Unless you are wealthy or just like to collect gadgets, there is no need to buy a lot of exercise equipment. A complete fitness program can be carried out with *no* equipment. If you learn to depend upon equipment, you may eventually feel that you cannot exercise unless you are at home or at a gym.
- If you do not like jogging or swimming, and you hate calisthenics, then the minimal equipment you may want to consider is a bicycle (regular or stationary), treadmill, or rowing machine for cardiovascular fitness; and a set of weights, pulleys, or isokinetic device for strength and endurance.
- Consult an expert if you want to know the effectiveness of a product. Individuals with college or university degrees in physical education, physical therapy, kinesiotherapy, and kinesiology should be able to give you good advice.
- Buy from a well-established, reputable company that will not disappear overnight and will back up warranties. Avoid mail-order products. If the product is not available in a retail store where it can be examined, you probably should not buy it.
- You get what you pay for. Buying an inexpensive, poorly produced product will result in dissatisfaction in the long run.

AMA Abbreviation for the American Medical Association.

The Facts about Health Clubs

> It is not necessary to join a club, spa, or salon to develop fitness, but if you are considering joining such an establishment, make your choice with care.

The consumer should observe these precautions before becoming a member of a club, spa, or salon:

- Do not expect "miraculous" results as advertised.
- Be prepared to haggle over price and to resist a very hard sell for a long-term contract.
- Choose a no-contract, pay-as-you-go establishment if possible. Otherwise, choose the shortest term contract available.
- If there is a contract, read the fine print carefully and look for:
  - the interest rate;
  - "confession of judgment" clauses waiving your right to defend yourself in court;
  - noncancelable clauses;
  - "holder-in-due-course" doctrines allowing the establishment to sell your contract to a collection agency;
  - a waiver of the establishment's liability for injury to you on the premises.
- Consult with an independent expert if you have questions about the programs offered by the establishment.
- Do not accept diets, drugs, or food supplements from the club. Your physician will prescribe these if they are needed.
- You do not have to conform to the program the club suggests for you. Do not perform dangerous exercises, or passive exercises, or participate in fraudulent "treatments." Choose only those activities that meet the criteria explained in this book.
- Refuse to be pestered by solicitations for new members.
- Make a trial visit to the establishment during the hours when you would normally expect to use the facility to determine if it is open, if it is overcrowded, if the equipment is available, if the attendants are selling rather than assisting, and if you would enjoy the company of the other patrons.
- Determine the qualifications of the personnel, especially of the individual responsible for your program. Is he or she an expert as defined previously?
- Make certain the club is a well-established facility that will not disappear overnight.
- Check its reputation with the Better Business Bureau in your area.
- Investigate the programs offered by the YMCA/YWCA, local colleges and universities, and municipal park and recreation departments. These agencies often have excellent fitness classes at lower prices than commercial establishments and usually employ qualified personnel. For weight loss, investigate franchised clubs, such as Weight Watchers or TOPS, or affiliate with a university or a hospital-based program.

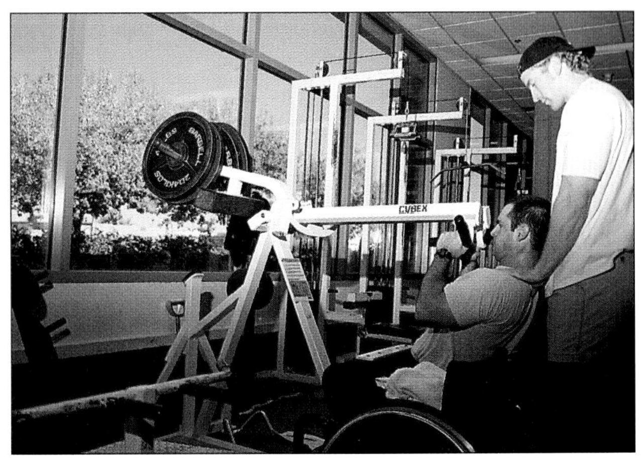

Visit a health club before you join.

The Facts about Dietary Supplements

> The burden of proof about the effectiveness of food supplements rests with the consumer.

The passage of the Dietary Supplements Health and Education Act in 1994 shifted the burden of providing assurances of product effectiveness from the FDA to the food supplement industry, which really means it shifted to you—the consumer. Food supplements are typically not considered to be drugs, so they are not regulated. Unlike drugs and medicines, food supplements need not be proven effective or even safe to be sold in stores. To be removed from stores, they must be proven ineffective or unsafe. This leaves consumers vulnerable to false claims. Many experts suggest that quackery has increased significantly since 1994 when the Act was passed.

The Act had at least one positive effect. Food supplement labeling must now be truthful and nonmisleading. Claims concerning disease prevention, treatment, or diagnosis must be substantiated in order to appear on the product. Unfortunately, the act did not limit false claims if they are not on the product label. The result has been the removal of claims from labels in favor of claims on separate literature often called "third-party" literature because the label makes no claims, and the seller makes no written claims (second party). Rather the seller provides claims in literature by other people (third party). The literature is distributed separately from the product, thus allowing sellers to make unsubstantiated claims for products. Also the law does not prohibit unproven verbal claims by sales people. A highly respected medical journal indicates that "alternative treatments should be subjected to scientific testing no less rigorous than that required for advocating unproven and potentially harmful treatments." However, as things currently stand it is up to the consumer to make decisions about the safety and effectiveness of food supplements so it is especially important to be well informed.

Current legislation does not provide protection to food supplement customers.

www.mhhe.com/phys_fit/webreview20 Click 03

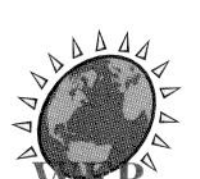

Since the Dietary Supplements Health and Education Act was passed in 1994, food supplement sales have doubled (from $8 to $16 billion a year). Common types of supplements include ergogenics, vitamins, minerals, and herbs or botanical supplements (e.g., St. John's Wort, ginseng, ginkgo). Recently the sales of supplements has leveled off, primarily because of increasing evidence of the danger of some supplements and the recent research showing the ineffectiveness of others. Among the adverse effects reported are lead poisoning, nausea, vomiting, diarrhea, abnormal heart rhythm, fainting, impotence, and lethargy. Over a six-year period 2,621 adverse events were reported to the FDA and 184 resulted in death.

www.mhhe.com/phys_fit/webreview20 Click 04

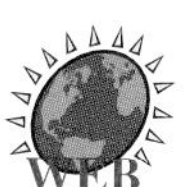

More than one half of American adults are unaware that food supplements are unregulated by the FDA or any governmental agency. An editorial in *USA Today* offered this comment: "The dirty secret of these unregulated 'natural' products is that their impact can vary widely from one person to another. Dosage strength can be wildly different from brand to brand, even batch to batch. Some can be downright dangerous."

In spite of the problems associated with lack of supplement regulations, a recent study in the New England Journal of Medicine indicates that nearly half of Americans routinely take supplements and slightly more than half believe in the value of the supplements. Interestingly, 44 percent believe that physicians know little or nothing about supplements.

The overwhelming majority (80 percent) believe that the Food and Drug Administration should review the safety of supplements before they are offered for sale. Also more than 60 percent believe that there are not enough rules to insure purity and accurate dosage amounts. A similar number of adults want more regulation on advertising claims to make sure that they are true.

USA Today (see Suggested Readings) notes that self-regulation within the industry has not worked well and suggests that the public will have more confidence in supplements "when they know independent experts, not just the hucksters, are watching out for their best interest."

Table 1 presents some questions that should be asked about food supplements. It would be wise to ask yourself these questions and to get answers before you consider using a food supplement.

The Facts about Fitness Books, Magazines, and Articles

All fitness books do not provide scientifically sound, accurate, and reliable information.

Because publishers are motivated by profit and publishing is a highly competitive field, the choice of material to be printed is often selected on the basis of how popular, famous, or attractive the author is, or how sensational or unusual his or her ideas are. Movie stars, models, TV personalities, and even Olympic athletes are rarely experts in biomechanics, anatomy and physiology, exercise, and other foundations of physical fitness. Having a good figure/physique, being fit, or having gone through a training program does not, in itself, qualify a person to advise others.

If you have read the facts presented in the other concepts, you should be able to distinguish between fact and fiction. To assist you further, however, there are 10 guidelines listed in Lab 20A. These might help you evaluate whether or not a book, magazine, or article on exercise and fitness is valid, reliable, and scientifically sound. If the answer to each of the questions is not "yes," then you should be suspicious of the material. If in doubt, ask one or more experts, or contact the American Alliance of Health, Physical Education, Recreation and Dance (AAHPERD) or the American College of Sports Medicine (ACSM) (see Web Review). These organizations will refer your question to an appropriate expert.

The Facts about Health Information on the Internet

All Internet websites do not provide scientifically sound, accurate, and reliable information.

The development of the Internet (World Wide Web) has made information more and more accessible to the masses. In fact a health goal for the nation—as outlined in *Healthy People 2010*—is to increase the proportion of households with access to the Internet with the specific intent of making reliable health information available to as many people as possible. While the development of the Internet has made an almost unlimited amount of health information accessible, it has also been the source of much misinformation, and even fraud.

The Federal Trade Commission (FTC) is a federal government agency charged with making sure that advertising claims for products are not false or misleading. In an effort to clean up websites, the FTC initiated "Operation Cure-All." As part of this operation, the FTC conducted two "Health Claim Surf Days" during which they identified 800 websites and usenet newsgroups with questionable content. The FTC sent mailers to these sites and 28 percent either

Table 1 Questions and Comments about Food Supplements

Questions	Comments
Does the government regulate this product to be sure that it is safe and effective?	Since 1994, food supplements can be sold without proof that they are effective. The government does not test food supplements to ensure effectiveness or safety. The FDA must prove the product to be harmful or ineffective to remove it from the market. It is much harder to prove a product ineffective than to provide evidence that it is effective.
Is there evidence to support claims for supplement?	The evidence should be based on research with normal people, not evidence based on a population of subjects who have medical problems or nutritional deficiencies. Third-party information often cites research out-of-context and based on inappropriate studies of atypical, not normal, people.
What are the active ingredients?	If the active ingredient really works, there will be research to show its effectiveness. Of course, if it works, then it is much like a medicine and has similar side effects. Sellers of supplements often suggest the product works, but that it has no side effects that are associated with medicines. Both cannot be true. For example, Cholestin is a variety of red yeast—a natural product. It contains lovastatin, the same active ingredients in medicines for lowering cholesterol. While the product works, it has now been banned by the FDA as an over-the-counter supplement because it has the same active ingredient as medicine and has the same side effects. The regulation of this product by the FDA has been challenged in the courts by the supplement industry. The decision of the courts will have consequences for future regulation of supplements.
What are the possible side-effects and risks of taking the supplement?	As noted above, if a product works as well as a medicine, it probably has the same side effects. If you know the active ingredient, you will know more about the side effects.
Are there possible interactions associated with taking the supplement?	When you take a medicine, you consult a physician or pharmacist about drug interactions. Supplements may interact with other supplements or medicines.
What are the long-term effects of taking the supplement?	Because supplements are not regulated, there has been little research about long-term effects of products. For example, melatonin is a hormone that is used for insomnia. Hormones have strong effects on the body and little is known about melatonin's long-term effects. Consider alternative solutions to long-term use of an unstudied supplement.
Are you sure the product is what it claims to be and that the size of the dose is appropriate?	U. S. Pharmacopeia (USP) is a private nonprofit organization that developed uniform standards for medicines and other health-care products. This organization sets standards for vitamins and minerals to assure quality and purity as well as appropriate size and strength of a standard unit of the product (dose size and strength). When standards are developed, the USP label will ensure that the product is what it says it is. As many as two or three dozen herbal products are currently being evaluated to determine appropriate dose size. Products with the USP label that fail to meet standards will be removed from stores. Without the USP label, you are at the mercy of the company that produces the product. The deaths associated with L-tryptophan, an amino acid supplement, occurred because of contaminants (Peak-X) in the unregulated product.
Who makes the product?	In the absence of regulations, the reputation of the company that makes the product is very important. Have complaints been made against the company? Have there been health problems with their products? How long has the company been in business? Large pharmaceutical companies are now beginning to sell supplements because of the high profit margin. Using a product from a large drug company is more likely to ensure that a product is what it is supposed to be but it does not ensure that the product is effective.
Is the cost worth the potential benefits?	The costs of dietary supplements are typically quite high. For example, protein supplements may cost as much as $1.00 a gram. The cost per gram in good food such as protein in a chicken breast is typically a few cents per gram. Most experts suggest that even the most effective supplements have relatively small effects at a very high cost.
Is the source of your information about the supplement reliable and accurate?	Avoid verbal information about products, especially information from the seller. Be wary of third-party literature or research in obscure journals. Be wary of those who discredit sound medical advice or information from regulatory agencies such as the FDA.

removed the claims or the website completely. In spite of the FTC efforts, there is still much health misinformation on the Web, leading one FTC official to suggest that ". . . miracle cures, once thought to have been laughed out of existence, have now found a new medium . . . on the Internet" (see Suggested Reading, NCAHF, 1999).

Another research study randomly selected 400 websites from 27,000 available on four different well-known search engines for a study of cancer. Nearly half had unverified information and 6 percent had major inaccuracies. Clearly, Internet users must be careful in selecting websites for obtaining fitness, health, and wellness information.

There are some general rules that can be followed to help you when you use the Web to obtain fitness, health, and wellness information. In general, government websites are good sources that contain sound information prepared by experts and based on scientific research. Government sites will typically include "gov" as part of the address. Professional organizations and universities can also be good sources of information. Organizations will typically have "org" and universities will typically have "edu" as part of the address. However, caution should still be used with organizations because it is easy to start an organization and obtain an "org" web address. Your greatest trust can be placed in the sites of stable organizations of long standing such as the AMA, the American Cancer Society, the American Heart Association, the American College of Sports Medicine, the National Council against Health Fraud, and the American Alliance for Health, Physical Education, Recreation and Dance, among others listed in this text. The AMA has recently developed extensive guidelines for health information on the Web (see Suggested Readings). The great majority of websites promoting health products have "com" in the title because these are commercial sites that are in business to make a profit. Because they are in business to make a profit, they are more inclined to contain information that is suspect or totally incorrect. Some "com" sites contain good information, for example, those listed at the end of each concept of this book. Nevertheless, it is important to evaluate, with special care, information found at "com" sites. The Tufts University School of Nutrition Science and Policy has developed a website that rates diet and health sites on the Internet. You may want to consult this website (http://navigator.tufts.edu). In Lab 20A, you can rate a website, using a checklist.

When selecting websites for inclusion at the end of each concept of the book, we used the same checklist as in Lab 20A. You will see that a majority of the sites listed are governmental and organizational sites. We do include some commercial sites but with some reservation. What we see when we evaluate a site may not be what you see when you use the site several weeks or months later. It is important that you evaluate all websites, using the criteria suggested here, including those listed at the end of each concept of this book.

Strategies for Action: The Facts

Being a good consumer requires time, information, and effort.

www.mhhe.com/phys_fit/webreview20 Click 05

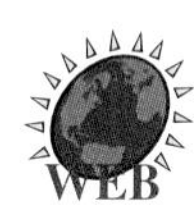

With time and effort, you can gain the information you need to make good decisions about products and services that you purchase. In Lab 20A, you will evaluate an exercise device, a food supplement, a magazine article, or a website. In Lab 20B, you will evaluate a health/wellness or fitness club. Taking the time to investigate a product will help you save money and help you avoid making poor decisions that affect your health, fitness, and wellness. The labs are designed to give you practice in being a good consumer. When you are making real decisions about products or services, it is a good idea to begin your investigation well in advance of the day when a decision is to be made. Sales people often suggest that "this offer is only good today." They know that people often make poor decisions when under time pressure, and they want you to make a decision today so that they won't lose a sale.

Web Review

Web review materials for Concept 20 are avail-

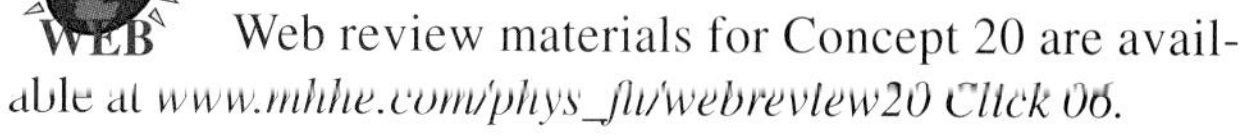
able at *www.mhhe.com/phys_fit/webreview20 Click 06.*

Agency for Health Care Policy and Research
www.ahcpr.gov

American Dietetics Association
www.eatright.org

American Medical Association Health Insight
www.ama-assn.org

Center for Science in the Public Interest
www.cspinet.org

Food and Drug Administration
www.fda.gov

Healthfinder
www.healthfinder.gov

Medscape
www.medscape.com

National Council Against Health Fraud
www.ncahf.org

Office of Dietary Supplements
http://ods.od.nih.gov

Quackwatch
www.quackwatch.com

Tufts University Nutrition Navigator
http://navigator.tufts.edu

U.S. Consumer Information Center
www.pueblo.gsa.gov

Suggested Readings

Berland, G. K. et al. "Health Information on the Internet: Accessibility, Quality, and Readability in English and Spanish." *Journal of the American Medical Association.* 285(20)(2001): 2612–2621.

Blendon, R. J. et al. "Americans' Views on the Use and Regulation of Dietary Supplements." *Archives of Internal Medicine.* 161(6)(2001): 805–810.

Catlin, D. H. et al. "Trace Contamination of Over-the-Counter Androstenedione and Postive Urine Test Results for a Nandrolone Metabolite." *Journal of the American Medical Association.* 284(20)(2000): 2618–2621.

Consumer Reports. "The Mainstreaming of Alternative Medicine." *Consumer Reports.* 65(5)(2000): 17–25.

Fetrow, C. W., and Avila, J. R. *Professional's Handbook of Complementary and Alternative Medicines.* Springhouse, PA: Springhouse Publications, 1999.

Gugliotta, G. "Health Concerns Grow Over Herbal Aids: As Industry Booms, Analysis Suggests Rising Toll in Illness and Death." *Washington Post.* 19 March 2000, A1+.

National Council Against Health Fraud. "FDA Guide to Supplements." *NCAHF Newsletter.* 22(2)(1999): 1–4.

National Council Against Health Fraud. "FTC Targets Internet Health Fraud." *NCAHF Newsletter.* 22(6)(1999): 1–2.

National Council Against Health Fraud. "National Surveys Produce Remarkable Findings on Alternative Health Practices and Dietary Supplement Misuse." *NCAHF Newsletter.* 23(2)(2000): 1–4.

National Council Against Health Fraud Newsletter. Published every other month, it contains articles that give objective information about health products and food supplements. NCAHF, P. O. Box 1276, Loma Linda, CA 92354.

Nutrition Business Journal. "Whatever Happened to Herbs?" *Nutrition Business Journal.* March 2001.

Park, R. L. *Voodoo Science: The Road from Foolishness to Fraud.* New York: Oxford University Press, 2000.

Porcari, J. P. "Pump Up Your Walking." *ASCM's Health and Fitness Journal.* 3(1)(1999): 25–29.

Shelton, R. C. et al. "Effectiveness of St. John's Wort in Major Depression." *Journal of the American Medical Association.* 285(15)(2001): 1978–1986.

USA Today. "Herbal Drug Bust." *USA Toady.* 10 May 2001, A14.

Winker, M. A. et al. "Guidelines for Medical and Health Information Sites on the Internet: Principles Governing AMA Web Sites." *Journal of the American Medical Association.* 283(12)(2000): 1600–1606.

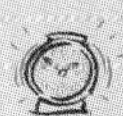

Physical Fitness News Update

As noted on the previous pages, many people use supplements and believe in their value. Their trust has eroded because of recent well-reported problems. Some of these recent problems are cited here.

- Herbal Medicines have been shown to cause postsurgical problems such as postoperative bleeding, irregular heart beat, and stroke (Echinacea, ephedra, garlic, ginseng, ginkgo, kava, St. John's Wort). A study at Texas Tech University showed that 7 out of 10 people failed to make their doctors aware of the fact that they were taking supplements. Supplements such as ephedra can have dangerous interactions with anesthetic drugs. Herbal supplements should be discontinued 2 to 3 weeks before surgery.
- The FDA mailed a letter to supplement companies warning them to cease making false, illegal, and unscientific claims about herbs and supplements added to foods. Examples include ginkgo, ginseng, and echinacea added to energy bars, bottled water, and other "sports" drinks.
- The body building/date rape drug GHB has been shown to be addicting and potentially deadly. Tom Gugliotta, an NBA starter, recently had a near fatal reaction to it.
- The FDA has asked makers of supplements to recall products containing comfrey because of damage to the liver and possible cancer-causing effect.
- Ephedra has been shown to be associated with heart attacks, stroke, and diabetes. Part of the danger is taking ephedra with other drugs, or food supplements that have similar effects. Lawsuits have been filed against ephedra suppliers since knowledge of the medical problems associated with its use were revealed.
- Even supplements commonly considered to be beneficial such as calcium can be potentially dangerous because current laws do not require that the content of supplements actually contain pure ingredients. A recent study showed that while the majority were lead-free, some nonprescription calcium supplements contain lead, a highly toxic substance.
- The FDA is working on the reclassification of several "over the counter" supplements to make them harder to get and easier to regulate. Substances shown to stimulate muscle growth will be considered for reclassification.
- Although there is no current evidence of harm, there is concern among USDA advisors that supplements containing brain and pituitary tissue (common in some "body building" supplements) may harbor mad cow disease.
- The first short-term study in the U.S. to study the effectiveness of St. John's Wort showed the supplement to be no more effective than a placebo in preventing depression over an eight-week period.
- Creatine is banned in France and the French Food Safety Agency suggests it may constitute a cancer risk. It is a legal supplement in the U. S. and is not banned by the International Olympic Committee. There is no long-term research to prove or disprove the claims.
- Some legal supplements have been implicated in positive drug tests of athletes and are now under study by the International Olympic Committee. Androstendione, for example, resulted in positive steroid tests in approximately half of the users.
- Water is not generally considered a food supplement, but the sale of water has become a big industry. A study by the World Wildlife Fund says that bottled water is no safer and no healthier than tap water in most industrialized nations. Even in less developed countries boiled tap water is a better option because it is safe and much less expensive. This is important because people in these countries have low incomes.

Lab 20B: Evaluating a Health/Wellness or Fitness Club

Name **Section** **Date**

Purpose: To practice evaluating a health club. (Various combinations of the words *health, wellness,* and *fitness* are often used for these clubs.)

Procedure:

1. Visit a club and pretend to be interested in becoming a member. (*Note:* Only one or two class members should go to each club to avoid suspicion.)
2. Listen carefully to all that is said and ask lots of questions (without exposing your real motives).
3. Look carefully all around you as you are given the tour of the facilities; ask what the exercises or the equipment does for you or ask leading questions such as, "Will this take inches off my hips?", etc.
4. As soon as you leave the club, rate it using Chart 1. Space is provided for notes in Chart 1.

Chart 1 Health Club Evaluation Questionnaire

Directions: Place an X over a yes or no answer. Make notes as necessary.	Yes	No	Notes
1. Were claims for improvement in weight, figure/physique, or fitness realistic?	○	○	
2. Was a long-term contract (1–3 years) encouraged?	○	○	
3. Was the sales pitch high-pressure to make an immediate decision?	○	○	
4. Were you given a copy of the contract to read at home?	○	○	
5. Did the fine print include objectionable clauses?	○	○	
6. Did they ask you about medical readiness?	○	○	
7. Did they sell diet supplements as a sideline?	○	○	
8. Did they have passive equipment?	○	○	
9. Did they have cardiovascular training equipment or facilities (cycles, track, pool, aerobic dance)?	○	○	
10. Did they make unscientific claims for the equipment, exercise, baths, or diet supplements?	○	○	
11. Were the facilities clean?	○	○	
12. Were the facilities crowded?	○	○	
13. Were there days and hours when facilities were open but would not be available to you?	○	○	
14. Were there limits on the number of minutes you could use a piece of equipment?	○	○	
15. Did the floor personnel closely supervise and assist clients?	○	○	
16. Were the floor personnel qualified "experts"?	○	○	
17. Were the managers/owners qualified "experts"?	○	○	
18. Has the club been in business at this location for a year or more?	○	○	

Results:

1. Score the chart as follows:
   A. Give one point for each "no" answer for items 2, 3, 5, 7, 8, 10, 12, 13, and 14 and place the score in the box. Total A ☐

   B. Give one point for each "yes" answer for items 1, 4, 6, 9, 11, and 18 and place the score in the box. Total B ☐

   Total A and B above and place the score in the box. Total A and B ☐

   C. Give one point for each "yes" answer on 15, 16, and 17 and place the score in the blank. Total C ☐
2. A total score of 12–15 points on items A and B suggests the club rates at least "fair" compared to other clubs.
3. A score of 3 on item C indicates that the personnel are qualified and suggests that you could expect to get accurate technical advice from the staff.
4. Regardless of the total scores, you would have to decide the importance of each item in the questionnaire to you personally, as well as evaluate other considerations such as cost, location, personalities of the clients and the personnel, and so on, to decide if this would be a good place for you or your friends to join.

Conclusions and Implications: In the space below, use several sentences to discuss your conclusion about the quality of this club and whether you think it would fit your needs if you wanted to belong.

Concept 21

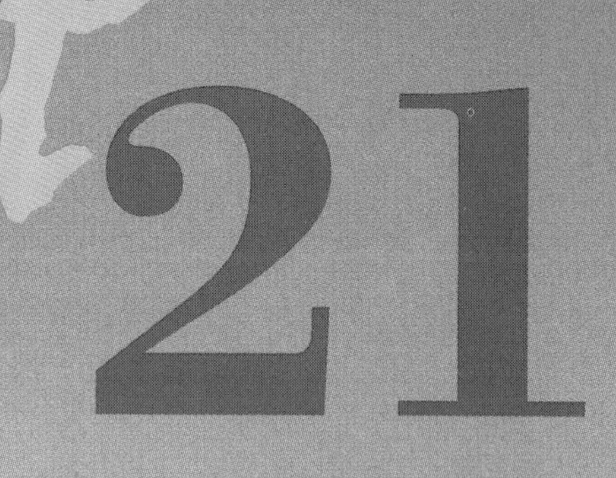

Toward Optimal Health and Wellness: Planning for Healthy Lifestyle Change

Using effective self-management techniques that promote healthy lifestyles can enhance fitness, health, and wellness for a lifetime.

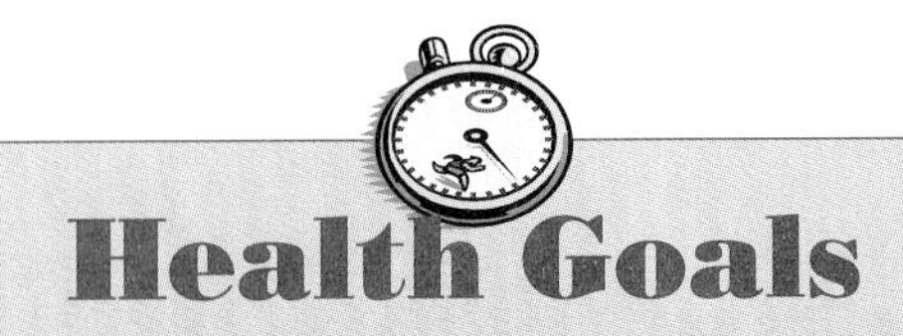

Health Goals

for year 2010

Increase quality and years of healthy life.

Increase healthy and active days.

Eliminate health disparities.

Increase adoption and maintenance of appropriate daily physical activity.

Promote health by improving dietary factors and nutritional status.

Promote healthy and safe communities.

Promote availability of high quality health information.

Increase availability of health care and counseling for mental health problems.

Avoiding destructive behaviors.

Introduction

The two primary health goals for the nation for the year 2010 are increasing the quality and years of life and eliminating health disparities so that all people can attain fitness, health, and wellness. The focus of this book has been on making changes in three priority lifestyles: performing adequate physical activity, eating well, and managing stress. In this concept, you will get information about other lifestyle changes that can affect health, fitness, and wellness and help all people achieve national health goals. You will have the opportunity to tie together all of the information presented in previous concepts to help you plan for a lifetime of healthy active living.

Increasing Years and Quality of Life: The Facts

Living a longer life is an important health goal.

Throughout this book, evidence has been presented to show how practicing healthy lifestyles can reduce risk of illness and contribute to longer life. You have learned that some of the factors that contribute to longer life and reduced risk of illness are out of your control (see Figure 1). Examples are heredity, poor medical care, and environmental factors. On the other hand, you know that healthy lifestyles are factors you can control and they have an enormous effect on health and length of life (see Figure 1).

It is important to note that virtually all people will be ill at some time in life. The key is to reduce the days of illness to a minimum. One of the specific goals for the nation is to increase the number of **healthy days** each of us experiences. Healthy days are typically measured using **self-rated health.**

Attaining wellness as evidenced by "quality of life" is a universal goal.

www.mhhe.com/phys_fit/webreview21 Click 01

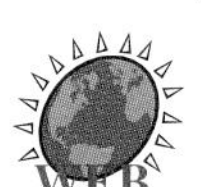

The focus of the national health goals for the year 2010 is to increase not only the years of life, but to increase the years of **quality of life.** Quality of life is an indicator of the positive component of health. Though the 2010 goals continue to emphasize treatment of illness and rehabilitation for people with disabilities, a new emphasis is placed on prevention of disease and disability and the promotion of wellness as indicated by quality of life. The Department of Health and Human Services uses various indicators to determine the extent to which the goal of increasing quality [illegible] years of healthy life has been achieved for all people. [illegible]ted in the previous section, one indicator is self-rated h[illegible] The intent is to increase the proportion of the popula[illegible]ho subjectively rate their health as good or better on m[illegible] of the year. If self-rated health is regularly good, a p[illegible] will have a high frequency of healthy days. Also of imp[illegible]e is having a high frequency of **activity days** or day[illegible] which you can do your normal activities without restrictio[illegible]

In summary, the goals for the nation and the goals of this book are to help readers achieve optimal health and wellness as evidenced by freedom from disease, the ability to function effectively on a daily basis, and a high quality of life including happiness and life satisfaction.

Community quality of life is important to personal quality of life.

Though national health goals focus on the individual, it is important to understand that community quality of life is also important. National goals have been directed at providing "livable" communities that provide an environment in which personal quality of life can thrive. Participation by citizens in community activities is essential if efforts to attain quality of life for all people are to be successful.

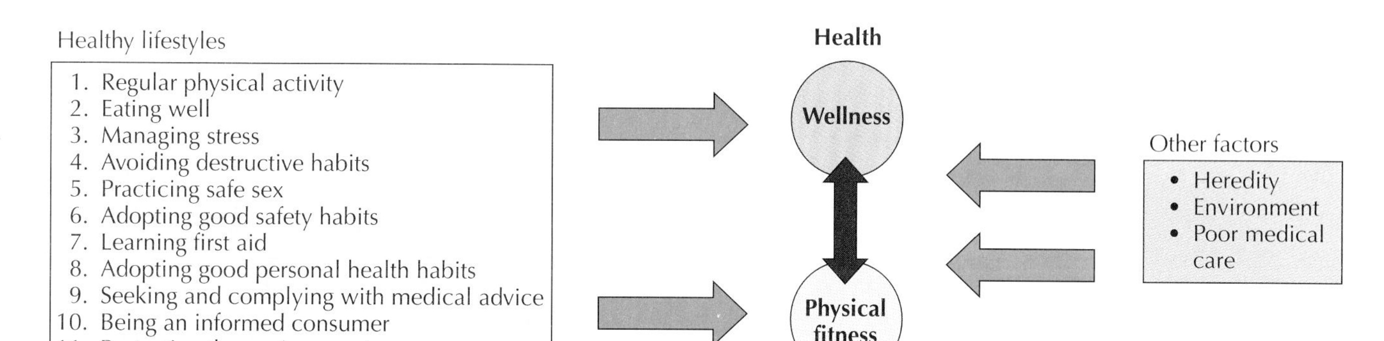

Figure 1
Factors influencing health, wellness, and physical fitness.

> Good fitness is important to both health and wellness.

Physical fitness is a state of being that results from healthy lifestyles, particularly regular physical activity. Fitness is neither health nor wellness, but possessing fitness enhances health and wellness. As noted throughout this book, having health-related physical fitness can help you reduce disease risk. Fitness is also crucial to wellness and quality of life. Evidence shows that fitness can help people to excel in performances that enhance quality of life. It allows you to do the daily work activities without fatigue and allows you to enjoy leisure time activities that enrich life. As people grow older, there are added benefits of fitness. Good fitness allows older adults to function independently in daily life activities such as driving a car and performing daily tasks without restriction.

Healthy Lifestyles: The Facts

> Adhering to healthy lifestyles is essential to increasing quality and years of healthy life.

Lifestyles and behaviors are in your control. If you make changes and adhere to them, good things will happen. Some of the important healthy lifestyles are listed in Figure 1 and are summarized in the following section.

Participating in Physical Activity Regularly

As noted throughout this book, regular physical activity is associated with the reduced risk of many diseases. Regular physical activity is a positive addiction. It is habit-forming, but the result of the habit is positive, not negative. Regular exercise can be fun and can improve the quality of life. It is interesting to note that people who exercise regularly are more likely to adopt other healthy lifestyles. For example, regular exercisers are more likely than sedentary individuals to visit a physician for preventive examinations, practice preventive dentistry, and wear seat belts.

Eating Properly (Good Nutrition)

Good eating habits can help you feel and look your best. Failure to eat properly can result in many health problems. It has been shown that six of the 10 leading causes of death in North America are linked to improper nutrition. Millions of teenagers and adults regularly modify

Activity Days A self-rating of the number of days (per week or month) a person feels that he/she can perform usual daily activities successfully and in good health.

Healthy Days A self-rating of the number of days (per week or month) a person considers himself or herself to be in good or better than good health.

Quality of Life A term used to describe wellness. An individual with quality of life can enjoy the activities of life with little or no limitation and can function independently. Individual quality of life requires a pleasant and supportive community quality of life.

Self-Rated Health A subjective measure of daily health and wellness.

their diet in an attempt to assume control of the way they look and their health. Unfortunately, many of these dietary modifications have a negative rather than positive impact on health. Making appropriate changes in eating patterns is the key. Eating properly is a goal that is achievable (see concepts on nutrition and managing diet and activity).

Managing Stress

Nearly 30 million professionals and executives who rank among the highest in annual earnings indicate that they would like to find a way to get away from their steady diet of stress and tension. Reducing stress in your life and learning to cope with stress are associated with feelings of well-being and an improved quality of life. Stress reduction is possible for most people with alterations in lifestyle (see concepts on stress and health and on stress management).

Avoiding Destructive Habits

Among the most destructive habits are the use of tobacco and alcohol and the abuse of drugs. Once they are adopted, these habits are exceptionally difficult to eliminate, but there are ways to help. These are lifestyle or health behaviors over which you have personal control, but breaking habits takes the assistance of others (see concepts on use and abuse of tobacco, alcohol, and drugs).

Practicing Safe Sex

Though sexually transmitted diseases (STDs) are not currently among the top 10 killers, they are the source of much pain and suffering. Healthy lifestyles are the key to prevention of the most common STDs (see concept on STDs).

Adopting Good Safety Habits

Accidents are a major cause of death in North America, accounting for nearly 5 percent of all deaths in the United States. In addition, they result in many disabilities and problems that can detract from good health and wellness. All accidents cannot be prevented, but it is possible to adopt habits that greatly reduce the risk of accidents. Deaths from automobile accidents can be greatly reduced by regular use of seat belts. The proper maintenance of play and work equipment can greatly reduce injury and death rates. Many children die each year from water-related accidents that can be prevented by proper supervision, the use of proper safety devices such as life jackets, and knowledge of cardiopulmonary resuscitation. Proper storage of guns, use of smoke alarms, proper use of ladders, and proper maintenance of cars, motorcycles, and bicycles can also reduce accident risk.

Learning First Aid

Many deaths could be prevented if those at the site of emergencies were able to administer first aid. Because they can prevent death, all people should be familiar with cardiopulmonary resuscitation (CPR) and the Heimlich maneuver for assisting a person who is choking. Many agencies give extensive classes in first aid taught by qualified experts. It is best to learn these procedures in such a class. First aid for minor injuries and poisoning and for control of bleeding are other important procedures.

Adopting Good Personal Health Behaviors

Many of the healthy lifestyles already discussed are good personal health habits. There are other simple personal health behaviors that are important to optimal health. These behaviors may be considered elementary because they are often taught in school and at home at a very young age. Still, there are many adults who fail to adopt these behaviors on a regular basis. Examples include regular brushing and flossing of the teeth; care of ears, eyes, and skin; proper sleep habits; proper innoculations for disease prevention; and good posture. Health behaviors that prevent sexually transmitted diseases are also important.

Seeking and Complying with Medical Advice

Some people purposely avoid seeking the advice of a physician because they fear that something may be wrong. This occurs in spite of the evidence that delay in treatment greatly increases the risk of death for many diseases that can be cured or controlled. In addition to medical exams for unhealthy people beginning exercise, regular preventive medical exams are important. After age 40, a yearly preventive exam is recommended for all people. Young adults probably need a regular medical examination less often, but a regular examination is important for all people to help in the early diagnosis of problems. For women (especially after age 40), regular self-examination for breast cancer is recommended, as are periodic mammograms and Pap tests. For men, regular testicular exams and a prostate test are recommended. Other important behaviors that should be considered are listed below:

- Be familiar with the symptoms of the most common medical problems in our culture.

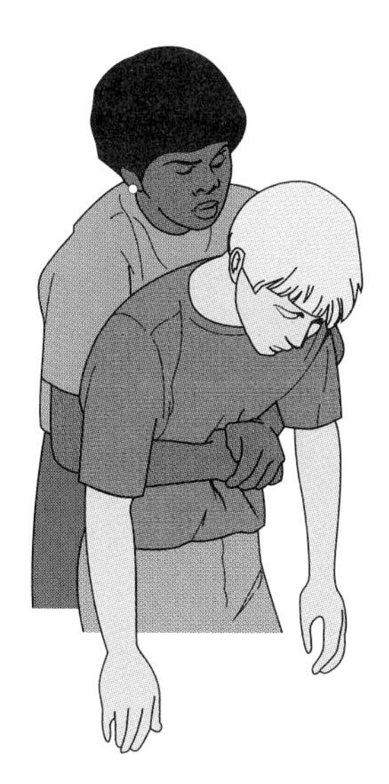

Learn first aid, such as the Heimlich maneuver.

- If symptoms are present, seek medical help. Many deaths could be prevented if the early warning signs of medical problems were heeded.
- If medical advice is given, comply. It is not uncommon for people to stop taking medicine when symptoms stop rather than taking the full amount of medicine prescribed.
- If you doubt the advice given, seek a second opinion.

Being an Informed Consumer

Each year too many people purchase health services and products that are ineffective and often dangerous. Extensive advertising of quack health products, often by celebrities, bombards all of us. It is important to investigate so-called health products and services of all kinds (see concept on quackery).

Protecting the Environment

A recent national poll indicated that 70 percent of the adult population felt that the public was not concerned enough about the environment. In fact, more than half felt that there was an immediate need to take drastic action to protect the environment. Concern for the environment has increased in recent years as indicated by the fact that more than eight of 10 households now indicate that they voluntarily recycle newspapers, glass, or aluminum. We have not been as actively involved in other lifestyle changes that would help protect the environment (e.g, carpool, reduce water use).

Unlike lifestyle behaviors such as regular physical activity or managing stress, behaviors that help protect the environment may not have immediate wellness benefits. Experts are quick to point out, however, that protecting the environment may be one of the most important things that we can do over time to guarantee quality of living for our children and the generations to come.

Managing Time and Priorities Effectively

Central to the concept of wellness are working efficiently and making a significant contribution to society. Working effectively requires a commitment of time. A social contribution requires time for special causes, and social wellness requires a commitment of time to family and friends. Similarly, each of the other dimensions of wellness requires a time commitment. A healthy lifestyle is one that allocates time efficiently to insure that appropriate time is allocated to appropriate priorities. Time and priority management can lead to behaviors that contribute to each wellness dimension, and ultimately to total wellness (see concept on stress management).

One positive lifestyle change often leads to another.

If you make one significant lifestyle change to enhance wellness you are likely to make other changes. For example, people who begin a regular physical activity program and adhere to it over a period of time are also likely to make modifications in diet and adopt effective stress-reduction procedures. People who smoke are more likely to stop if they have been successful in becoming a regular exerciser or a healthy eater.

The wellness lifestyle seems to be contagious. The key is to start slowly to increase the chance of success. Remember, a critical goal for the year 2010 is increasing quality of life for all people. This is best accomplished by altering lifestyles in a consistent and regular manner. The nation's health leaders believe that a commitment by each individual combined with scientific knowledge, professional skills, community support, and political effort will enable each of us to achieve our potential to live full, active lives.

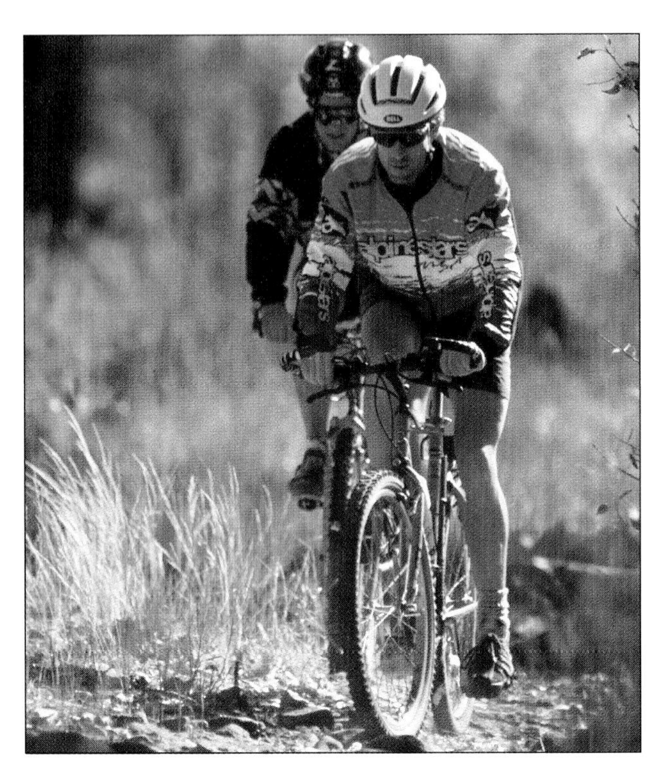

Making one lifestyle change, such as becoming more physically active, can lead to other healthy lifestyle changes.

Adhering to behaviors supported by scientific principles will do a lot to promote optimal wellness. But health promotion is also an art. Accordingly, pursuit of optimal wellness requires social and personal purpose. For example, interactions with friends, family, and community contribute to wellness, as do expressing and receiving love, having hope of better things to come, having a sense of charity to promote the community good, and having a personal sense of purpose.

Being compassionate, understanding, and supportive of family, friends, and coworkers will strengthen the bonds in your relationships and contribute to higher levels of social wellness. Meaningful relationships cannot be formed overnight; instead, they require persistent effort over an extended period of time. Similarly, to gain high levels of spiritual wellness, dedication and commitment to the principles of your particular religion or spiritual doctrine are necessary. Spiritual enlightenment and understanding cannot be attained without committed effort and focus on these behaviors.

The basic truth in all of these examples is that you can't get something for nothing. The benefits of wellness require continued commitments and efforts, but the benefits are well worth the effort. The "products" are health, wellness, and physical fitness. These outcomes occur when you do the "processes" of healthy lifestyle behaviors associated with each of the dimensions of wellness summarized in Table 1.

The Art of Achieving Health and Wellness: The Facts

Having insight to the different dimensions of wellness can help you adopt healthy lifestyles.

www.mhhe.com/phys_fit/webreview21 Click 02

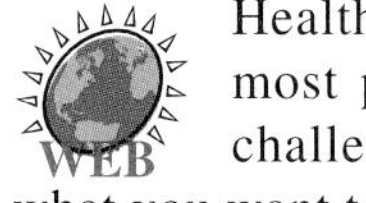

Health, including wellness, is something that most people desire, but achieving it is more challenging. Having a clear understanding of what you want to achieve in the areas of health and wellness can also help you change behavior to achieve your personal goals. The American Journal of Health Promotion defines health promotion as the "science and art of helping people change their lifestyle to move toward a state of optimal health." Adopting the healthy lifestyles discussed in the previous section of this concept would constitute adherence to the science of health promotion.

Strategies for Action: The Facts

Sometimes bad things happen to good people, but good things are likely to happen to those who make an effort to alter lifestyles.

Healthy lifestyle adherence is under your control. But all factors that influence your fitness, health, and wellness are not under your control. As noted on several occasions in previous concepts, factors such as heredity and quality of health services are not always in your personal control. Even people who do all of the right things will have health problems. Still, the best way to make a difference in your own health and wellness is to take control of the things over which you have control. Making an effort to control these factors is the closest thing to the proverbial fountain of youth.

Table 1 Dimensions of Wellness: Processes and Products

Dimension of Wellness	Process or Behavior	Product or Outcome
Physical wellness	Pursuing behaviors that are conducive to good physical health (being physically active and maintaining a healthy diet).	Development of good physical fitness and good physical health that provides some freedom from disease.
Social wellness	Being supportive of family, friends, and co-workers and practicing good communication skills.	Development of a strong social support system and satisfying relationships.
Emotional wellness	Balancing work and leisure and responding proactively to challenging or stressful situations.	Development of a positive outlook on life and freedom from emotional illness and stress.
Intellectual wellness	Challenging yourself to continually learn and improve in your work and personal life.	Development of satisfying career, hobbies, or pursuits that provides a sense of meaning or purpose.
Spiritual wellness	Praying, meditating, or reflecting on life.	Development of a philosophy or spiritual relationship that guides your life's pursuits.
Total wellness	Taking responsibility for your own health and happiness.	Quality of life.

Adopting a new way of thinking can help you achieve health, fitness, and wellness.

The determination as to whether a person is healthy, fit, or well is often subjective. The tendency of many is to make comparisons to other people. Such comparisons often result in setting personal standards that are impossible to achieve. Trying to achieve the body fatness of a model seen on TV is not realistic nor healthy for most people. Expecting to be able to perform like a professional athlete is not something that most of us can achieve. It is for this reason that the standards for fitness, health, and wellness in this book are based on health criteria rather than comparative criteria. As you began your study on this book, you were introduced to the HELP philosophy. Adhering to this philosophy can help you adopt a new way of thinking. This philosophy suggests that each person should use health (H) as the basis for making decisions rather than comparisons to others. This is something that everyone (E) can do for a lifetime (L). This allows each of us to set personal (P) goals that are realistic and possible for each person to attain.

The new way of thinking simply allows each of us to be successful on our own terms rather than comparing ourselves to others in ways that make success impossible. As you set personal health, fitness, and wellness goals, consider using a new way of thinking.

Assessing your current stage of change for a variety of lifestyles will help you determine goals for the future.

www.mhhe.com/phys_fit/webreview21 Click 03

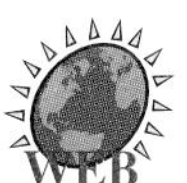

The stages of change model described in the first concept provides the basis for assessing your current behaviors related to a variety of lifestyles. Research suggests that people can be at a level of maintenance for one behavior and at a precontemplation level for another. In Labs 21A and 21B, you will have the opportunity to rate your current stage of change for a variety of lifestyle behaviors.

Table 2 Self-Management Skills

Skill	Description
Self-assessment	The ability to administer and interpret assessments of health, fitness, and wellness.
Self-monitoring skills	The ability to keep records of your adherence to activity, good eating, or other lifestyles.
Goal setting	The ability to set realistic and attainable goals for modifying lifestyles.
Planning skills	The ability to plan for healthy lifestyles based on personal self-assessments and goals.
Balancing attitudes	The ability to develop more good than bad attitudes about healthy lifestyles.
Overcoming barriers	The ability to practice healthy lifestyles even when barriers make it difficult.
Consumer skills	The ability to make good consumer decisions based on the facts rather than misinformation.
Finding social support	The ability to find support from other people.
Preventing relapse	The ability to prevent relapsing into unhealthy lifestyles after making positive changes.
Coping skills	The ability to cope with stressful situations and to adopt a positive outlook on life.
Managing time	The ability to use time wisely to achieve personal goals.
Performance skills	The ability to perform skills that enhance fitness and health, such as sports and recreation skills and stress-management skills.

Self-management skills can help you adopt and adhere to healthy lifestyles.

In earlier concepts you learned about a variety of self-management skills. These skills are summarized again in Table 2. If you are to alter your behaviors to improve fitness, health, and wellness, it is important that you practice these self-management skills. You have had the opportunity to practice them in a variety of labs in this book.

Self-management skills have been shown to very effective. They are based on sound theory and research. You may want to review these skills and the theories on which they are based (see concept on self-management). You will use many of the self-management skills to develop comprehensive lifetime physical activity plans and to make plans to change to other healthy lifestyles.

Self-planning is one of the most important self-management skills.

In a number of labs, you have had the opportunity to plan for a variety of different physical activities in the physical activity pyramid. In Lab 21A, you will plan a comprehensive physical activity program using self-management skills you have practiced previously. In this case, you will plan for all types of activities in the pyramid. In Lab 21B you will use self-management skills to plan for changing other lifestyles. The steps in program planning for physical activity were described in a previous concept. These steps are reviewed in Table 3. They can be used in planning for other healthy lifestyles as well (see Lab 21B).

In the end, it is what you do that counts!

Throughout this book, lifestyle modification has been endorsed as a means of achieving optimal health, fitness, and wellness. An underlying and consistent thread in all of the concepts has been an emphasis on the behavior rather than the outcome. This philosophy is best expressed as "focusing on the process instead of the product." *If you do the process, the product follows,* to the extent that is possible for a person with your heredity. Develop a plan and stick to it.

Sometimes lifestyle changes cannot be made without the assistance of others.

As already noted, support of friends and family can be very important in helping you to accomplish lifestyle changes. However, there are some lifestyle changes that may require the assistance of a professional. If your attempts to change your lifestyle meet with failure, don't set yourself up for repeated failure. Get help!

Table 3 Steps in Program Planning

1. Clarify your reason for making a lifestyle change.
2. Identify your needs using self-assessment.
3. Set realistic and achievable goals.
4. Select the lifestyles you plan to change.
5. Prepare a written plan.
6. Keep records of progress.

Most colleges have programs through their health center that provide free, confidential assistance or referral. Many businesses now have Employee Assistance Programs (EAP). The programs have counselors who will help you or your family members find help with a particular problem. The EAP staff are dedicated to help you without revealing personal information to your employer. These programs have a strong record for helping people with problems ranging from small to very serious, such as drug addiction or smoking cessation. Many other programs and support groups are now available to help you change your lifestyle. For example, most hospitals and many health organizations now have hotlines that provide you with referral services for establishing healthy lifestyles.

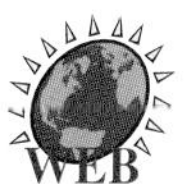

Web Review

Web review materials for Concept 21 are available at *www.mhhe.com/phys_fit/webreview21 Click 04.*

American College Health Association
www.acha.org

American Dietetics Association
www.eatright.org

Health Canada Online
www.hc_sc.gc.ca

Health Canada-Physical Activity Guide
www.hc_sc.gc.ca/hppb/paguide

Healthfinder
www.healthfinder.gov

Healthy People 2010
www.health.gov/healthypeople

Mayo Clinic Web Site
www.mayoclinic.com

Morbidity and Mortality Weekly Reports
www.cdc.gov/mmwr

National Institute of Alcohol Abuse and Alcoholism
www.niaaa.nih.gov

National Institute of Drug Abuse
www.nida.nih.gov

National Institute of Environmental Health Sciences
www.niehs.nih.gov

U.S. Consumer Information Center
www.pueblo.gsa.gov

World Health Organization
www.who.int

Suggested Readings

American College of Sports Medicine. *ACSM's Guidelines for Exercise Testing and Exercise Prescription.* 6th ed. Philadelphia: Lippincott, Williams and Wilkins, 2000.

Armbruster, B. and Gladwin, L. A. "More than Fitness for Older Adults." *ACSM's Health and Fitness Journal.* 5(2)(2001): 6–12.

Blair, S. N. et al. *Active Living Every Day.* Champaign, IL: Human Kinetics, 2001.

Booth, F. W. et al. "Waging War on Modern Chronic Disease: Primary Prevention through Exercise Biology." *Journal of Applied Physiology.* 88(2000):774–787.

Breslow, L. "From Disease Prevention to Health Promotion." *Journal of the American Medical Association.* 281(11)(1999):1030–1033.

Corbin, C. B., and Pangrazi, R. P. (Editors). *Towards a Better Understanding of Physical Fitness and Activity.* Scottsdale, AZ: Holcomb-Hathaway, 1999.

Corbin, C. B., Pangrazi, R. P., and Franks, B. D. "Definitions: Health, Fitness, and Physical Activity." *President's Council on Physical Fitness and Sports Research Digest.* 3(9)(2000):1–8.

Payne, W. A., and Hahn, D. B. *Understanding Your Health.* 6th ed. St. Louis: McGraw-Hill, 2000.

Spain, C. G., and Franks, B. D. "Healthy People 2010: Physical Activity and Fitness." *President's Council on Physical Fitness and Sports Research Digest.* 2(3)(2001): 1–16.

U.S. Department of Health and Human Services. *Healthy People 2010.* 2nd ed. With *Understanding and Improving Health* and *Objectives for Improving Health.* 2 vols. Washington, DC: U.S. Government Printing Office, November 2000.

U.S. Department of Health and Human Services. *Physical Activity and Health: A Report of the Surgeon General.* Atlanta: U.S. Department of Health and Human Services, 1996.

World Health Organization. *World Health Report 2000.* Geneva: World Health Organization, 2000.

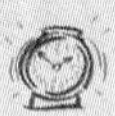

Physical Fitness News Update

A major goal of this text is to help college students gain the knowledge and self-management skills necessary to make informed decisions about health, fitness, wellness, and healthy lifestyles. We know, from the information presented in the first concept of this book, that people in Western culture are living longer. The following facts reveal the extent to which people have been successful in improving the quality of life in our culture.

- A recent global survey places the United States as the third "happiest" country in the world, after Denmark and Australia. Canada was not listed in the top ten. Self-confidence, not money, is the most often cited source of happiness. In general, most Americans indicate that they feel self-reliant and optimistic, and generally "feel good" about themselves.
- The types of news stories having the greatest interest among adults are those about health. Nearly half of all adults say they "follow closely" stories about health. Health is ranked above issues such as Washington events, people, local events, and sports.
- Seventy-eight percent of adults say they are satisfied with their standard of living and the things they can buy or do.
- Americans are not just living longer, they are healthier in old age. A recent study shows that older adults are spending less time in hospitals and nursing homes. The authors of the study suggest that better overall health among older adults is the reason. Another poll indicates that among adults 65 and over, 45 percent say that they are enjoying the best years of their lives.
- On a less positive note, the World Health Organization ranks the overall performance of the health care systems of Canada as 30th and the United States as 37th in the world. This occurs in spite of the fact that the United States is number 1 and Canada number 10 in per capita spending.

Appendix A

Metric Conversion Chart

Approximate Conversions from Metric to Traditional Measures

Length

centimeters to inches: cm × .39 = in
meters to feet: m × 3.3 = ft
meters to yards: m × 1.09 = yd
kilometers to miles: km × 0.6 = mi

Mass (Weight)

grams to ounces: g × 0.0352 = oz
kilograms to pounds: kg × 2.2 = lbs

Area

square centimeters to square inches: $cm^2 \times 0.16 = in^2$
square meters to square feet: $m^2 \times 11.11 = ft^2$
square meters to square yards: $m^2 \times 1.02 = yd^2$

Volume

milliliters to fluid ounces: ml × 0.03 = fl oz
liters to quarts: l × 1.06 = qt
liters to gallons: l × 0.264 = gal

Approximate Conversions from Traditional to Metric Measures

Length

inches to centimeters: in × 2.54 = cm
feet to meters: ft × .3048 = m
yards to meters: yd × 0.92 = m
miles to kilometers: mi × 1.6 = km

Mass (Weight)

ounces to grams: oz × 28.41 = gm
pounds to kilograms: lbs × 0.45 = kg

Area

square inches to square centimeters: $in^2 \times 6.5 = cm^2$
square feet to square meters: $ft^2 \times 0.09 = m^2$
square yards to square meters: $yd^2 \times 0.76 = m^2$

Volume

fluid ounces to milliliters: fl oz × 29.573 = ml
quarts to liters: qt × 0.95 = l
gallons to liters: gal × 3.8 = l

Appendix B

Metric Conversions: Selected Charts and Tables

Chart 1 Twelve-Minute Run Test (Scores in Meters)

	Men (Age)			
Classification	**17–26**	**27–39**	**40–49**	**50+**
High-performance zone	2880+	2560+	2400+	2240+
Good fitness zone	2480–2779	2320–2559	2240–2399	2000–2239
Marginal zone	2160–2479	2080–2319	2000–2239	1760–1999
Low zone	< 2160	< 2080	< 2000	< 1760
	Women (Age)			
Classification	**17–26**	**27–39**	**40–49**	**50+**
High-performance zone	2320+	2160+	2000+	1840+
Good fitness zone	2000–2319	1920–2159	1840–1999	1680–1839
Marginal zone	1840–1999	1680–1919	1600–1839	1520–1679
Low zone	< 1840	< 1680	< 1600	< 1520

Chart 2 Isometric Strength Rating Scale (kg)

Classification	Left Grip	Right Grip	Total Score
Men			
High-performance zone	57+	61+	118+
Good fitness zone	45–56	50–60	95–117
Marginal zone	41–44	43–49	84–94
Low zone	<41	<43	<84
Women			
High-performance zone	34+	39+	73+
Good fitness zone	27–33	32–38	59–72
Marginal zone	20–26	23–31	43–58
Low zone	<20	<23	<43

Suitable for use by young adults between 18 and 30 years of age. After 30, an adjustment of 0.5 of 1 percent per year is appropriate because some loss of muscle tissue typically occurs as you grow older.

Chart 3 Power Rating Scale

Classification	Men	Women
Excellent	68 cm+	60 cm+
Very good	53–67 cm	48–59 cm
Good	42–52 cm	37–47 cm
Fair	31–41 cm	27–36 cm
Poor	<32 cm	<27 cm

Chart 4 Reaction Time Rating Scale

Classification	Score in inches	Score in centimeters
Excellent	More than 21"	53+
Very good	19"–21"	48–52
Good	16"–18 3/4"	41–47
Fair	13"–15 3/4"	33–40
Poor	Below 13"	<33

Chart 5 Speed Rating Scale

Classification	Men		Women	
	Yards	Meters	Yards	Meters
Excellent	24+	22+	22+	20+
Very good	22–23	20–21.9	20–21	18–19.9
Good	18–21	16.5–19.9	16–19	14.5–17.9
Fair	16–17	14.5–16.4	14–15	13–14.4
Poor	<16	<14.5	<14	<13

Appendix C

Calorie Guide to Common Foods

Beverages	
Coffee (black)	0
Coke (12 oz.)	137
Hot chocolate, milk (1 cup)	247
Lemonade (1 cup)	100
Limeade, diluted to serve (1 cup)	110
Soda, fruit flavored (12 oz.)	161
Tea (clear)	0

Breads and Cereals	
Bagel (1 half)	76
Biscuit (2″ × 2″)	135
Bread, pita (1 oz.)	80
Bread, raisin (1/2″ thick)	65
Bread, rye	55
Bread, white enriched (1/2″ thick)	64
Bread, whole wheat (1/2″ thick)	55
Bun (hamburger)	120
Cereals, cooked (1/2 cup)	80
Corn flakes (1 cup)	96
Corn grits (1 cup)	125
Corn muffin (2 1/2″ diam.)	103
Crackers, graham (1 med.)	28
Crackers, soda (1 plain)	24
English muffin (1 half)	74
Macaroni, with cheese (1 cup)	464
Muffin, plain	135
Noodles (1 cup)	200
Oatmeal (1 cup)	150
Pancakes (1–4″ diam.)	59
Pizza (1 section)	180
Popped corn (1 cup)	54
Potato chips (10 med.)	108
Pretzels (5 small sticks)	18
Rice (1 cup)	225
Roll, plain (1 med.)	118
Roll, sweet (1 med.)	178
Shredded wheat (1 med. biscuit)	79
Spaghetti, plain cooked (1 cup)	218
Tortilla (1 corn)	70
Waffle (4 1/2″ × 5″)	216

Dairy Products	
Butter, 1 pat (1 1/2 tsp.)	50
Cheese, cheddar (1 oz.)	113
Cheese, cottage (1 cup)	270
Cheese, cream (1 oz.)	106
Cheese, Parmesan (1 tbsp.)	29
Cheese, Swiss natural (1 oz.)	105
Cream, sour (1 tbsp.)	31
Frozen custard (1 cup)	375
Frozen yogurt, vanilla (1 cup)	180
Ice cream, plain (prem.) (1 cup)	350
Ice cream soda, choc. (large glass)	455
Ice milk (1 cup)	184
Ices (1 cup)	177
Milk, chocolate (1 cup)	185
Milk, half-and-half (1 tbsp.)	20
Milk, malted (1 cup)	281
Milk, skim (1 cup)	88
Milk, skim dry (1 tbsp.)	28
Milk, whole (1 cup)	166
Sherbet (1 cup)	270
Softserve cone (med.)	335
Whipped topping (1 tbsp.)	14
Yogurt (1 cup)	150

Desserts and Sweets	
Cake, angel (2″ wedge)	108
Cake, chocolate (2″ × 3″ × 1″)	150
Cake, plain (3″ × 2 1/2″)	180
Chocolate, bar	200–300
Chocolate, bitter (1 oz.)	142
Chocolate, sweet (1 oz.)	133
Chocolate, syrup (1 tbsp.)	42
Cocoa (1 tbsp.)	21
Cookies, plain (1 med.)	75
Custard, baked (1 cup)	283
Doughnut (1 large)	250
Gelatin, dessert (1 cup)	155
Gelatin, with fruit (1 cup)	170
Gingerbread (2″ × 2″ × 2″)	180
Jams, jellies (1 tbsp.)	55
Pie, apple (1/7 of 9″ pie)	345
Pie, cherry (1/7 of 9″ pie)	355
Pie, chocolate (1/7 of 9″ pie)	360
Pie, coconut (1/7 of 9″ pie)	266
Pie, lemon meringue (1/7 of 9″ pie)	302
Sugar, granulated (1 tsp.)	27
Syrup, table (1 tbsp.)	57

Fruit	
Apple, fresh (med.)	76
Applesauce, unsweetened (1 cup)	184
Avocado, raw (1/2 peeled)	279
Banana, fresh (med.)	88
Cantaloupe, raw (1/2, 5″ diam.)	60
Cherries (10 sweet)	50
Cranberry sauce, unsweetened (1 tbsp.)	25
Fruit cocktail, canned (1 cup)	170
Grapefruit, fresh (1/2)	60
Grapefruit juice, raw (1 cup)	95
Grape juice, bottled (1/2 cup)	80
Grapes (20–25)	75
Nectarine (1 med.)	88
Olives, green	72
Olives, ripe (10)	105
Orange, fresh (med.)	60
Orange juice, frozen diluted (1 cup)	110
Peach, fresh (med.)	46
Peach, canned in syrup (2 halves)	79
Pear, fresh (med.)	95
Pears, canned in syrup (2 halves)	79
Pineapple, crushed in syrup (1 cup)	204
Pineapple (1/2 cup fresh)	50
Prune juice (1 cup)	170
Raisins, dry (1 tbsp.)	26
Strawberries, fresh (1 cup)	54
Strawberries, frozen (3 oz.)	90
Tangerine (2 1/2″ diam.)	40
Watermelon, wedge (4″ × 8″)	120

Meat, Fish, Eggs	
Bacon, drained (2 slices)	97
Bacon, Canadian (1 oz.)	62
Beef, hamburger chuck (3 oz.)	316
Beef, pot pie	560
Beef steak, sirloin or T-bone (3 oz.)	257
Beef and vegetable stew (1 cup)	185
Chicken, fried breast (8 oz.)	210
Chicken, fried (1 leg and thigh)	305
Chicken, roasted breast (2 slices)	100
Chili, without beans (1 cup)	510
Chili, with beans (1 cup)	335
Egg, boiled	77
Egg, fried	125
Egg, scrambled	100
Fish and chips (2 pcs. fish; 4 oz. chips)	275
Fish, broiled (3″ × 3″ × 1/2″)	112
Fish stick	40
Frankfurter, boiled	124
Ham (4″ × 4″)	338
Lamb (3 oz. roast, lean)	158
Liver (3″ × 3″)	150
Luncheon meat (2 oz.)	135
Pork chop, loin (3″ × 5″)	284
Salmon, canned (1 cup)	145
Sausage, pork (4 oz.)	510
Shrimp, canned (3 oz.)	108
Tuna, canned (1/2 cup)	185
Veal, cutlet (3″ × 4″)	175

Nuts and Seeds	
Cashews (1 cup)	770
Coconut (1 cup)	450
Peanut butter (1 tbsp.)	92
Peanuts, roasted, no skin (1 cup)	805
Pecans (1 cup)	752
Sunflower seeds (1 tbsp.)	50

Sandwiches (2 slices of bread—plain)	
Bologna	214
Cheeseburger (small McDonald's)	300
Chicken salad	185
Egg salad	240
Fish filet (McDonald's)	400
Ham	360
Ham and cheese	360
Hamburger (small McDonald's)	260
Hamburger, Burger King Whopper	600
Hamburger, Big Mac	550
Hamburger (McDonald's Quarter Pounder)	420
Peanut butter	250
Roast beef (Arby's Regular)	425

Sauces, Fats, Oils	
Catsup, tomato (1 tbsp.)	17
Chili sauce (1 tbsp.)	17
French dressing (1 tbsp.)	59
Margarine (1 pat)	50
Mayonnaise (1 tbsp.)	92

Mayonnaise-type (1 tbsp.)	65
Vegetable, sunflower, safflower oils (1 tbsp.)	120
Soup, Ready to Serve (1 cup)	
Bean	190
Beef noodle	100
Cream	200
Tomato	90
Vegetable	80
Vegetables	
Alfalfa sprouts (1/2 cup)	19
Asparagus (6 spears)	22
Bean sprouts (1 cup)	37
Beans, green (1 cup)	27
Beans, lima (1 cup)	152
Beans, navy (1 cup)	642
Beans, pork and molasses (1 cup)	325
Broccoli, fresh cooked (1 cup)	60
Cabbage, cooked (1 cup)	40
Cauliflower (1 cup)	25
Carrot, raw (med.)	21
Carrots, canned (1 cup)	44
Celery, diced raw (1 cup)	20
Coleslaw (1 cup)	102
Corn, sweet, canned (1 cup)	140
Corn, sweet (med. ear)	84
Cucumber, raw (6 slices)	6
Lettuce (2 large leaves)	7
Mushrooms, canned (1 cup)	28
Onions, french fried (10 rings)	75
Onions, raw (med.)	25
Peas, field (1/2 cup)	90
Peas, green (1 cup)	145
Pickles, dill (med.)	15
Pickles, sweet (med.)	22
Potato, baked (med.)	97
Potato, french fried (8 sticks)	155
Potato, mashed (1 cup)	185
Radish, raw (small)	1
Sauerkraut, drained (1 cup)	32
Spinach, fresh, cooked (1 cup)	46
Squash, summer (1 cup)	30
Sweet pepper (med.)	15
Sweet potato, candied (small)	314
Tomato, cooked (1 cup)	50
Tomato, raw (med.)	30

Due to space limitations it is not possible to list the nutrient content of all commercially available foods. There are a variety of valuable web-based resources that can be accessed to obtain more detailed lists of foods or complete dietary analyses. The Nutrition Department at Tufts University has developed a web page called Nutrition Navigators (http://www.navigator.tufts.edu/) that reviews the quality of various nutrition-related websites. The list below highlights a few of the dietary analysis programs that received favorable reviews from the Nutrition Navigator website. These resources are recommended for students interested in learning about the nutrient content of foods not listed in appendices C and D. Directly consulting the Nutrition Navigator site may bring up additional sites that may be useful as well.

Cyberdiet—http://www.cyberdiet.com/

This website, developed by a team of registered dietitians, offers a variety of information about nutrition. The database of commonly used foods (http://www.cyberdiet.com/ni/htdocs/index.html) can be quickly searched for dietary information. An advantage of this database is that it allows you to search by various categories of foods and quickly view and compare foods in a similar category.

Diet Analysis Web Page—http://dawp.anet.com/

This diet analysis site lets you enter the foods you've eaten over the course of a day, and then, based on the RDA, reports a complete nutritional review of your diet. Tufts Nutrition Navigator gives this site a rating of "better than most."

Fast Food Finder—http://www.olen.com/food/

This online analysis program, developed with support from the Minnesota Attorney General's Office, allows you to obtain dietary information about nearly all items available from fast food chains.

Nutrition Analysis Tool—http://www.nat.uiuc.edu

This diet analysis program, developed by the University of Illinois Department of Food Science/Nutrition, provides a nutrient analysis of foods by searching foods within the USDA database.

Sante Food Database—http://www.nightcrew.com/sante7000/sante7000_search.cfm

This website program provides a nutrient analysis of over 7,248 foods that are listed in the U.S. Department of Agriculture (USDA) database. The report provides a listing of over 29 nutrients for each food.

Appendix D

Calories of Protein, Carbohydrates, and Fats in Foods*

Food No./Food Choice	Total Calories	Protein Calories	Carbohydrate Calories	Fat Calories
Breakfast				
1. Scrambled Egg (1 lg)	111	29	7	75
2. Fried Egg (1 lg)	99	26	1	72
3. Pancake (1–6^W^)	146	19	67	58
4. Syrup (1 T)	60	0	60	0
5. French Toast (1 slice)	180	23	49	108
6. Waffle (7-inch)	245	28	100	117
7. Biscuit (medium)	104	8	52	44
8. Bran Muffin (medium)	104	11	63	31
9. White Toast (slice)	68	9	52	7
10. Wheat Toast (slice)	67	14	52	6
11. Peanut Butter (1 T)	94	15	11	68
12. Yogurt (8 oz. plain)	227	39	161	27
13. Orange Juice (8 oz.)	114	8	100	6
14. Apple Juice (8 oz.)	117	1	116	0
15. Soft Drink (12 oz.)	144	0	144	0
16. Bacon (2 slices)	86	15	2	70
17. Sausage (1-link)	141	11	0	130
18. Sausage (1 patty)	284	23	0	261
19. Grits (8 oz.)	125	11	110	4
20. Hash Browns (8 oz.)	355	18	178	159
21. French Fries (reg.)	239	12	115	112
22. Donut Cake	125	4	61	60
23. Donut Glazed	164	8	87	69
24. Sweet Roll	317	22	136	159
25. Cake (medium slice)	274	14	175	85
26. Ice Cream (8 oz.)	257	15	108	134
27. Cream Cheese (T)	52	4	1	47
28. Jelly (T)	49	0	49	0
29. Jam (T)	54	0	54	0
30. Coffee (cup)	0	0	0	0
31. Tea (cup)	0	0	0	0
32. Cream (T)	32	2	2	28
33. Sugar (t)	15	0	15	0
34. Corn Flakes (8 oz.)	97	8	87	2
35. Wheat Flakes (8 oz.)	106	12	90	4
36. Oatmeal (8 oz.)	132	19	92	21
37. Strawberries (8 oz.)	55	4	46	5
38. Orange (medium)	64	6	57	1
39. Apple (medium)	96	1	86	9
40. Banana (medium)	101	4	95	2
41. Cantaloupe (half)	82	7	73	2
42. Grapefruit (half)	40	2	37	1
43. Custard Pie (slice)	285	20	188	77
44. Fruit Pie (slice)	350	14	259	77
45. Fritter (medium)	132	11	54	67
46. Skim Milk (8 oz.)	88	36	52	0
47. Whole Milk (8 oz.)	159	33	48	78
48. Butter (pat)	36	0	0	36
49. Margarine (pat)	36	0	0	36

Food No./Food Choice	Total Calories	Protein Calories	Carbohydrate Calories	Fat Calories
Lunch				
1. Hamburger (reg. FF)	255	48	120	89
2. Cheeseburger (reg. FF)	307	61	120	126
3. Doubleburger (FF)	563	101	163	299
4. 1/4 lb. Burger (FF)	427	73	137	217
5. Doublecheese Burger (FF)	670	174	134	362
6. Doublecheese Baconburger (FF)	724	138	174	340
7. Hot Dog (FF)	214	36	54	124
8. Chili Dog (FF)	320	51	90	179
9. Pizza, Cheese (slice FF)	290	116	116	58
10. Pizza, Meat (slice FF)	360	126	126	108
11. Pizza, Everything (slice FF)	510	179	173	158
12. Sandwich, Roast Beef (FF)	350	88	126	137
13. Sandwich, Bologna	313	44	106	163
14. Sandwich, Bologna-Cheese	428	69	158	201
15. Sandwich, Ham-Cheese (FF)	380	91	133	156
16. Sandwich, Peanut Butter	281	39	118	124
17. Sandwich, PB and Jelly	330	40	168	122
18. Sandwich, Egg Salad	330	40	109	181
19. Sandwich, Tuna Salad	390	101	109	180
20. Sandwich, Fish (FF)	432	56	147	229
21. French Fries (reg. FF)	239	12	115	112
22. French Fries (lg. FF)	406	20	195	191
23. Onion Rings (reg. FF)	274	14	112	148
24. Chili (8 oz.)	260	49	62	148
25. Bean Soup (8 oz.)	355	67	181	107
26. Beef Noodle Soup (8 oz.)	140	32	59	49
27. Tomato Soup (8 oz.)	180	14	121	45
28. Vegetable Soup (8 oz.)	160	21	107	32
29. Small Salad, Plain	37	6	27	4
30. Small Salad, French Dressing	152	8	50	94
31. Small Salad, Italian Dressing	162	8	28	126
32. Small Salad, Bleu Cheese	184	13	28	143
33. Potato Salad (8 oz.)	248	27	159	62
34. Cole Slaw (8 oz.)	180	0	25	155
35. Macaroni and Cheese (8 oz.)	230	37	103	90
36. Taco Beef (FF)	186	59	56	71
37. Bean Burrito (FF)	343	45	192	106
38. Meat Burrito (FF)	466	158	196	112
39. Mexican Rice (FF)	213	17	160	36
40. Mexican Beans (FF)	168	42	82	44
41. Fried Chicken Breast (FF)	436	262	13	161
42. Broiled Chicken Breast	284	224	0	60
43. Broiled Fish	228	82	32	114
44. Fish Stick (1 stick FF)	50	18	8	24
45. Fried Egg	99	26	1	72
46. Donut	125	4	61	60
47. Potato Chips (small bag)	115	3	39	73
48. Soft Drink (12 oz.)	144	0	144	0

*Notes:

1. FF by a food indicates that it is typical of a food served in a fast food restaurant.
2. Your portions of foods may be larger or smaller than those listed here. For this reason you may wish to select a food more than once (i.e., two hamburgers) or select only a portion of a serving (i.e., divide the calories in half for a half portion).
3. An oz. equals an ounce or 28.4 grams.
4. T = Tablespoon and t = teaspoon.

The principal reference for the calculation of values used in this appendix were the *Nutritive Value of Foods,* published by the United States Department of Agriculture, Washington, D.C., Home and Gardens Bulletin, No. 72, although other published sources were consulted, including Jacobson, M., and S. Fritschner, *The Fast-Food Guide* (an excellent source of information about fast foods), New York, Workman Publishing Company.

Food No./Food Choice	Total Calories	Protein Calories	Carbohydrate Calories	Fat Calories
49. Apple Juice (8 oz.)	117	1	116	0
50. Skim Milk (8 oz.)	88	36	52	0
51. Whole Milk (8 oz.)	159	33	48	78
52. Diet Drink (12 oz.)	0	0	0	0
53. Mustard (t)	4	0	4	0
54. Catsup (t)	6	0	6	0
55. Mayonnaise (T)	100	0	0	100
56. Fruit Pie	350	14	259	77
57. Cheese Cake	400	56	132	212
58. Ice Cream (8 oz.)	257	15	108	134
59. Coffee (8 oz.)	0	0	0	0
60. Tea (8 oz.)	0	0	0	0
Dinner				
1. Hamburger (reg. FF)	255	48	120	89
2. Cheeseburger (reg. FF)	307	61	120	126
3. Doubleburger (FF)	563	101	163	299
4. 1/4 lb. Burger (FF)	427	73	137	217
5. Doublecheese Burger (FF)	670	174	134	362
6. Doublecheese Baconburger (FF)	724	138	174	412
7. Hot Dog (FF)	214	36	54	124
8. Chili Dog (FF)	320	51	90	179
9. Pizza, Cheese (slice FF)	290	116	116	58
10. Pizza, Meat (slice FF)	360	126	126	108
11. Pizza, Everything (slice FF)	510	179	173	158
12. Steak (8 oz.)	880	290	0	590
13. French Fried Shrimp (6 oz.)	360	133	68	158
14. Roast Beef (8 oz.)	440	268	0	172
15. Liver (8 oz.)	520	250	52	218
16. Corned Beef (8 oz.)	493	242	0	251
17. Meat Loaf (8 oz.)	711	228	35	448
18. Ham (8 oz.)	540	178	0	362
19. Spaghetti, No Meat (13 oz.)	400	56	220	124
20. Spaghetti, Meat (13 oz.)	500	115	230	155
21. Baked Potato (medium)	90	12	78	0
22. Cooked Carrots (8 oz.)	71	12	59	0
23. Cooked Spinach (8 oz.)	50	18	18	14
24. Corn (one ear)	70	10	52	8
25. Cooked Green Beans (8 oz.)	54	11	43	0
26. Cooked Broccoli (8 oz.)	60	19	26	15
27. Cooked Cabbage	47	12	35	0
28. French Fries (reg. FF)	239	12	115	112
29. French Fries (lg. FF)	406	20	195	191
30. Onion Rings (reg. FF)	274	14	112	148
31. Chili (8 oz.)	260	49	62	148
32. Small Salad, Plain	37	6	27	4
33. Small Salad, French Dressing	152	8	50	94
34. Small Salad, Italian Dressing	162	8	28	126
35. Small Salad, Bleu Cheese	184	13	28	143
36. Potato Salad (8 oz.)	248	27	159	62
37. Cole Slaw (8 oz.)	180	0	25	155
38. Macaroni and Cheese (8 oz.)	230	37	103	90
39. Taco Beef (FF)	186	59	56	71
40. Bean Burrito (FF)	343	45	192	106
41. Meat Burrito (FF)	466	158	196	112
42. Mexican Rice (FF)	213	17	160	36
43. Mexican Beans (FF)	168	42	82	44
44. Fried Chicken Breast (FF)	436	262	13	161

Food No./Food Choice	Total Calories	Protein Calories	Carbohydrate Calories	Fat Calories
45. Broiled Chicken Breast	284	224	0	60
46. Broiled Fish	228	82	32	114
47. Fish Stick (1 stick FF)	50	18	8	24
48. Soft Drink (12 oz.)	144	0	144	0
49. Apple Juice (8 oz.)	117	1	116	0
50. Skim Milk (8 oz.)	88	36	52	0
51. Whole Milk (8 oz.)	159	33	48	78
52. Diet Drink (12 oz.)	0	0	0	0
53. Mustard (t)	4	0	4	0
54. Catsup (t)	6	0	6	0
55. Mayonnaise (T)	100	0	0	100
56. Fruit Pie (slice)	350	14	259	77
57. Cheese Cake (slice)	400	56	132	212
58. Ice Cream (8 oz.)	257	15	108	134
59. Custard Pie (slice)	285	20	188	77
60. Cake (slice)	274	14	175	85
Snacks				
1. Peanut Butter (1 T)	94	15	11	68
2. Yogurt (8 oz. plain)	227	39	161	27
3. Orange Juice (8 oz.)	114	8	100	6
4. Apple Juice (8 oz.)	117	1	116	0
5. Soft Drink (12 oz.)	144	0	144	0
6. Donut, Cake	125	4	61	60
7. Donut, Glazed	164	8	87	69
8. Sweet Roll	317	22	136	159
9. Cake (medium slice)	274	14	175	85
10. Ice Cream (8 oz.)	257	15	108	134
11. Soft Serve Cone (reg.)	240	10	89	134
12. Ice Cream Sandwich Bar	210	40	82	88
13. Strawberries (8 oz.)	55	4	46	5
14. Orange (medium)	64	6	57	1
15. Apple (medium)	96	1	86	9
16. Banana (medium)	101	4	95	2
17. Cantaloupe (half)	82	7	73	2
18. Grapefruit (half)	40	2	37	1
19. Celery Stick	5	2	3	0
20. Carrot (medium)	20	3	17	0
21. Raisins (4 oz.)	210	6	204	0
22. Watermelon (4″ × 6″ slice)	115	8	99	8
23. Chocolate Chip Cookie	60	3	9	48
24. Brownie	145	6	26	113
25. Oatmeal Cookie	65	3	13	49
26. Sandwich Cookie	200	8	112	80
27. Custard Pie (slice)	285	20	188	77
28. Fruit Pie (slice)	350	14	259	77
29. Gelatin (4 oz.)	70	4	32	34
30. Fritter (medium)	132	11	54	67
31. Skim Milk (8 oz.)	88	36	52	0
32. Diet Drink	0	0	0	0
33. Potato Chips (small bag)	115	3	39	73
34. Roasted Peanuts (1.3 oz.)	210	34	25	151
35. Chocolate Candy Bar (1 oz.)	145	7	61	77
36. Choc. Almond Candy Bar (1 oz.)	265	38	74	164
37. Saltine Cracker	18	1	1	16
38. Popped Corn	40	7	33	0
39. Cheese Nachos	471	63	194	214

See Note in Appendix C for additional nutrition information on the Web.

Appendix E

Canada's Food Guide to Healthy Eating

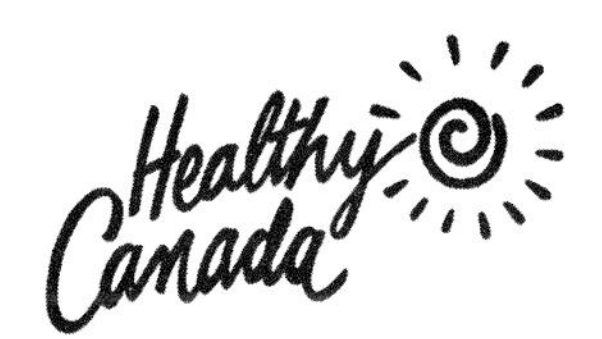

Health and Welfare Canada Santé et Bien-être social Canada

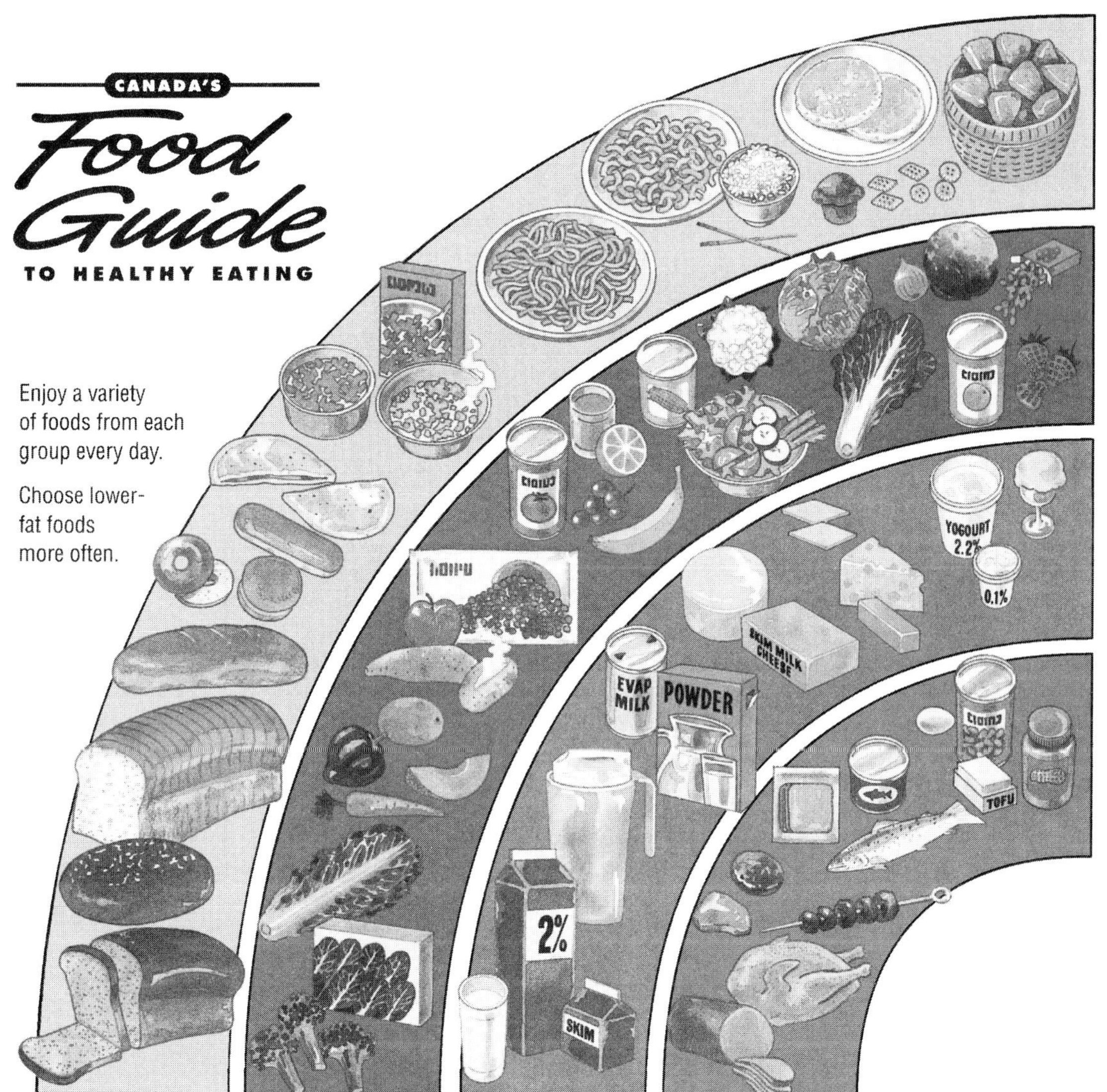

Grain Products
Choose whole grain and enriched products more often.

Vegetables & Fruit
Choose dark green and orange vegetables and orange fruit more often.

Milk Products
Choose lower-fat milk products more often.

Meat & Alternatives
Choose leaner meats, poultry and fish, as well as dried peas, beans and lentils more often.

Canada

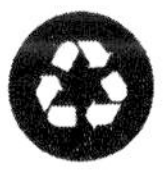

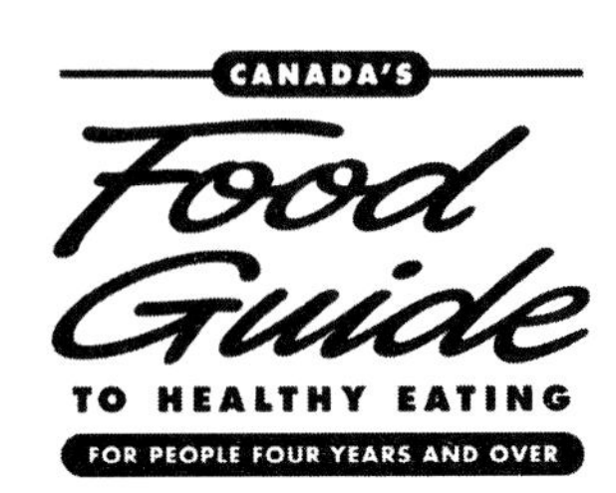

Different People Need Different Amounts of Food

The amount of food you need every day from the 4 food groups and other foods depends on your age, body size, activity level, whether you are male or female and if you are pregnant or breast-feeding. That's why the Food Guide gives a lower and higher number of servings for each food group. For example, young children can choose the lower number of servings, while male teenagers can go to the higher number. Most other people can choose servings somewhere in between.

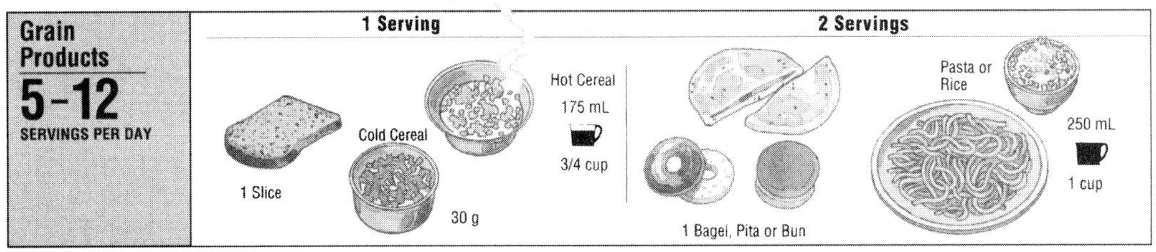

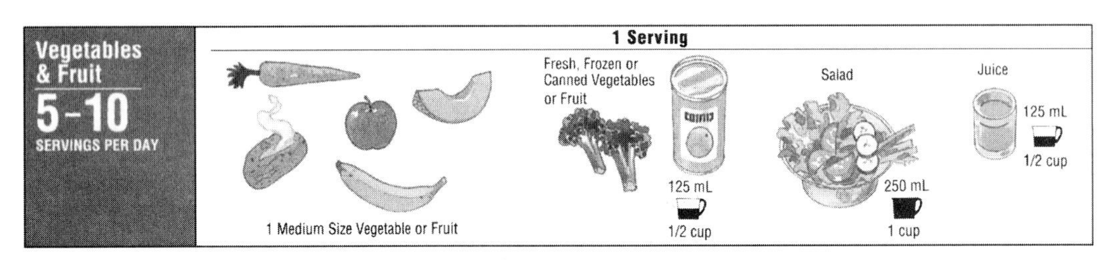

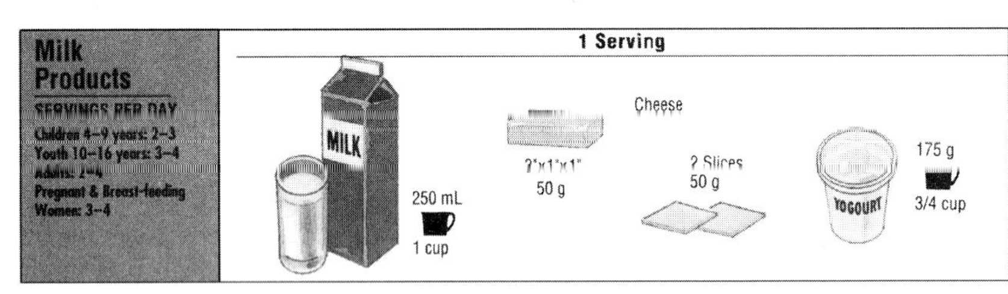

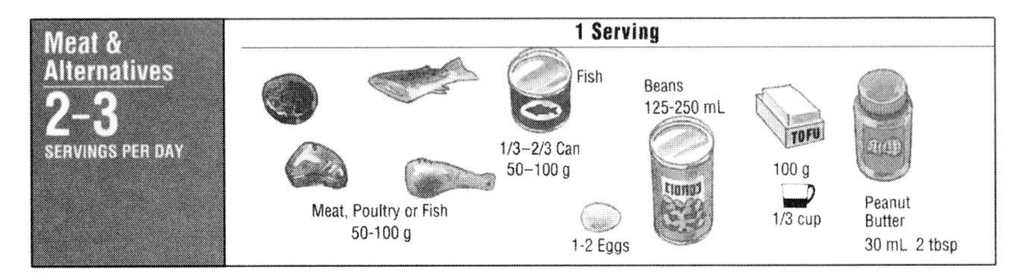

Other Foods

Taste and enjoyment can also come from other foods and beverages that are not part of the 4 food groups. Some of these foods are higher in fat or Calories, so use these foods in moderation.

Enjoy eating well, being active and feeling good about yourself. That's VITALITY

ISBN 0-662-19648-1

Selected References

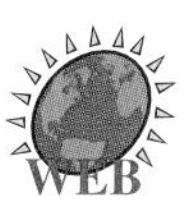

www.mhhe.com/hper/physed/corbin/
Additional references available at this address.

ACSM's Health and Fitness Journal. 2(2)(1998): entire issue. This issue contains 11 articles dealing with the health benefits of physical activity.

Agosti, R. "Reduce Risk of Activity Induced Injury." *ACSM's Health and Fitness.* 2(2)(1998):28.

Albert, C. M. et al. "Fish Consumption and Risk of Sudden Cardiac Death." *Journal of the American Medical Association.* 279(1)(1998):23.

Albert, C. M. et al. "Triggering of Sudden Death from Cardiac Causes by Vigorous Exertion." *New England Journal of Medicine.* 243(19)(2000): 1355–1361.

Alcohol 101 Research Results: National Data Analyses. *Century Council* (1998).

Alderman, M. H. et al. "Dietary Sodium Intake and Mortality." *Lancet.* 351(9105)(1998):781.

Allison, D. B. et al. "Annual Deaths Attributable to Obesity in the United States." *Journal of the American Medical Association.* 282(1999):1538.

Almeida, S. A. et al. "Epidemiological Patterns of Musculoskeletal Injuries and Physical Training." *Medicine and Science in Sports and Exercise.* 31(8)(1999): 1176.

Alter, M. J. *Science of Flexibility.* Champaign, IL: Human Kinetics, 1996.

American Academy of Orthopaedic Surgeons, Schenck, R. C. (ed.). *Athletic Training and Sports Medicine.* (3rd ed.). Chicago, IL: AAOS, 2000.

American Cancer Society. *Cancer Statistics 1999.* www.cancer.org/cancerinfo/specific.a8p.

American College of Sports Medicine. *ACSM's Guidelines for Exercise Prescription and Testing* (6th ed.). Philadelphia: Lippincott, Williams and Wilkins, 2000.

American College of Sports Medicine. "Creatine Supplementation: Current Content." (www.acsm.org)

American College of Sports Medicine and American Dietetics Association. "Joint Statement on Diabetes Mellitus and Exercise." *Medicine and Science in Sports and Exercise.* 29(12)(1997):992.

American College of Sports Medicine. "Exercise and Physical Activity for Older Adults." *Medicine and Science in Sports and Exercise.* 30(6)(1998):992.

American College of Sports Medicine. "Position Stand on Exercise and Fluid Replacement." *Medicine and Science in Sports and Exercise.* 28(1)(1996):i.

American College of Sports Medicine. "Position Stand on Heat and Cold Illness During Distance Running." *Medicine and Science in Sports and Exercise.* 28(12)(1996):i.

American College of Sports Medicine. "The Recommended Quantity and Quality of Exercise for Developing and Maintaining Cardiorespiratory and Muscular Fitness in Healthy Adults." *Medicine and Science in Sports and Exercise.* 22(1990):2.

American College of Sports Medicine. "The Recommended Quantity and Quality of Exercise for Developing and Maintaining Cardiorespiratory and Muscular Fitness and Flexibility in Healthy Adults." *Medicine and Science in Sports and Exercise.* 30(6)(1998):975.

American College of Sports Medicine. *ACSM's Guidelines for Exercise Prescription and Testing* (6th ed.). Philadelphia: Lippincott, Williams and Wilkins, 2000.

American Dietetics Association. "Fat Replacers—ADA Position." *Journal of the American Dietetics Association.* 98(1998):463.

American Dietetics Association. "Vegetarian Diets—Position of ADA." *Journal of the American Dietetics Association.* 97(1997):1317.

American Dietetics Association. "Weight Management—Position of ADA." *Journal of the American Dietetics Association.* 97(1997):71.

American Heart Association. "A Statement on Exercise: Benefits and Recommendations for Physical Activity Programs for All Americans." *Circulation.* 91(1995): 580.

American Heart Association. *1999 Heart & Stroke Statistical Update.* www.amhrt.org/catalog/scientifc-catpage70.html

American Opinion in the 20th Century. *USA Today,* 31 December 1999, 11A and 29A.

Andersen, R. E. et al. "Effects of Lifestyle Activity vs. Structured Aerobic Exercise in Obese Women." *Journal of the American Medical Association.* 281(4)(1999): 335.

Anderson, R. E. "Exercise, an Active Lifestyle, and Obesity: Making an Exercise Prescription Work." *The Physician and Sports Medicine.* 27(10)(1999):41.

Androstenedione et al: "Nonprescription Steroids." *The Physician and Sports Medicine.* 26(11)(1998):15.

Angell, M., and Kassirer, J. P. "Alternative Medicine: The Risks of Untested and Unregulated Remedies." *New England Journal of Medicine.* 339(12)(1998):839.

Ang-Lee, M. K., Moss, J., and Yuan, C. "Herbal Medicines and Perioperative Care." *Journal of the American Medical Association.* 286(1)(2000): 208–216.

Appel, L. J. et al. "Effect of Dietary Patterns on Serum Homocysteine." *Circulation.* 102(2000):852.

Armbruster, B., and Gladwin, L. A. "More Fitness for Older Adults." *ACSM's Health and Fitness Journal.* 5(2)(2001): 6–12.

Armsey, T. D., and Green, G. A. "Nutrition Supplements: Science vs. Hype." *The Physician and Sports Medicine* 25(6)(1997):76.

Artal, P., and Sherman, C. "Exercise During Pregnancy: Safe and Beneficial for Most." *The Physician and Sports Medicine.* 27(8)(1999):51.

Audran, M. et al. "Effects of Erythropoetin Administration in Training Athletes and Possible Indirect Detection in Doping Control." *Medicine and Science in Sports and Exercise.* 31(5)(1999):639.

Babbitt, D. "Training Theory: Periodization." *American Track and Field* (1998), Summer.

Babyak, M. et al. "Exercise Treatment for Major Depression: Maintenance of Therapeutic Benefit at 10 Months." *Psychosomatic Medicine,* 62(5)(2000): 633–638.

Baechle, T. R., and Earle, R. W. (eds.) *Essentials of Strength Training and Conditioning* (2nd ed.). Champaign, IL: Human Kinetics, 2000

Barnard, J.R. "A Carbohydrate Diet to Prevent and Control Coronary Heart Disease: Pritikin was Right." *ACSM's Health and Fitness Journal.* 3(3)(1999):23.

Barnard, R.J. "The Heart Needs a Warm-Up Time." *The Physician and Sports Medicine.* 4(1976):40.

Bassett, D. R., Cureton, A. L., and Ainsworth, B. E. "Measurement of Daily Walking Distance—Questionnaire versus Pedometer." *Medicine and Science in Sports and Exercise* 32(5)(2000):1018.

Beck, B. R., and Shoemaker, M. R. "Osteoporosis: Understanding Key Risk Factors and Therapeutic Options." *The Physician and Sports Medicine.* 28(2)(2000):67–81.

Berland, G. K. et al. "Health Information on the Internet: Accessibility, Quality, and Readability in English and Spanish." *Journal of the American Medical Association.* 285(20)(2001): 2612–2621.

Benson, H. "Mind-Body Pioneer." *USA Today,* 1 June 2001.

Bhasin, S. "Testosterone Replacement and Resistance Exercise in HIV-infected Men with Weight Loss and Low Testosterone Levels." *Journal of American Medical Association.* 283(6)(2000):763.

Biermann, J. S. et al. "Evaluation of Cancer Information on the Net." *Cancer.* 86(3)(1999):381.

Biermann, J. S., Fetrow, C. W., and Avila, J. R. *Professional Handbook of Complementary and Alternative Medicines.* Springhouse, PA: Springhouse Publications, 1999.

Biddle, S. J. H., and Fox, K. R. "Motivation for Physical Activity and Weight Management." *International Journal of Obesity.* 22 (Supplement 2)(1998):S:39.

Bindman, R. et.al. "Multistate Evaluation of Anonymous HIV Testing and Access to Medical Care." *Journal of the American Medical Association.* 280(16)(1998):1416.

Bird, C. E. "Gender, Household Labor, and Psychological Distress: The Impact of the Amount and Division of Housework." *Journal of Health and Social Behavior.* 40(1999):32.

Blair, S. N. et al. *Active Living Every Day.* Champaign, IL: Human Kinetics, 2001.

Blair, S. N., and Bouchard, C. "Physical Activity and Obesity: ACSM Consensus Conference." *Medicine and Science in Sports and Exercise.* 31(11S)(1999):S497.

Blair, S. N., and Jackson, A. S. "A Guest Editorial to Accompany Physical Fitness and Activity as Separate Heart Disease Risk Factors: A Meta-analysis." *Medicine and Science in Sports and Exercise.* 33(5)(2001): 762–764.

Blendon, R. J. et al. "Americans' Views on the Use and Regulation of Dietary Supplements." *Archives of Internal Medicine.* 161(6)(2001): 805–810.

Blonna, R. *Coping with Stress in a Changing World.* St. Louis: McGraw-Hill, 1999.

Boden, D. et al. "HIV-1 Drug Resistance in Newly Infected Individuals." *Journal of the American Medical Association.* 282(12) (2000):1135.

Booth, F. et al. "Waging War on Modern Chronic Disease." *Journal of Applied Physiology.* 88(2)(2000):774.

Bouchard, C. et al. *Genetics of Fitness and Physical Performance.* Champaign, IL: Human Kinetics, 1997.

Bouchard, C. "Physical Activity and Health: Introduction to the Dose-Response Symposium." *Medicine and Science in Sports and Exercise.* 33(6)(supplement)(2001): S347–350.

Bova, A. A., and Sherman, C. "Active Control of Hypertension." *The Physician and Sports Medicine.* 26(4)(1998):45.

Brandon, L. J. et al. "Strength Training for Older Adults." *ACSM's Health and Fitness Journal.* 4(6)(2000): 13–28.

Brehm, B. A. "Maximizing the Psychological Benefits of Physical Activity." *ACSM's Health and Fitness Journal.* 4(6)(2000): 7–11.

Breslow, L. "From Disease Prevention to Health Promotion." *Journal of the American Medical Association.* 281(11)(1999):1030.

Brill, P. A., Macera, C. A., Davis, D. R., Blair, S. N., and Gordon, N. "Muscular Strength and Physical Function." *Medicine and Science in Sports and Exercise.* 32(2)(2000): 412.

Broocks, A. et al. "Comparison of Aerobic Exercise, Clomipramine, and Placebo in the Treatment of Panic Disorder." *American Journal of Psychiatry.* 155(5)(1998): 603–609.

Buckwalter, J. A. "Decreased Mobility in the Elderly: The Exercise Antidote." *The Physician and Sports Medicine.* 25(9)(1997):138.

Burke, E. et al. *Long-Distance Cycling: Build the Strength, Skills and Confidence to Ride as Far as You Want.* Emmaus, PA: Rodale Press, 2000.

Burney, M. W., and Brehm, B. A. "The Female Athlete Triad." *Journal of Physical Education, Recreation and Dance.* 69(9)(1998):29.

Burns, D. D. *The Feeling Good Handbook.* (revised ed.) Plume/Penguin Books: New York:1999.

Burstein, G. R. et al. "Incident Chlamydia Trachomatis Infections Among Inner City Adolescent Females." *Journal of the American Medical Association.* 280(6)(1999):521.

Cailliet, R. *Knee Pain and Disability.* 3d ed. Philadelphia: F.A. Davis, Co., 1992.

Cailliet, R. *Low Back Pain Syndrome.* 5th ed. Philadelphia: F.A. Davis, Co., 1994.

Cailliet, R. *Neck and Arm Pain.* 3d ed. Philadelphia: F.A. Davis, Co., 1991.

Cailliet, R. *Shoulder Pain.* 3d ed. Philadelphia: F.A. Davis, Co., 1995.

Campaigne, B. N. "Exercise and Type I Diabetes." *ACSM's Health and Fitness Journal.* 2(4)(1998):35.

Campaigne, B. N. "Provide Physical Activity Precautions for Clients with Diabetes." *ACSM's Health and Fitness.* 2(2)(1998):18.

Canto, J. G. et al. "Prevalence, Clinical Characteristics, and Mortality among Patients with Myocardial Infarction Presenting without Chest Pain." *Journal of the American Medical Association.* 283(24)(2000):3223.

Carpenter, C. C. J. et al. "Antiretroviral for HIV Infection in 1998: Updated Recommendations." *Journal of the American Medical Association.* 280(1)(1998):78.

Carpenter, D. M., and Nelson, B. W. "Low Back Strengthening for the Prevention and Treatment of Low Back Pain." *Medicine and Science in Sports and Exercise.* 31(1)(1999):18.

Cataldo, D., and Heyward, V. H. "Pinch an Inch: A Comparison of Several High-quality and Plastic Skinfold Calipers." *ACSM's Health and Fitness Journal.* 4(3)(2000):12.

Catlin, D. H. et al. "Trace Contamination of Over-the-Counter Androstenedione and Positive Urine Test Results for a Nandrolone Metabolite." *Journal of the American Medical Association.* 284(20)(2000): 2618–2621.

Cavadini, C., Siega-Riz, A. M., and Popkin, B. M. "U.S. Adolescent Food Intake Trends from 1965 to 1996." *Archives of Disease in Childhood.* 83(2000):18.

Centers for Disease Control and Prevention. "Cigarette Smoking among Adults—United States." *Morbidity and Mortality Weekly Reports.* 18(43)(1999):993.

Centers for Disease Control and Prevention. "Cigarette Smoking among High School Students—United States." *Morbidity and Mortality Weekly Reports.* 18(47)(1998):229.

Centers for Disease Control and Prevention. "The Cost Effectiveness of Screening for Type II Diabetes." *Journal of the American Medical Association.* 280(20)(1999):1957.

Centers for Disease Control and Prevention. "Prevalence of Leisure-Time Physical Activity among Overweight Adults—United States, 1998." *Morbidity and Mortality Weekly Reports.* 49(15):32.

Centers for Disease Control and Prevention. "Ten Great Public Health Accomplishments—United States 1900—1999." *Morbidity and Mortality Weekly Reports.* 48(12)(2000): 241.

Chase, L. A., Corbin, C. B., and Rutherford, W. "Self Measured vs Expert-Measured Skinfolds of College Aged Females." *J. British Journal of Physical Education:* Research Supplement. 12(1992):9.

Cherkin, D. C. et al. "A Comparison of Physical Therapy, Chiropractic Manipulation and Providing of an Educational Book for Treatment of Patients with Low Back Pain." *New England Journal of Medicine.* 339(15) (1998):1021.

Chevront, S. N. "The Zone Diet and Athletic Performance." *Sports Medicine.* 27(1999):214.

Chewning, B., Yu, T., and Johnson, J. "T'ai chi—Part 2: Effects on Health." *ACSM's Health and Fitness Journal.* 4(3)(2000):17.

Chewning, B., Yu, T., and Johnson, J. "T'ai chi: Ancient Exercise for Contemporary Life." *ACSM's Health and Fitness Journal.* 4(2)(2000):21.

Ciocca, M. "Pneumothaorx in a Weight Lifter." *The Physician and Sports Medicine.* 28(4)(2000):97.

Chu, D. A. *Jumping Into Plyometrics*, 2e. Champaign, IL: Human Kinetics, 1998.

Clark, J. R. "Sexually Transmitted Disease: Detection, Differentiation, and Treatment." *The Physician and Sports Medicine.* 25(1)(1997):76.

Clark, K. "Replacing Fat: Have We Managed a Miracle?" *ACSM's Health and Fitness Journal.* 3(2)(1999):22.

Clark, K. "Water, Sports Drinks, Juice, or Soda?" *ACSM's Health and Fitness Journal.* 2(5)(1998):41.

Clarkson, P. M. "The Skinny on Weight Loss Supplements and Drugs: Winning the War Against Fat." *ACSM's Health and Fitness Journal.* 2(4)(1998):18.

Cochran, S. *Complete Conditioning for Martial Arts.* Champaign, IL: Human Kinetics, 2001.

Cohne, O. J., and Fauci, A. S. "HIV/AIDS in 1998: Gaining the Upper Hand." *Journal of the American Medical Association.* 280(1)(1998):87.

Colberg, S. R. "Exercise: A Diabeters 'Cure' for Many." *ACSM's Health and Fitness Journal.* 5(2)(2001): 20–26.

Colberg, S. R., and Swain, D. P. "Exercise and Diabetes Control." *The Physician and Sports Medicine.* 28(4)(2000): 63.

Cole, C. R. et al. "Heart Rate Recovery after Submaximal Exercise Testing as a Predictor of Mortality in Cardiovascularly Healthy Cohort." *Annals of Internal Medicine.* 132(7)(2000):552.

Coleman, E. "AHA Dietary Guidelines." *Sports Medicine Digest.* 22(2000): 133. www.sportsmedicinedigest.com

Coleman, E. "Carbohydrate Unloading." *The Physician and Sports Medicine.* 25(2)(1997):97.

Consumer Reports "The Mainstreaming of Alternative Medicine." *Consumer Reports.* 65(5)(2000):17.

Contreras-Vidal, J. L., Van Den Heuvel, C. E., Teulings, H. L., and Stelmach, G. E. "Adaptations Visuo-motirices Chez les Utilisateurs de Tabac Sans Fumée. *Nicotine & Tobacco Research.* 1(1999):219.

Corbin, C. B., and Pangrazi, R. P. (Editors), *Towards a Better Understanding of Physical Fitness and Activity.* Scottsdale, AZ: Holcomb-Hathaway, 1999.

Corbin, C. B., and Pangrazi, R. P. "Physical Activity Pyramid Rebuffs Peak Exercise." *ACSM's Health and Fitness Journal.* 2(1)(1998):12.

Corbin, C. B., and Pangrazi, R. P. "What You Need to Know about the Surgeon General's Report on Physical Activity and Health." In Corbin, C. B., and Pangrazi, R. P. *Towards an Understanding of Physical Fitness and Activity.* Scottsdale, AZ: Holcomb-Hathaway, 1999.

Corbin, C. B., and Pangrazi, R. P. *Physical Activity for Children: A Statement of Guidelines.* Reston, VA: National Association for Physical Education and Sports, 1998.

Corbin, C. B., Pangrazi, R. P., and Franks, B. D. "Definitions: Health, Fitness, and Physical Activity." *President's Council on Physical Fitness and Sport Research Digest.* 3(9)(2000):1.

Corbin, C.B., and R. Lindsey. *Fitness for Life.* 4th ed. Champaign, IL:Human Kinetics, 2002.

Corbin, D. E. (ed.). *Perspectives: Stress Management.* Boulder, CO: Coursewise Publishing Co., 1999.

Courneya, K. S., Mackey, J. R., and Jones, L. W. "Coping with Cancer: Can Exercise Help?" *The Physician and Sports Medicine.* 28(5)(2000):49.

Cox, F. D. *The Aids Booklet.* St. Louis: McGraw-Hill, 2000.

Crawford, D. A., Jeffery, R. W., and French, S. A. "Television Viewing, Physical Interactivity, and Obesity." *International Journal of Obesity and Related Metabolic Disorders.* 23(4)(1999):437–440.

Crespo, C. J. et al. "Prevalence of Physical Inactivity and Its Relation to Social Class in U. S. Adults." *Medicine and Science in Sports and Exercise.* 31(12)(1999):1821.

Curry, S. J. et al. "Use and Cost Effectiveness of Smoking Cessation Services under Four Insurance Plans in an HMO." *New England Journal of Medicine.* 339(10)(1998):673.

Dagnone, R. R. et al. "Reduction in Obesity and Related Comorbid Conditions after Diet-Induced Weight Loss or Exercise-Induced Weight Loss In Men." *Annals of Internal Medicine.* 133(2)(2000): 92–103.

Davidson, M. H. et al. "Weight Control and Risk Factor Reduction in Obese Subjects Treated for 2 Years with Orlistat." *Journal of the American Medical Association.* 280(3)(1999):281.

Davis, M. et al. *The Relaxation and Stress Reduction Workbook.* (5th ed.) Oakland, CA: New Harbinger, 2000.

DeMarco, H. M. et al. "Pre-Exercise Carbohydrate Meals: Application of the Glycemic Index." *Medicine and Science in Sports and Exercise.* 31(1)(1999):164.

de Lorgirel, M. et al. "Mediterranean Diet, Traditional Risk Factors and the Rate of Cardiovascular Complications after Myocardial Infarction." *Circulation.* 99(1999):779.

Dembo, L., and McCormick, K. M. "Exercise Prescription to Prevent Osteoporosis" *ACSM's Health and Fitness Journal.* 4(1)(2000): 32.

Dement, W. C., and Vaughan, C. *The Promise of Sleep: A Pioneer In Sleep Medicine Explores the Vital Connection between Health, Happiness, and a Good Night's Sleep.* Delacorte Press: New York: 1999.

Detels, R. et al. "Effects of Potent Antiretroviral Therapy on the Time to AIDS in Men Known to Have HIV Infection Duration." *Journal of the American Medical Association.* 280(17)(1998):1497.

Diaz-Mitoma, F. et al. "Oral Famciclovir for Suppression of Recurrent Genital Herpes." *Journal of the American Medical Association.* 280(10)(1998):887.

DiBello, V. et al. "Effects of Anabolic-Androgenic Steroids on Weight-Lifters' Myocardium: An Ultrasonic Videodensitometric Study." *Medicine and Science in Sports and Exercise.* 31(4)(1999):514.

DiClemente, R. J. "Prevention of Sexually Transmitted Infections among Adolescents: A Clash of Ideology and Science." *Journal of the American Medical Association.* 279(19)(1998):1574.

Dietary Guidelines and Your Diet. Hyattsville, MD: USDA, 1992, No. HG–232, 1–11.

"Diet Riot." *People,* 12 June 2000, 104.

DiFranza, J. R. et al. "RJR Nabisco's Cartoon Camel Promotes Camel Cigarettes to Children." *Journal of American Medical Association.* 266(22)(1991):3149.

Dillingham, T. R. "Lumbar Supports for Prevention of Low Back Pain in the Workplace." *Journal of the American Medical Association.* 279(22)(1998):1826.

Dimeo, F. et al. "Aerobic Exercise As Therapy for Cancer Fatigue." *Medicine and Science in Sports and Exercise.* 30(4)(1998):475.

Disabella, V., and Sherman, C. "Exercise for Asthma Patients." *The Physician and Sports Medicine.* 26(6)(1998):75.

Dishman, R.K., (ed.) *Advances in Exercise Adherence.* Champaign, IL: Human Kinetics Publishers, 1994.

Dobs, A. S. "Is There a Role for Anabolic Steroids in Medical Practice?" *Journal of the American Medical Association.* 281(14)(1999):1326.

Drinkwater, B. "Teach Osteoporosis Prevention Through Physical Activity." *ACSM's Health and Fitness.* 2(2)(1998):12.

Drossman, D. A. et al. "Effects of Coping on Health Outcome among Women with Gastrointestinal Disorders." *Psychosomatic Medicine.* 62(3)(2000):309.

"Drug Ecstasy Could Cause Brain Damage." *Orange County Register,* 15 Sept. 1995.

Dudley, R. A. et al. "Selective Referrals to High-Volume Hospitals: Estimating Potentially Unavoidable Deaths." *Journal of the American Medical Association.* 283(9)(2000):1159.

Dunn, A. L. et al. "Comparison of Lifestyle and Structured Interventions to Increase Physical Activity and Cardiorespiratory Fitness."

Journal of the American Medical Association. 281(1999):327.
Dunn, A. L. et al. "Lifestyle Physical Activity Intervention." *American Journal of Preventive Medicine.* 15(1998):398.
Dunn, A. L. et al. "Comparison of Lifestyle and Structured Interventions to Increase Physical Activity and Cardiorespiratory Fitness." *Journal of the American Medical Association.* 281(4)(1999):327.
Durak, E. "The Use of Exercise in the Cancer Recovery Process." *ACSM's Health and Fitness Journal.* 5(1)(2001): 6–10.
Dwyer, J.T., and Rippe, J.M. *Lifestyle Nutrition.* Malden, MA: Blackwell Science, 2000.
"Early Breast Cancer Trialists' Collaborative Group. Tamoxifen for Early Breast Cancer." *Lancet.* 351(1998):1510.
Earnest, C. P. "Dietary Androgen Supplements." *The Physician and Sports Medicine.* 29(5)(2001): 63–79.
Ebbens, W. P., and Jensen, R. L. "Strength Training for Women." *The Physician and Sports Medicine.* 26(5)(1998):86.
Eckert, D. M. et al. "Inhibitinf HIV-1 Entry." *Cell.* 99(1999):103.
Eikelboom, J. M. et al. "Homocysteine and Cardiovascular Disease." *Annals of Internal Medicine.* 131(1999):363.
Eisenberg, D. M. "Trends in Alternative Medicine in the US 1990–1997." *Journal of the American Medical Association.* 280(18)(1998):1569.
Eisner, M. D. et al. "Bartenders' Respiratory Health After Establishment of Smoke-Free Bars and Taverns." *Journal of the American Medical Association.* 280(22)(1998):1909.
Elkin, P. L. "Effects of Diet and Exercise on Cholesterol Levels." *New England Journal of Medicine.* 339(21)(1998):552.
Engel, J. P. "Long Term Suppression of Genital Herpes." *Journal of the American Medical Association.* 280(10)(1998):928.
Engels, H. J. et al. "An Empirical Evaluation of the Prediction of Maximal Heart Rate." *Research Quarterly for Exercise and Sport.* 69(1)(1998):94.
Englehardt, M. et al. "Creatine Supplementation in Endurance Sports." *Medicine and Science in Sports and Exercise.* 30(7)(1998):1123.
Epstein, L. H., and Roemmich, J. N. "Reducing Sedentary Behavior: Role Modifying Physical Activity." *Exercise and Sport Sciences Reviews.* 29(3)(2002): 103–108.
Erickson, S. M., and Sevier, T. L. "Osteoporosis in Active Women." *The Physician and Sports Medicine.* 25(11)(1997):61.
Etnier, J. L. et al. "The Influence of Physical Fitness and Exercise Upon Cognitive Functioning: A Meta Analysis." *The Journal of Sport and Exercise Psychology.* 19(3)(1997):249.
Evans, W. J. "Exercise Training Guidelines for the Elderly." *Medicine and Science in Sports and Exercise.* 31(1)(1999):12.
Farrel, S. W. et al. "Influences of Cardiorespiratory Fitness Levels and Other Predictors of Cardiovascular Disease Mortality in Men." *Medicine and Science in Sports and Exercise.* 30(6)(1998):899.
Farzadegen, H. et al. "Sex Difference in HIV-1 Load and Progression of AIDS." *Lancet.* 352(9139)(1998):1510.
"Fat for Life." *Newsweek,* 3 July 2000, 40.
Feigenbaum, M. S., and Pollock, M. L. "Strength Training: Rationale for Current Guidelines for Adult Fitness Programs." *The Physician and Sports Medicine.* 25(2)(1997):44.
Feigenbaum, M. S., and Pollock, M. L. "Prescription of Resistance Training for Health and Disease." *Medicine and Science in Sports and Exercise.* 31(1)(1999):38.
Fetrow, C. W., and Avila, J. R. *Professional Handbook of Alternative Medicines.* Springhouse, PA: Springhouse Publications, 1999.
Fiore, M. C. et al. "Clinical Practice Guideline for Treating Tobacco Use and Dependence: A U. S. Public Health Service Report." *Journal of the American Medical Association.* 283(24)(2000):3244.
Fischer, P. M. et al. "Brand Logo Recognition by Children Aged 3 to 6 Years. Mickey Mouse and Old Joe the Camel." *Journal of the American Medical Association.* 266(22)(1991):3145.
Fogelholm, M. et al. "Assessment of Energy Expenditure in Overweight Women." *Medicine and Science in Sports and Exercise.* 30(8)(1998):1191.
Fontanarosa, P. B. "Alternative Medicine Meets Science." *Journal of the American Medical Association.* 280(18)(1998):1618.
Foy, S. F. et al. "Seven-Step Guide to Motivating Clients." *ACSM's Health and Fitness.* 2(2)(1998):5.
Francis, P. R. et al. "An Electromyographical Approach to the Evaluation of Abdominal Exercises." *ACSM's Health and Fitness Journal.* 5(4)(2001): 8+.
Franklin, B. A. "A Common Misunderstanding About Heart Rate and Exercise." *ACSM's Health and Fitness.* 2(1)(1998):18–19.
Franklin, B. A. "Homocysteine: A New Risk Factor for Heart Disease." *ACSM's Health and Fitness.* 2(4)(1998):43.
Franklin, B. A. "Prevent Cardiac Events During Physical Activity." *ACSM's Health and Fitness.* 2(2)(1998):8.
Franklin, B. A. "Pumping Iron: Rationale, Benefits, Safety, and Prescription." *ACSM's Health and Fitness Journal.* 2(5)(1998):12.
Frankovich, R. J. et al. "In-Line Skating Injuries." *The Physician and Sports Medicine.* 29(4)(2001): 57–65.
Franks, B. D. "Individualized Recommendations for Physical Activity." In Corbin, C. B., and Pangrazi, R. P. *Towards an Understanding of Physical Fitness and Activity.* Scottsdale, AZ: Holcomb-Hathaway, 1999.
Franks, B. D. et al. "Physical Activity Intensity: How Much Is Enough?" *ACSM's Health and Fitness.* 1(6)(1997):14.
Fredrickson, B. "Cultivating Positive Emotions to Optimize Health and Well-Being." *Prevention and Treatment.* 3(2000):321.
Fredricson, M., Guillet, M., and Devenedicits, L. "Innovative Solutions to Iliotibial Band Syndrome." *The Physician and Sports Medicine.* 28(2)(2000):52.
Fuchs, C. S. et al. "Dietary Fiber and Risk of Colorectal Cancer in Women." *New England Journal of Medicine.* 340(4)(1999):169.
Gaesser, G.A. "Thinness and Weight Loss: Beneficial or Detrimental to Longevity?" *Medicine and Science in Sports and Exercise.* 31(8)(1999):1118.
Gaydos, C. A. "Chlamydia Trachomatis Infections in Female Military Recruits." *New England Journal of Medicine.* 339(11)(1998):739.
George, J. D., Fellingham, G. W., and Fisher, A. G. "A Modified Version of the Rockport Fitness Walking Test for College Men and Women." *Research Quarterly for Exercise and Sport.* 69(2)(1998):205.
Gill, D. L. *Psychological Dynamics of Sport and Exercise.* 2nd ed. Champaign, IL: Human Kinetics, 2000.
Girdano, D., and Everly, G. *Controlling Stress and Tension.* 6th ed. Needham, MA: Allyn and Bacon, 2000.
Golding, L. A. "Engage Older Adults in Physical Activity." *ACSM's Health and Fitness.* 2(2)(1998):24.
Goldman, L. K., and Glantz, S. A. "Evaluation of Antismoking Campaigns." *Journal of the American Medical Association.* 279(10)(1998):772.
Gollan, J. *Paper Presented at the 33rd Annual Convention of the Association for the Advancement of Behavior Therapy.* Toronto, November 1999.
Golomb, L. M. et al. "Primary Dysmenorrhea and Physical Activity." *Medicine and Science in Sports and Exercise.* 30(6)(1998):906.
Gould, R. H. *Tennis Anyone?* St. Louis: McGraw-Hill, 2000.
Gouzoulis-Mayfrank, E. et al. "Impaired Cognitive Performance in Drug-Free Users of Recreational Ecstasy (MDMA)." *Journal of Neurology and Neurosurgical Psychiatry.* 68(2000):19.
Grady, D. "A Silent Killer Returns: Doctors Rethink Tactics to Lower Blood Pressure." *New York Times,* 14 July 1998, F1.

Grandal, N. A. et al. "Effects of Sodium Restriction on Blood Pressure and Other Factors." *Journal of the American Medical Association.* 279(17)(1998):1383.

Graves, J.E. et al. "Physiological Responses to Walking with Hand Weights, Wrist Weights and Ankle Weights." *Medicine and Science in Sports and Exercise.* 20(1988):265.

Greenberg, J. S. *Comprehensive Stress Management.* (7th ed.) St. Louis: McGraw-Hill, 2002.

Greenberg, W., Cohen, N., and Juraska, J. "New Neurons in Old Brains: Learning to Survive." *Nature Neuroscience.* 2(3)(1999):178.

Gugliotta, G. "Health Concerns Grow Over Herbal Aids: As Industry Booms, Analysis Suggests Rising Toll in Illness and Death." *Washington Post,* 19 March 2000, A1+.

Gulick, R. M. "HIV Treatment Strategies: Planning for the Long Term." *Journal of the American Medical Association.* 279(12)(1998):957.

Gunderson, L. "Faith and Healing." *Annals of Internal Medicine.* 132(2)(2000):169.

Guo, H. R. et al. "Back Pain Prevalence in U. S. Industry and Estimates of Lost Workdays." *American Journal of Public Health.* 89(1999):1029.

Haddock, B. L. et al. "Cardiorespiratory Fitness and Cardiovascular Disease Risk Factors in Postmenopausal Women." *Medicine and Science in Sports and Exercise.* 30(6)(1998):1893.

Hagg, R. S. et al. "Improved Survival Among HIV Infected Individuals Following Initiation of Antiretroviral." *Journal of the American Medical Association.* 279(67)(1998):450.

Hales, D. "What Everyone Should Know About Breast Cancer." *Parade.* 31 January 1999, 4–7.

Hall, A. *The Essential Backpacker: A Complete Guide for the Foot Traveler.* St. Louis: McGraw-Hill, 2001.

Hallstrom, A. et al. "Cardiopulmonary Resuscitation by Chest Compression Alone or with Mouth-to-Mouth Ventilation." *The New England Journal of Medicine.* 342(21)(2000):1546.

Hambrecht, R. "Effects of Exercise Training on Left Ventricular Function and Peripheral Resistance in Patients with Chronic Heart Failure." *Journal of the American Medical Association.* 283(23)(2000): 3095.

Hannula, D. *The Swim Coaching Bible.* Champaign, IL: Human Kinetics, 2001.

Harris, W. S. et al. "A Randomized, Controlled Trial of the Effects of Remote, Intercessory Prayer on Outcomes in Patients Admitted to the Coronary Care Unit." *Archives of Internal Medicine.* 159(19)(1999):2273.

Hartgens, F. et al. "Androgenic-Anabolic Steroid-Induced Body Changes in Strength Athletes." *The Physician and Sports Medicine.* 29(1)(2001): 49–66.

Hatano, Y. "Prevalence and Use of Pedometer." *Research Journal for Walking.* 1(1997):45.

Hatzidimitriou, G., McCann, U. D., and Ricaurte, G. A. "Altered Serotonin Innervation Patterns in the Forebrain of Monkeys Treated with (+/–)3,4 Methylenedioxymethamphetamine Seven Years Previously: Factors Influencing Abnormal Recovery." *Journal of Neuroscience.* 19(12)(1999):5096.

Haussenblas, H. A. et al. "Applications of the Theories of Reasoned Action and Planned Behaviors: A Meta Analysis." *The Journal of Sport and Exercise Psychology.* 19(1997):36.

Hawley, J. A. "Fat Burning During Exercise: Can Ergogenics Change the Balance?" *The Physician and Sports Medicine.* 26(9)(1998):56.

He, J. et al. "Dietary Sodium Intake and Subsequent Risk of Cardiovascular Disease in Overweight Adults." *Journal of the American Medical Association.* 282(21)(1999):2027.

Hill K. L. *Frameworks for Sports Psychologists: Enhancing Sports Performance.* Champaign, IL: Human Kinetics, 2000.

Hirsch, M. S. et al. "Antiretroviral Drug Testing in Adults with HIV Infection." *Journal of the American Medical Association.* 279(24)(1998):1984.

Hjelm, J., and Johnson, R. C. "Spiritual Health: An Annotated Bibliography." *Journal of Health Education.* 27(1996):248–252.

Hoeger, W.W.K., and Hopkins, D.R. "A Comparison of the Sit-and-Reach and the Modified Sit-and-Reach in the Measurement of Flexibility in Women." *Research Quarterly for Exercise and Sport.* 31(June 1992):191–95.

Holmes, M. D. et al. "Association of Dietary Intake of Fat and Fatty Acids with Risk of Breast Cancer." *Journal of the American Medical Association.* 281(1999):914.

Holt, S. "Mechanics of Machines: Selecting the Right Piece of Equipment." *Fitness Management.* July 2001, 56+.

"Homocystein and Heart Disease: A Culprit or Just a Suspect?" *The Physician and Sports Medicine.* 27(7)(1999):13.

Honein, M. A. et al. "Impact of Folic Acid Fortification of the U. S. Food Supply on the Occurrence of Neural Tube Defects." *Journal of the American Medical Association.* 285(23)(2001): 3022.

Hopkins, D.R., and Hoeger W.W.K. "A Comparison of the Sit-and-Reach Test and the Modified Sit-and-Reach Test in the Measurement of Flexibility for Males." *Journal of Applied Sport Science Research.* 6(1992):7–10.

Howard, G. "Cigarette Smoking and Progression of Atherosclerosis." *Journal of the American Medical Association.* 279(2)(1998):119.

Howley, E. T., and Franks, B. D. *Health Fitness Instructor's Handbook.* (3rd ed.). Champaign, IL: Human Kinetics, 1997.

Hu, F. B. et al. "Trends in the Incidence of Coronary Heart Disease and Changes in Diet and Lifestyle in Women." *New England Journal of Medicine.* 343(2000):530.

Hudd, S. et al. "Stress at College: Effects on Health Habits, Health Status, and Self-Esteem." *College Student Journal.* 34(2)(2000): 217–227.

Hulley, S. et al. "Randomized Trial of Estrogen and Progestin for Secondary Prevention of CHD in Post Menopausal Women." *Journal of the American Medical Association.* 280(7)(1998):605.

Humphries, B. et al. "Effects of Exercise Intensity on Bone Density, Strength, and Calcium Turnover in Older Women." *Medicine and Science in Sports and Exercise.* 32(6)(2000):1043.

Hunter et al. "Resistance Training Increases Total Energy Expenditure and Free-Living Activity in Older Adults." *Journal of Applied Physiology.* 89(3)(2000): 977–984.

Hutchins, G. M. "Dietary Supplements Containing Ephedra Alkaloids." *The New England Journal of Medicine.* 344(14)(2001): 1095–1097.

Irbarren, C. et al. "Calcification of the Aeortic Arch." *Journal of the American Medical Association.* 283(21)(2000):2810.

Ives, J. C., and Sosnoff, J. "Beyond the Mind-Body Exercise Hype." *The Physician and Sports Medicine.* 28(3)(2000):67.

Jacobs, E. J., Thun, M. J., and Apicella, L. F. "Cigar Smoking and Death from Coronary Heart Disease in a Prospective Study of U.S. Men." *Archives of Internal Medicine.* 159(20)(1999):2413.

Jacobson, M. F., and Brownell, K. D. "Small Taxes on Soft Drink and Snack Foods to Promote Health." *American Journal of Public Health.* 90(6)(2000):854.

Jaeger, T. M. *Swimming.* St. Louis: McGraw-Hill, 1999.

Jakicic, J. M. et al. "Effects of Intermittent Exercise and Use of Home Exercise Equipment on Adherence, Weight Loss, and Fitness in Overweight Women." *Journal of the American Medical Association.* 282(1999):1554.

Johnson, E. "Aquatic Exercise For Better Living on Land." *ACSM's Health and Fitness Journal.* 2(3)(1998):16.

Johnston, L. D., O'Malley, P. M., and Bachman, J. G. "The Monitoring of the National Survey Results on Adolescent Drug Use: Overview of Key Findings, 1999" (*NIH Publication No. 00-4690*). (2000) Rockville, MD: National Institute on Drug Abuse.

Jonas, W. B. et al. "Alternative Medicine: Learning from the Past, Examining the

Present, Advancing to the Future." *Journal of the American Medical Association.* 280(18)(1998):1616.

Jones, C. S., Christenson, C., and Young, M. "Weight Training Injury Trends: A 20-Year Survey." *The Physician and Sports Medicine.* 28(7)(2000):61.

Jones, B. T., Corbin, W. R., and Fromme, K. "A Review of Expectancy Theory and Alcohol Consumption." *Addiction.* 96(1)(2000): 57–72.

Jung, A. P., and Nieman, D. C. "An Evaluation of Home Exercise Equipment Claims: Too Good to Be True." *ACSM's Health and Fitness.* 4(5)(2000):14.

Kahn, H. S. et al. "Increased Cancer Mortality Following a History of Non-Melanoma Skin Cancer." *Journal of the American Medical Association.* 280(10)(1998):910.

Kamber, M. et al. "Creatine Supplementation—Part 1: Performance, Clinical Chemistry, and Muscle Volume." *Medicine and Science in Sports and Exercise.* 31(12)(1999):1763.

Kamb, M. L. et al. "Efficacy of Risk Reduction Counseling to Prevent HIV and STDs." *Journal of the American Medical Association.* 280(13)(1998):1161.

Kant, A. K. et al. "A Prospective Study of Diet Quality and Mortality in [illegible] *the American Medical Association.* 283(16)(2000):2109.

Katz, W. A., and Sherman, C. "Exercise for Osteoporosis." *The Physician and Sports Medicine.* 26(2)(1998):43.

Katz, W. A., and Sherman, C. "Osteoporosis: The Role of Exercise in Optimal Management." *The Physician and Sports Medicine.* 26(2)(1998):33.

Katzmarzyk, T. et al. "Fitness, Fatness and Estimated Coronary Heart Disease Risk: The Heritage Family Study." *Medicine and Science in Sports and Exercise.* 33(4)(2001): 585–590.

Kenyon, G.S. "Six Scales for Assessing Attitudes Toward Physical Activity." *Research Quarterly.* 39(1968):566.

Kesaniemi, Y. A. et al. "Dose-response Issues Concerning Physical Activity and Health." *Medicine and Science in Sports and Exercise.* 33(6)(supplement)(2001): S347–350.

Kestenbaum, R. *The Ultralight Backpacker: The Complete Guide to Simplicity and Comfort on the Trail.* St. Louis: McGraw-Hill, 2001.

King, D. S. et al. "Effects of Oral Androstenedione and Serum Testosterone and Adaptations to Resistance Training in Young Men." *Journal of the American Medical Association.* 281(21)(1999):2020.

Knudson, D. V., Magnusson, P., and McHugh, M. "Current Issues in Flexibility Fitness." *President's Council on Physical Fitness and Sports Research Digest.* 3(10)(2000): 1–8.

Knudsen, D. V. "Stretching During Warm-up: Do We Have Enough Evidence?" *Journal of Physical Education, Recreation and Dance.* 70(7)(2000):24.

Knudson, D. "Stretching: From Science to Practice." *Journal of Physical Education, Recreation and Dance.* 69(3)(1998):38.

Knudsen, D. V., Magnusson, P., and McHugh, M. "Current Issues in Flexibility Fitness" *President's Council on Physical Fitness and Sports Research Digest.* 2(10)(2000):1.

Kobashigawa, J. A. et al. "A Controlled Trial of Exercise Rehabilitation After Heart Transplant." *New England Journal of Medicine.* 340(4)(1999):272.

Koop, C. E. et al. "Reinventing American Tobacco Policy." *Journal of the American Medical Association.* 279(7)(1998):550.

Korber, B. "Timing the Ancestor of HIV-1 Pandemic Strains." *Science.* 288(2000):1789.

Kottke, F.J. et al. *Krusen's Handbook of Physical Medicine and Rehabilitation.* 4th ed. Philadelphia: W. B. Saunders Co., 1990.

Kraus, H., and W. Raab. *Hypokinetic Disease.* Springfield, IL: Charles C. Thomas, 1961.

Krauss, D. *Mastering Your Inner Game.* Champaign, IL: Human Kinetics, 2000.

Krauss, R. M. et al. "AHA Dietary Guidelines [illegible] Revision 2000: A Statement for Health-Care Professionals from the Nutrition Committee of the American Heart Association." *Circulation.* 102(2000): 2284–99.

Kreider, R. B., Fry, A. C., and O'Toole, M. L. *Overtraining in Sport.* Champaign, IL: Human Kinetics, 1998.

Kreis, R. et al. "Creatine Supplementation—Part 2: In Nivo Magnetic Resonance Spectroscopy." *Medicine and Science in Sports and Exercise.* 31(12)(1999):1770.

Kreketos, A. D. et al. "Effects of Aerobic Fitness on Fat Oxidation and Body Fatness." *Medicine and Science in Sports and Exercise.* 32(4)(2000):805.

Kromhout, D. "Fish Consumption and Sudden Cardiac Death." *Journal of the American Medical Association.* 279(1)(1998):65.

Kuehl, K., Goldberg, L., and Elliot, D. "Response: Long-term Oral Creatine Supplementation Does Not Impair Renal Function in Healthy Athletes." *Medicine and Science in Sports and Exercise.* 32(1)(1999):248–249.

Kujala, U. M. et al. "Relationship of Leisure Time Physical Activity and Mortality." *Journal of the American Medical Association.* 279(6)(1998):440.

Kuritzky, L., and White, J. "Extend Yourself for Back Relief." *The Physician and Sports Medicine.* 25(1)(1998):65.

Kuritzky, L., and White, J. "Low Back Pain." *The Physician and Sports Medicine.* 25(1)(1998):56.

Landers, D. "The Influence of Exercise on Mental Health." In Corbin, C. B., and Pangrazi, R. P. (ed.). *Towards a Better Understanding of Physical Fitness and Activity.* Scottsdale, AZ: Holcomb-Hathaway, 1999, Chapter 16.

Layne, J. E., and Nelson, M. E. "The Effects of Progressive Resistance Training on Bone Density: A Review." *Medicine and Science in Sports and Exercise.* 31(1)(1999):25.

Leder, B. et al. "Oral Androstenedione Administration and Serum Testosterone Concentrations in Young Men." *Journal of the American Medical Association.* 283(6)(2000):779.

Lee, C. D., Blair, S. N., and Jackson, A. S. "Cardiorespiratory Fitness, Body Composition, and All-Cause and Cardiovascular Disease Mortality in Men." *American Journal of Clinical Nutrition.* 69(1999):373.

Lee, C. D., Jackson, A. S., and Blair, S. N. "US Weight Guidelines: It Is Also Important to Consider Cardiorespiratory Fitness." *International Journal of Obesity.* 22(supplement 2)(1998):S2.

Lee, I. "Exercise and Physical Health: Cancer and Immune Function." *Research Quarterly for Exercise and Sport.* 66(1995):286.

Lee, I., and Paffenbarger, R. S. "Preventing Coronary Heart Disease: The Role of Physical Activity." *The Physician and Sports Medicing.* 29(2)(2001): 37–52.

Leutholtz, B. C. "Exercise Can Reduce Incidence and Severity of Hypertension." *ACSM's Health and Fitness.* 2(5)(1998):36.

Levine, J. A. et al. "Role of Nonexercise Activity in Fat Burning in Humans." *Science.* 283(5399)(1998):212.

Li, R. et al. "Trends in Fruit and Vegetable Consumption Among Adults in the United States." *American Journal of Public Health.* 90(2000): 777–781.

Liao, Y. et al. "Quality of the Last Year of Life of Older Adults." *Journal of the American Medical Association.* 283(4)(2000):512.

Libonati, J. R. "The Heart of the Matter: Myocardial Adaptations to Exercise." *ACSM's Health and Fitness Journal.* 3(4)(1999):19.

Lichtenstein, P. et al. "Effects of Different Forms of Dietary Hydrogenated Fats on Serum Lipoprotein Cholesterol Levels." *New England Journal of Medicine.* 340(25)(1999):1933.

Lichtenstein, P. et al. "Environmental and Heritable Factors in the Causation of Cancer." *New England Journal of Medicine.* 343(2)(2000):78.

Liemohn, W. et al. "Criterion Related Validity of the Sit and Reach Test." *Journal of Strength and Conditioning Research.* 8(1994):91.

Liemohn, W., Haydu, T., and Phillips, D. "Questionable Exercises." *President's Council on*

Physical Fitness and Sports Research Digest. 3(8)(1999):1.

Lindeman, A. K. "Quest for Ideal Weight: Cost and Consequences." *Medicine and Science in Sports and Exercise.* 31(8)(1999):1135.

Litt, A. S. *The College Student's Guide to Eating Well on Campus.* Bethesda, MD: Tulip Hill Press, 2000.

Lohman, T. G., Houtkooper, L. H., and Going, S. B. "Body Fat Measurement Goes Hi-Tech." *ACSM's Health and Fitness Journal.* 1(1)(1997):18–21.

Long, J., and Hodgson, M. *The Complete Hiker.* 2nd ed. St. Louis: McGraw-Hill, 2000.

Lori, F. et al. "Structured Treatment Interruptions to Control HIV-1 Infection." *Lancet* 354(2000):287.

Lovett, R. *The Essential Touring Cyclist: A Complete Guide for the Bicycle Traveler.* 2nd ed. St. Louis: McGraw-Hill, 2001.

Lovett, R., and Petersen, P. *The Essential Cross-Country Skier.* St. Louis: McGraw-Hill, 2000.

Loy, S. F. et al. "Easy Grip on Body Composition Measures." *ACSM's Health and Fitness.* 2(5)(1998):16.

Ludwig, D. S. et al. "Dietary Fiber, Weight Gain, and Cardiovascular Disease Risk Factors in Young Adults." *Journal of the American Medical Association.* 282(1999):1539.

Lyman, S. A. et al. "Date Rape Drugs a Growing Concern." *Journal of Health Education.* 29(5)(1998):271.

Maddux, J. E. "Habit, Health, and Happiness." *Journal of Sport & Exercise Psychology.* 19(1997):331.

Magill, R.A. *Motor Learning: Concepts and Applications.* 5th ed. Dubuque, IA: McGraw-Hill, 1998.

Manilow, M. R., Bostom, A. G., and Krauss, R. M. "Homocysteine, Diet and Cardiovascular Disease: A Statement for Health Care Professionals from the Nutrition Committee of the American Heart Association." *Circulation.* 99(1)(1999):178.

Manore, M., and Thompson, J. *Sport Nutrition for Health and Performance.* Champaign, IL: Human Kinetics, 2000.

Manore, M. M., and Thompson, J. A. *Sport Nutrition for Health and Performance.* Champaign, IL: Human Kinetics, 2000.

Manore, M. M., Barr, S. I., and Butterfield, G. E. "Position of the American Dietetic Association: Nutrition and Athletic Performance." *Journal of the American Dietetic Association,* 5(1)(2001): 1543–1556.

Manore, M. M. "Vitamins and Minerals. Part I: How Much Do You Need?" *ACSM's Health and Fitness Journal.* 5(1)(2001): 33–36.

Manore, M. M. "Vitamins and Minerals. Part II: Who Needs Supplements?" *ACSM's Health and Fitness Journal.* 5(3)(2001): 33–36.

Manore, M. M. "Vitamins and Minerals. Part III: Can You Get Too Much?" *ACSM's Health and Fitness Journal.* 5(5)(2001): 26–28.

Manson, J. E. et al. "A Prospective Study of Walking as Compared to Vigorous Exercise in the Prevention of Coronary Heart Disease in Women." *New England Journal of Medicine.* 34(1999):650.

Manson, W. C. et al. "A Perspective Study of Walking as Compared with Vigorous Exercise in the Prevention of Coronary Heart Disease in Women." *New England Journal of Medicine.* 341(9)(1999): 650–658.

Mantzoros, C. S. "The Role of Leptin in Human Obesity and Disease." *Annals of Internal Medicine.* 130(8)(1999):671.

Marcus, B. H. et al. "The Efficacy of Exercise as an Aid for Smoking Cessation in Women: A Randomized Controlled Trial." *Archives of Internal Medicine.* 159(11)(1999): 1229–1234.

Mark, D. B. "Sex Bias in Cardiovascular Care: Should Women Be Treated More Like Men?" *Journal of the American Medical Association.* 283(5)(2000):659.

Marrugat, J. et al. "Mortality Differences Between Men and Women Following First Myocardial Infarction." *Journal of the American Medical Association.* 280(16)(1998):1405.

Martin D. R. "Athletic Shoes: Finding a Good Match." *The The Physician and Sports Medicine.* 25(9)(1997):138.

Martin, D. R. "How to Steer Patients Toward the Right Sport Shoe." *The Physician and Sports Medicine.* 25(9)(1997):138.

Maruta, T., Colligan, R. C., Malinchoc, M., and Offord, K. P. "Optimists vs. Pessimists: Survival Rate among Medical Patients over a 30-year Period." *Mayo Clinic Proceedings.* 75(2)(2000):140.

Mayer-Davis, E. J. et al. "Intensity and Amount of Physical Activity in Relation to Insulin Sensitivity." *Journal of the American Medical Association.* 279(9)(1998):669.

Mayers, D. L. et al. "Drug-Resistant HIV-1: The Virus Strikes Back." *Journal of the American Medical Association.* 279(24)(1998):2000.

Mayo Clinic. "Optimism, Pessimism and Mortality." *Mayo Clinic Proceedings.* 75(2000):133.

McAuley, E., and Blissmer, B. "Self-Efficacy Determinants and Consequences of Physical Activity." *Exercise and Sport Sciences Reviews.* 28(2)(2000):85.

McCann, U. D. et al. "Positron Emission Tomographic Evidence of Toxic Effect of MDMA ("Ecstasy") on Brain Seratonin Neurons in Human Beings." *The Lancet.* 352(1998):1433.

McCulley, K. S. "Homocysteine, Folate, Vitamin B6 and Cardiovascular Disease." *Journal of the American Medical Association.* 279(5)(1998):392.

McCullough, M. E. et al. "Religious Involvement and Mortality: A Meta-Analytic Review." *Health Psychology.* 19(3)(2000):211.

McGill, S. M. "Low Back Stability." *Exercise and Science Reviews.* 29(1)(2001): 26–31.

McMurray, R. G. et al. "Is Physical Activity or Aerobic Power More Influential on Reducing Cardiovascular Disease Risk Factors?" *Medicine and Science in Sports and Exercise.* 30(10)(1998):1521.

Medicine and Science in Sports and Exercise. "Dose-Response Issues Concerning Physical Activity and Health: An Evidence-Based Symposium." *Medicine and Science in Sports and Exercise.* 33(6)(2001), entire issue.

Metcalf, L. et al. "Postmenopausal Women and Exercise for Prevention of Osteoporosis." *ACSM's Health and Fitness Journal.* 5(3)(2001): 6–14.

Miller, L. *Advanced Inline Skating.* St. Louis: McGraw-Hill, 2000.

Miller, L. *Get Rolling: A Beginner's Guide to Inline Skating.* 2nd ed. St. Louis: McGraw-Hill, 1998.

Miller, W. C. "How Effective Are Traditional Dietary and Exercise Interventions for Weight Loss?" *Medicine and Science in Sports and Exercies.* 31(8)(1999):1129.

Mitchell, T. L., and Gibbons, L. W. "Controlling Blood Lipids: A Practical Role for Diet and Exercise." *The Physician and Sports Medicine.* 26(10)(1998):41.

Mokdad et al. "The Spread of the Obesity Epidemic in the United States." *Journal of the American Medical Association.* 282(1999): 1519.

Morbidity and Mortality Weekly Reports. Published Weekly by the Centers for Disease Control and Prevention, Provides Updated Information on Health, Available on the WEB at *www.cdc.gov.epo/mmwr/mmwr.html.*

Morey, M. C. et al. "Physical and Functional Limitations in Community Dwelling Older Adults." *Medicine and Science in Sports and Exercise.* 30(5)(1998):715.

Morgan, G. T., and McGlynn, G. H. *Cross-Training for Sports.* Champaign, IL: Human Kinetics, 1997.

Morrey, M. A., and Hensrud, D. D. "Risk of Medical Events in Supervised Health and Fitness Facilities." *Medicine and Science in Sports and Exercise.* 31(9)(1999):1233–1236.

Moss, A. J. et al. "Thrombogenic Factors and Recurrent Coronary Events." *Circulation.* 99(1999):2517.

Moulson, G. "The Longest Workday: It's in the U.S." *Associated Press.* 6 September 1999.

Mujika, I. et al. "Creatine Supplementation and Sprint Performance of Soccer Players." *Medicine and Science in Sports and Exercise.* 32(2)(2000):518.

Nagle, D. L. et al. "The Mahogany Protein Is a Receptor Involved in the Suppression of Obesity." *Nature.* 398(1999):148.

Narod, S. A. et al. "Oral Contraception and the Risk of Ovarian Cancer." *New England Journal of Medicine.* 339(7)(1998):424.

National Center for Health Statistics. *Health, United States, 1998: With Socioeconomic Statistics and Health Chartbook.* Hyattsville, MD: National Center for Health Statistics, 1998.

National Cholesterol Education Program. "Executive Summary of the Third Report of the National Cholesterol Education Program Expert Panel on Detection, Evaluation, and Treatment of High Blood Cholesterol in Adults." *Journal of the American Medical Association.* 285(2001): 2486–2497.

National Council Against Health Fraud Newsletter. Published every other month it contains articles that give objective information about health products and food supplements. NCAHF, P. O. Box 1276, Loma Linda, CA 92354.

National Council Against Health Fraud . "FDA Guidelines to Supplements." *NCAHF Newsletter.* 22(2)(1999):4.

National Council Against Health Fraud . "FTC Targets Internet Health Fraud." *NCAHF Newsletter.* 22(6)(1999):1.

National Council Against Health Fraud . "National Surveys Produce Remarkable Findings on Alternative Health Practices and Dietary Supplements." *NCAHF Newsletter.* 23(2)(2000):1.

National Institutes of Health Developmental Panel. "Acupuncture." *Journal of the American Medical Association.* 280(17)(1998):1518.

National Institutes of Health. "Interventions to Prevent HIV Risk Behaviors." *NIH Consensus Statement.* 15(2)(1997):1.

National Institute on Alcohol Abuse and Alcoholism. *Tenth Special Report to the U.S. Congress on Alcohol and Health from the Secretary of Health and Human Services.* Bethesda, MD: National Institute on Alcohol Abuse and Alcoholism, 2000.

National Institutes on Drug Abuse. *Principles of Drug Abuse Treatment: A Research-Based Guide.* National Institute on Drug Abuse (NIH Publication No. 99-4180)(1999).

National Institutes on Drug Abuse. *The Sixth Triennial Report to Congress on Drug Abuse and Addiction Research: 25 Years of Discovery to Advance the Health of the Public.* National Institutes on Drug Abuse, 1999.

New England Journal of Medicine Sounding Board. "Fortification of Foods with Folic Acid: How Much Is Enough?" *New England Journal of Medicine.* 343(2000):1442.

Newton, F. "The Stressed Out Student—How Can We Help?" *On Campus* (1998).

Nieman, D. C. "Does Exercise Alter Immune Function and Respiratory Infections?" *President's Council on Physical Fitness and Sports Research Digest.* 3(13)(2001): 1–8.

Nieman, D. C. "Exercise Soothes Arthritis: Joint Effects." *ACSM's Health and Fitness Journal.* 4(3)(2000):20.

Nortier, J. L. et al. "Urothelial Carcinoma Associated with the Use of a Chinese Herb." *New England Journal of Medicine.* 342(23) (2000):1686.

Nutrition Business Journal. "Whatever Happened to Herbs?" *Nutrition Business Journal.* March, 2001.

Ortal, M., and Sherman, C. "Exercise Against Depression." *The Physician and Sports Medicine.* 26(10)(1998):55.

Osness, W. H. "Exercise and the Older Adult." Reston, VA: AAHPERD, 1998.

Osness, W., and Mulligan, L. "Physical Activity and Depression in Older Adults." *Journal of Physical Education, Recreation and Dance.* 69(9)(1998):16.

Otis, C. L. "Too Slim, Amenorrheic, Fracture Prone: The Female Athlete Triad." *ACSM's Health and Fitness Journal.* 2(1)(1998):20.

Otis, C. L., Drinkwater, B., Johnson, M., Loucks, A., and Wilmore, J. "ACSM Position Stand on the Female Athlete Triad." *Medicine and Science in Sports and Exercise.* 29(5)(1997):i.

Painter, K. "Drug Cuts AIDS Death Nearly in Half." *USA Today.* 8 October 1998, 1A.

Park, R. L. *Voodoo Science: The Road from Foolishness to Fraud.* New York: Oxford University Press, 2000.

Parkkari, J. et al. "A Controlled Trial of the Health Benefits of Regular Walking on a Golf Course." *American Journal of Medicine.* 109(2)(2000): 102–108.

Patrick, D. "Drug Czar Pushing for Fast Definition of Performance Drug." *USA Today.* 19 May 1999, 14.

Payne, V. G. et al. "Resistance Training in Children and Youth: A Meta Analysis." *ACSM's Health and Fitness.* 2(3)(1998):11.

Payne, W. A., and Hahn, D. B. *Understanding Your Health.* 6th ed. St. Louis: McGraw-Hill, 2000.

Pescatello, L. S., and Murphy, D. "Lower Intensity Physical Activity is Advantageous for Fat Distribution and Blood Glucose Among Viscerally Obese Older Women." *Medicine and Science in Sports and Exercise.* 30(9) (1998):1408.

Peterson, J. "10 Ways to Avoid Heat-Related Conditions While Exercising." *ACSM's Health and Fitness Journal.* 2(3)(1998):48.

Peterson, J. A., Bryant, C. X., and Franklin, B. A. "50 Nifty Ways to Reduce Fat in Your Diet." *Fitness Management.* 14(11) (1998):40.

Peterson, K. S. "Smoke and Marriage Don't Always Go Together." *USA Today.* 28 December 1998, 1D.

Picciotto, M. R., Zoli, M., and Rimondini, R. "Acetylcholine Receptors Containing the Beta2 Subunit Are Involved in the Reinforcing Properties of Nicotine." *Nature.* 391 (1998):173.

Pierce, J. P. et al. "Tobacco Industry Promotion of Cigarettes and Adolescent Smoking." *Journal of the American Medical Association.* 279(7)(1998):511.

Pinger, R., Payne, W. A., Hahn, D. B., and Hahn, E. J. *Drugs: Issues for Today.* 3rd ed. St. Louis: WCB/McGraw-Hill, 1998.

Plowman, S.A. "Physical Fitness and Healthy Low Back Pain Function." In Corbin, C.B., and Pangrazi, R.P. (eds.), *Towards a Better Understanding of Physical Fitness and Activity.* Scottsdale, AZ: Halcomb-Hathaway, 1999, Chapter 13.

Plunkett, B. T., and Hopkins, W. G. "Investigation of the Side Pain Stitch Induced by Running after Fluid Ingestion." *Medicine and Science in Sports and Exercise.* 31(8)(1999): 1169.

Pollock, M. J., and Evans, W. J. "Resistance Training for Health and Disease." *Medicine and Science in Sports and Exercise.* 31(1) (1999):10.

Pollock, M. L., and Vincent, K. R. "Resistance Training for Health." In Corbin, C. B., and Pangrazi, R. P. (eds.). *Towards a Better Understanding of Physical Fitness and Activity.* Scottsdale, AZ: Holcomb-Hathaway, 1999, Chapter 14.

Poortmans, J. R. et al. "Long-term Oral Creatine Supplementation Does Not Impair Renal Function in Healthy Athletes." *Medicine and Science in Sports and Exercise.* 31(8)(2000): 1108.

Pope, H. G. et al. "Body Image Perceptions among Men in Three Countries." *American Journal of Psychiatry.* 157(8)(2000):1297.

Pope, H. G. et al. "Muscle Dysmorphia: An Underrecognized Form of Body Dysmorphic Disorder." *Psychosomatics.* 38(6)(1997):548.

Pope, R. P. et al. "A Randomized Study of Preexercise Stretching for Prevention of Lower-limb Injury" *Medicine and Science in Sports and Exercise.* 31(2)(2000):271.

Porcari, J. P. "Pump Up Your Walking." *ASCM's Health and Fitness Journal.* 3(1)(1999):25.

Potter, J. D. "Fiber and Colorectal Cancer: Where to Now?" *New England Journal of Medicine.* 340(3)(1999):223.

Powell, K. E. et al. "Injury Rates from Walking, Gardening, Weightlifting, Outdoor Bicycling, and Aerobics." *Medicine and Science in Sports and Exercise.* 30(8)(1998):1246.

Pratt, M. "Benefits of Lifestyle Activity vs. Structured Exercise." *Journal of the American Medical Association.* 281(4)(1999):375.

Pronk, N. P., Tan, A. W. H., and O'Conner, P. "Obesity, Fitness, Willingness to Communicate and Health Care Cost." *Medicine and Science in Sports and Exercise.* 31(11)(1999): 1535.

Pryor, E. *Keep Moving: Fitness Through Aerobics and Step.* 4th ed. St. Louis: McGraw-Hill, 2000.

Questioning 40/40/30: A Guide to Understanding Sports Nutrition Advice. A 22-page booklet published jointly by the American College of Sport Medicine, the American Dietetics Association, the Women's Sports Foundation and the Cooper Institute for Aerobics Research, 1997.

Quittner, J. "High-tech Walking." *Time.* 24 July 2000, 77.

Radcliffe, J., and Farentinos, R. *High-Powered Plyometrics.* Champaign, IL: Human Kinetics, 1999.

Raglin, J., and Bardukas, A. "Overtraining in Athletes: The Challenge of Prevention—A Consensus Statement." *ACSM's Health and Fitness Journal.* 3(2)(1999):27.

Raisz, L. G., and Prestwood, K. M. "Estrogen and the Risk of Fracture—New Data—New Quest." *New England Journal of Medicine.* 339(11)(1998):767.

Ransdell, L. B., Snow, H., and Ostlund, D. "Metabolic Syndrome X: Postmenopausal Women's Hidden Nemesis." *Journal of Women and Aging.* 9(1)(1997):53.

Reeves, R. K., Laskowski, E. R., and Smith, J. "Weight Training Injuries: Part I." *The Physician and Sport Medicine.* 26(2)(1998):54.

Reeves, R. K., Laskowski, E. R., and Smith, J. "Weight Training Injuries: Part II." *The Physician and Sports Medicine.* 26(3)(1998):46.

Reginster, J. Y. et al. "Long-term Effects of Glucosamine Sulphate on Osteoarthritis Progression." *Lancet.* 357(9252)(2001): 251–256.

Reibe, D., and Nigg, C. "Setting the State for Healthy Living." *ACSM's Health and Fitness.* 2(3)(1998):11.

Reim, E. B. et al. "Folate and Vitamin B6 from Diet and Supplements in Relation to Risk of CHD Among Women." *Journal of the American Medical Association.* 279(5)(1998):359.

Rexrode, K. M. et al. "Abdominal Adiposity and Coronary Heart Disease in Women." *Journal of the American Medical Association.* 28(21)(1999):1843.

Rice, V. H. (ed.) *Handbook of Stress, Coping and Health.* Thousand Oaks, CA: Sage Publications, 2000.

Rico-Sanz, H., and Mendez Marco, M. T. "Creatine Enhances Oxygen Uptake and Performance During Alternating Intensity Exercise." *Medicine and Science in Sports and Exercise.* 32(2)(2000):379.

Ridker, P. M. et al. "C-Reactive Protein and Other Markers of Inflammation in the Prediction of Heart Disease in Women." *New England Journal of Medicine.* 342(12)(2000):836.

Rigotti, N. A. "U.S. College Students' Use of Tobacco Products: Results of a National Survey." *Journal of the American Medical Association.* 284(6)(2000):699.

Roberts, G. *Advances in Motivation in Sports and Exercise.* Champaign, IL: Human Kinetics, 2001.

Roche, A. F., Hyemsfield, S. B., and Lohman, T. G. *Human Body Composition.* Champaign, IL: Human Kinetics, 1996.

Roitman, J. L. (ed.) *ACSM's Resource Manual for Guidelines for Exercise Testing and Prescription.* 3rd ed. Baltimore: Williams & Wilkins, 1998.

Roizen, M. F., and Stephenson, E. A. "Want to Live Longer? Here's Exactly How!" *Prevention.* 1 April 2000.

Rosamond, W. D. et al. "Trends in the Incidence of Myocardial Infarction and the Mortality Due to CHD." *New England Journal of Medicine.* 339(13)(1998):861.

Rosenberg, P. S., and Biggar, R. J. "Trends in HIV Incidence Among Young Adults in the US." *Journal of the American Medical Association.* 279(23)(1998):1894.

Rosenfeld, I. "Acupuncture Goes Mainstream (Almost)." *Parade.* 16 August 1998,10.

Rosenfeld, I. "For A Good Nights Sleep." *Parade.* 25 October 1998, 8.

Rosenfeld, I. "New Treatments (HIV/AIDS), Renewed Hope." *Parade.* 23 July 2000, 4.

Rosenfeld, I. "Stay Safe: Know Your STDs." *Parade.* 6 August 2000, 8.

Rosenfeld, I. "What is Normal Cholesterol Anyway?" *Parade.* 12 July 1998, 4.

Ross, R. "Mechanisms of Disease: Atherosclerosis and Inflammatory Disease?" *Journal of the American Medical Association.* 340(3)(1999):115.

Rubin, R. "Measuring Up is Tricky." *USA Today.* 10 June 1998, D1.

Ruowei, L. et al. "Trends in Fruit and Vegetable Consumption among Adults in 16 U.S. States." *American Journal of Public Health.* 90(2000):777.

Russell, R. M. et al. "Modified Food Guide Pyramid for People over Seventy Years of Age." *The Journal of Nutrition.* 129(1999):751.

Rutherford, M. et al. "Pal Power: If Friends Are Gifts We Give Ourselves, It's Good to Be Greedy. Hold On to What You've Got-and Grab Some More." *Time.* 13 November 2000.

Sabol, S. Z. et al. "A Genetic Association for Cigarette Smoking." *Health Psychology.* 18(1)(1999):7.

Sallis, J. F. "Influences of Physical Activity on Children, Adolescents, and Adults or Determinants of Physical Activity." In Corbin, C. B., and Pangrazi, R. P. (ed.). *Towards a Better Understanding of Physical Fitness and Activity.* Scottsdale, AZ: Holcomb-Hathaway, 1999, Chapter 4.

Sallis, J. F., and Owen, N. "Determinants of Physical Activity." Chap. 7 in *Physical Activity and Behavioral Medicine.* Thousand Oaks, CA: Sage, 1999.

Sallis, J. F. et al. "Environmental and Policy Intervention to Promote Physical Activity." *American Journal of Preventive Medicine.* 15(1998):379.

Sallis, R., and Chassay, C. M. "Recognizing and Treating Common Cold-induced Injury in Outdoor Sports." *Medicine and Science in Sports and Exercise.* 31(10)(1999):1367.

Saris, W. H. M. "Fit, Fat and Fat Free: The Metabolic Effects of Weight Control." *International Journal of Obesity.* 22(Supplement 22)(1998):S15.

Schatzkin, A. et al. "Lack of Effect of a Low-Fat, High-Fiber Diet on the Recurrence of Colorectal Adenomas." *New England Journal of Medicine.* 342(2000):1149.

Schilling, B. K. et al. "Creatine Supplementation and Health Variables." *Medicine and Science in Sports and Exercise.* 33(2)(2001): 183–188.

Schniffing, L. "Can Exercise Gadgets Motivate Patients?" *The Physician and Sports Medicine.* 29(1)(2001): 15–18.

Schnirring, L. "New Formula Estimates Maximal Heart Rate." *The Physician and Sports Medicine.* 29(7)(2001): 13–14.

Schwellnus, M. P. "Skeletal Muscle Cramps During Exercise." *The Physician and Sports Medicine.* 27(12)(1999):1019.

Schwartz, A. L. et al. "Exercise Reduces Daily Fatigue in Women with Breast Cancer Receiving Chemotherapy." *Medicne and Science in Sports and Exercise.* 33(5)(2001): 718–723.

Seligman, M. E. *Learned Optimism: How to Change Your Mind and Your Life*. New York: Pocket Books, 1998.

Seligman, M. E. P. "Building Human Strength: Psychology's Forgotten Mission." *APA Monitor*. 29(1)(1998):2.

Serdula, M. K. et al. "Prevalence of Attempting Weight Loss and Strategies for Controlling Weight." *Journal of the American Medical Association*. 282(4)(1999):1353.

Shangold, M. M. (1998). "Beyond the Exercise Prescription: Making Exercise as Way of Life." *The Physician and Sports Medicine*. 26(11)(1998):35.

Shairer, C. et al. "Menopausal Estrogen and E-Progestin Replacement Therapy and Breast Cancer Risk." *Journal of the American Medical Association*. 283(4)(2000):485.

Shelton, R. C. et al. "Effectiveness of St. John's Wort in Major Depression." *Journal of the American Medical Association*. 285(15)(2001): 1978–1986.

Shephard, R. J., and Shek, P. N. "Exercise, Immunity and Susceptibility to Infection." *The Physician and Sports Medicine*. 27(6)(1999): 47–71.

Shepard, R. J. "Exercise in the Heat." *The Physician and Sports Medicine*. 29(6)(2001). 21–31.

Shephard, R. J. "Preparing for Physical Activity." In Corbin, C. B., and Pangrazi, R. P. (ed.). *Towards a Better Understanding of Physical Fitness and Activity*. Scottsdale, AZ: Holcomb-Hathway, 1999, Chapter 1.

Shipple, B. "Treating Low Back Pain: Exercise Knowns and Unknowns." *The Physician and Sports Medicine*. 25(8)(1997):67.

Shirreffs, S. M., and Maughan, R. J. "Rehydration and Recovery of Fluid Balance after Exercise." *Exercise and Sport Sciences Reviews*. 28(1)(2000): 27.

Shrier, I., and Gosseal, K. "Myths and Truths of Stretching." *The Physician and Sports Medicine*. 28(8)(2000):57.

Simons-Morton, D. G. et al. "Effects of Interventions in Health Care Settings on Physical Activity or Cardiovascular Fitness." *American Journal of Preventive Medicine*. 15(1998):413.

Smith, A. D. "The Fit Woman in the 21st Century." *The Physician and Sports Medicine*. 26(1998):23.

Smith, B. J. "Promoting Physical Acitivty in General Practice: A Controlled Trial of Written Advice and Information Mateirals." *British Journal of Sports Medicine*. 34(4)(2000): 262–267.

Smith, J. K. "Exercise and Atherogenesis." *Exercise and Sports Science Reviews*. 29(2)(2001):49–53.

Spain, C. G., and Franks, B. D. "Healthy People 2010: Physical Activity and Fitness." *President's Council on Physical Fitness and Sports Research Digest*. 3(13)(2001): 1–16.

Sparling, P. B., and Millard-Stafford, M. "Keeping Sports Participants Safe in Hot Weather." *The Physician and Sports Medicine*. 27(7)(1999):27.

Sparling, P. B. et al. "Development of a Cadence Curl-up Test for College Students." *Research Quarterly for Exercise and Sport*. 68(1)(1997):110.

Srundy, S. M. et al. "Physical Activity in the Prevention and Treatment of Obesity and its Comorbidities: Evidence Report of Independent Panel to Assess the Role of Physical Activity in the Treatment of Obesity and its Comorbidities." *Medicine and Science in Sports and Exercise*. 31(11)(1999):1493.

Stampfer, M. J. et al. "Primary Prevention of Coronary Heart Disease in Women through Diet and Lifestyle." *New England Journal of Medicine*. 343(2000):16.

Staszewski, S. et al. "Efavirenz Plus Zidovudine and Lamivudine, Efavirenz Plus Indinavir, and Indinavir Plus Zidovudine and Lamivudine in the Treatment of HIV-1 Infection in Adults." *New England Journal of Medicine*. 341(25)(1999):1865.

Steffen-Batey, L. et al. "Changes in Level of Physical Activity and Risk of All-Cause Mortality and Reinfarction." *Circulation*. 102(18)(2000): 2204–2209.

Stephanick, M. L. et al. "Effects of Diet and Exercise in Men and Postmenopausal Women with Low Levels of HDL Cholesterol and High Levels of LDL." *New England Journal of Medicine*. 340(1)(1999):12.

Strawford, A. et al. "Resistance Exercise and Supraphysiologic Androgen Therapy in Eugonadal Men with HIV-related Weight Loss." *Journal of the American Medical Association*. 281(14)(1999):1282.

"Supplements Dodge Regulation." *USA Today*. 23 November 1998, 22A.

Studdert, D. M. "Medical Malpractice: Implications of Alternative Medicine." *Journal of the American Medical Association*. 280(1998):1610.

Stuhr, R. M. "Strategies for Beating the Barriers to Exercise for Women." *ACSM's Health and Fitness Journal*. 2(5)(1998):20.

Surgeon General's Office. *Surgeon General's Report on Physical Activity and Health*. Washington, DC: U.S. Government Printing Office, 1996.

Taddei, S. et al. "Physical Activity Prevents Age-Related Impairments in Nitric Oxide Availability in Elderly Athletes." *Circulation*. 101(2000):2896.

Talbot, L. A., Metter, E. J., and Fleg, J. L. "Leisure-time Physical Activities and Their Relationship to Cardiovascular Fitness in Healthy Men and Women 18–95 Years." *Medicine and Science in Sports and Exercise*. 32(2)(2000):417.

Tanaka, H., Monahan, K. D., and Seals, D. R. "Age-predicted Maximal Heart Rate Revisited." *Journal of the American College of Cardiology*. 37(1)(2001): 153–156.

Tate, D. F., Wing, R. R., and Winett, R. A. "Using Internet Technology to Deliver a Behavioral Weight Loss Program." *Journal of the American Medical Association*. 285(2001): 1172.

Terbizan, D. J., and Strand, B. "How Much Exercise?" *Fitness Management*. 14(9)(1998):32.

"Thigh Cream Fails Test." *National Council Against Health Fraud Newsletter*. 18(1995).

Thomas, D. Q. et al. "Nasal Strips and Mouthpieces Do Not Effect Power Output During Anaerobic Exercise." *Research Quarterly for Exercise and Sport*. 69(2)(1998):201.

Thomis, M. A. I. et al. "Strength Training: Importance of Genetic Factors." *Medicine and Science in Sports and Exercise*. 30(5)(1998):725.

Thompson, P. D. "Cardiovascular Risks of Exercise." *The Physician and Sports Medicine*. 29(4)(2001): 33–47.

Thompson, S. R., Weber, M. M., and Brown, L. B. "The Relationship Between Health and Fitness Magazine Readings and Eating-Disordered Weight-Loss Methods Among High School Girls." *American Journal of Health Education*. 32(3)(2001): 133–138.

Tofler, I. R. et al. "Physical and Emotional Problems of Elite Female Gymnasts." *New England Journal of Medicine*. 335(4)(1998):281.

Townsend, C. *The Advanced Backpacker: A Handbook of Year Round, Long-Distance Hiking*. St. Louis: McGraw-Hill, 2001.

Townsend, C. *The Backpacker's Pocketguide*. St. Louis: McGraw-Hill, 2001.

Turner, E. E. et al. "Psychological Benefits of Physical Activity Are Influenced by the Social Environment." *Journal of Sport and Exercise Psychology*. 19(2)(1997):119.

U. S. Department of Health and Human Services. *Healthy People 2010*. (Conference Edition in Two Volumes). Washington, DC: USDHHS, 2000.

U.S. Department of Health and Human Services. *Healthy People 2010 Objectives: Draft for Comment*. Washington, DC: U.S. Department of Health and Human Services, 1998.

U.S. Department of Health and Human Services. *Healthy People 2010*. 2nd ed. With "Understanding and Improving Health" and "Objectives for Improving Health." 2 vols.

Washington, DC: U. S. Government Printing Office, November 2000.

U.S. Department of Health and Human Services. *Reducing Tobacco Use: A Report of the Surgeon General.* Atlanta: CDC, National Center for Chronic Disease Prevention and Health Promotion, Office of Smoking and Health, 2000.

USA Today. "Herbal Drug Bust." *USA Today.* 8 June 2001.

Uusitalo, A. L. "Overtraining." *The Physician and Sports Medicine.* 29(5)(2001): 35–50.

Van Loan, M. D. "Do You Restrict Your Food Intake? The Implications of Food Restriction on Bone Health." *ACSM's Health and Fitness Journal.* 5(1)(2001): 11-14.

Van Loan, M. D. "What Makes Good Bones: Factors Affecting Bone Health." *ACSM's Health and Fitness Journal.* 2(4)(1998):27.

Volek, J. S. "Update: What We Know About Creatine." *ACSM's Health and Fitness Journal.* 3(3)(1999):27.

Volek, J. S. et al. "Performance and Muscle Fiber Adaptations to Creatine Supplementation and Heavy Resistance Training." *Medicine and Science in Sports and Exercise.* 31(8)(1999):19.

von Poppel, H. "Lumbar Supports and Education for Prevention of Low Back Pain in Industry." *Journal of the American Medical Association.* 279(27)(1998):1789.

Walker, L. S. et al. "Chromium Picolinate Effects On Body Composition and Muscular Performance in Wrestlers." *Medicine and Science in Sports and Exercise.* 30(12) (1998):1730.

Wallace, J. P. "Exercise Can Reduce High Blood Pressure." *ACSM's Health and Fitness.* 2(1)(1998):29.

Wallman, H. "Low Back Pain: Is It Really All Behind You? An Excellent 7-Step Abdominal Strengthening Program." *ACSM's Health and Fitness.* 2(5)(1998):30.

Walters, P. H. "Back to the Basics: Strengthening the Neglected Lower Back." *ACSM's Health and Fitness Journal.* 4(4)(2000):19.

Wannamethee, S. G. et al. "Physical Activity and Mortality in Older Men with Diagnosed Coronary Heart Disease." *Circulation.* 102(12)(2000): 1358–1363.

Wannamethee, S. G. et al. "Physical Activity and Mortality in Older Men with Diagnosed Coronary Heart Disease." *Circulation.* 102(2000):1358.

Wardlaw, G. M. *Contemporary Nutrition.* 5th ed. St. Louis: McGraw-Hill, 2002.

Warlaw, G. M. *Contemporary Nutrition.* 4th ed. St. Louis: McGraw-Hill, 2000.

Wechsler, H. "What Colleges Are Doing about Student Binge Drinking: A Survey of College Administrators." *Journal of American College Health.* 48(2000):219–226.

Wechsler, H. et al. "Increased Level of Cigarettes Use Among College Students: A Cause for National Concern." *Journal of the American Medical Association.* 280(19)(1998):1673.

Wechsler, H., Lee, J. E., Kuo, M., and Lee, H. "College Binge Drinking in the 1990s: A Continuing Problem." Results of the Harvard School of Public Health 1999 College Alcohol Study. *Journal of American College Health.* 48(2000):199.

Wei, M. et al. "Low Cardiorespiratory Fitness and Inactivity as Predictors of Mortality in Men with Type 2 Diabetes." *Annals of Internal Medicine.* 132(8)(2000):605.

Wei, M. et al. "Relationship between Low Cardiorespiratory Fitness and Morbidity in Normal Weight, Overweight, and Obese Men," *Journal of the American Medical Association.* 282(1999):1547.

Weiler, J. M. et al. "Effects of Fexofenadine, Diphenhydramine, and Alcohol on Driving Performance. A Randomized, Placebo-controlled Trial in the Iowa Driving Simulator." *Annals of Internal Medicine.* 132(2000):354.

Weisfuse, I. B. "Gonorrhea Control and Antimicrobial Resistance." *Lancet.* 352(9107) (1998):928.

Weiss, P. H. "Sleep Facts." *ACSM's Health and Fitness Journal.* 4(6)(2000): 17–19.

Welk, G. J. et al. "The Utility of the Digi-Walker Step Counter to Assess Daily Physical Activity Patterns." *Medicine and Science in Sports and Exercise.* 32 (9 Supplement) (2000):S481–488

Welk, G. J., and Blair, S. N. "Physical Activity Protects Against the Health Risk of Obesity." *President's Council on Physical Fitness and Sports Research Digest.* 3(12)(2000): 1–8.

Wells, C. L. "Physical Activity and Cancer Prevention: Focus on Breast Cancer." *ACSM's Health and Fitness Journal.* 3(1)(1999):13.

Werner, R. M., and Pearson, T. A. "What's So Passive about Passive Smoking? Secondhand Smoke as a Cause of Atherosclerotic Disease." *Journal of the American Medical Association.* 279(2)(1998):157–8.

Wescott, W. L. "How Long? How Often?" *Fitness Management.* 14(7)(1998):48.

Wescott, W. L., and Baechle, T. R. *Strength Training for Seniors.* Champaign, IL: Human Kinetics, 1999.

Whaley, M. H. et al. "Physical Fitness and Clustering of Risk Factors Associated with Metabolic Syndrome." *Medicine and Science in Sports and Exercise.* 31(2)(1999): 287.

Whitehead, J. R. "Physical Activity and Intrinsic Motivation." In Corbin, C. B., and Pangrazi, R. P. (eds.). *Towards a Better Understanding of Physical Fitness and Activity.* Scottsdale, AZ: Holcomb-Hathaway, 1999, Chapter 5.

Wilde, B. E., Sidman, C. L., and Corbin, C. B. "A 10,000 Step Count as a Physical Activity Standard for Sedentary Women." *Research Quarterly for Exercise and Sport.* (72)(1)(2002): 411–414.

Williams, M. "Nutrition Ergogenics and Sport Performance." In Corbin, C. B., and Pangrazi, R. P. (eds.). *Towards a Better Understanding of Physical Fitness and Activity.* Scottsdale, AZ: Holcomb-Hathaway, 1999, Chapter 22.

Williams, M. *Nutrition for Health, Fitness and Sports.* 6th ed. St. Louis:McGraw-Hill, 2002.

Williams, M. H., Kreider, R. B., and Branch, J. D. *Creatine: The Power Supplement.* Champaign, IL: Human Kinetics, 1999.

Williams, P. T. "Physical Fitness and Activity as Separate Heart Disease Risk Factors: A Meta-analysis." *Medicine and Science in Sports and Exercise.* 33(5)(2001): 754–761.

Williams, R., and Williams, V. *Anger Kills: 17 Strategies for Controlling Hostility That Can Harm You.* New York: Harper Collins, 1999.

Wilmore, J. H. "Exercise, Obesity and Weight Control." In Corbin, C. B., and Pangrazi, R. P. (eds.). *Towards a Better Understanding of Physical Fitness and Activity.* Scottsdale, AZ: Holcomb-Hathaway, 1999, Chapter 16.

Wilmore, J. H., and Costill, D. L. *Physiology of Sport and Exercise.* 2nd ed. Champaign, IL: Human Kinetics, 1999.

Wilson, J. et al. "Effects of Walking Poles on Lower Extremity Gait Mechanics." *Medicine and Science in Sports and Exercise.* 33(1)(2001): 142–147.

Wilt, T. J. "Saw Palmetto Extracts for Treatment of Benign Prostatic Hyperplasia." *Journal of the American Medical Association.* 280(18)(1998):1604.

Winker, M. A. et al. "Guidelines for Medical and Health Information Sites on the Internet: Principles Governing AMA Web Sites." *Journal of the American Medical Association.* 283(12)(2000): 1600–1606.

Winkle, J., and Ozumn, J. *Teaching Martial Arts for Fitness and Fun.* Champaign, IL: Human Kintetics, 2001.

Winkley, M. A. et al. "Ethnic and Socioeconomic Differences in Cardiovascular Disease Risk Factors." *Journal of the American Medical Association.* 280(4) (1998):356.

Wolk, A. "Long-term Intake of Dietary Fiber and Decreased Risk of Coronary Heart Disease among Women." *Journal of the American Medical Association.* 281(21)(1999): 1998.

World Health Organization. *Obesity: Preventing and Managing the Global Epidemic.* Geneva: World Health Organization, 2000.

World Health Organization. *World Health Report 2000.* Geneva: World Health Organization, 2000.

Yesalis, C. E., and Cowart, V. S. *The Steroids Game.* Champaign, IL: Human Kinetics, 1998.

Young, J. C. "Exercise and Type II Diabetes." *ACSM's Health and Fitness.* 2(3)(1998):24.

Youngstedt, S. D. "Does Exercise Truly Enhance Sleep?" *The Physician and Sports Medicine.* 25(10)(1997):72.

Zamula, E. "Back Talk: Advice for Suffering Spines." *FDA Consumer.* 23(1989):28.

Zielbauer, P. "New Campus High: Illicit Prescription Drugs." *New York Times.* 24 March 2000.

Zvosec, D. L. et al. "Adverse Events, Including Death, Associated with the Use of 1,4-Butanediol." *The New England Journal of Medicine.* 344(2)(2001): 87–94.

Credits

Photos

Concept 1

CO1: © James Kay/Adstock Photos, p. 7 top left: © Charles B. Corbin, p. 7 top right: © Vic Bider/Photo Edit, p. 7 bottom right: © Bonnie Kamin/Photo Edit, p. 7 middle left: © David Young Wolff/Photo Edit, p. 7 bottom left, p. 8 top left: © David R. Frazier Photolibrary, p. 8 top middle: © Vic Bider/Photo Edit, p. 8 top right: Kevin Syms/David R. Frazier Photolibrary, p. 8 bottom left: Corel, p. 8 bottom middle: © Scott Stallard/The Image Bank, p. 8 bottom right: © David R. Frazier Photolibrary, p. 10: © David Frazier Photolibrary, p. 13: © Tony Freeman/Photo Edit

Concept 2

CO2: © Mark Ahn, p. 24: © Bob Daemmrich/Stock Boston, p. 28: © Tom McCarthy/Photo Edit

Concept 3

CO3: © Charles B. Corbin

Concept 4

CO4: © Kevin Syms/David R. Frazier Photolibrary, p. 53: © David Young Wolff/Photo Edit

Concept 5

CO5: © Richard Price/FPG, p. 62: © Charles B. Corbin, p. 65: © David Madison, p. 69: © Charles B. Corbin

Concept 6

CO6: © David Young Wolff/Photo Edit, p. 86: © Charles B. Corbin

Concept 7

CO7: ©Esbin Anderson/The Image Works, p. 97: Joaquin Palting/© Digital Imagery by PhotoDosc, Inc., p. 99 left: © David Frazier Photolibrary, p. 99 right: Myrleen Ferguson/Photo Edit

Concept 8

CO8: © Tefe Rakle/The Image Bank, p. 113 left: © Charles B. Corbin, p. 113 right: © Mark Ahn, p. 125 © Charles B. Corbin

Concept 9

CO9: © Corel, p. 132: © Keri Weatherly/Corbis, p. 136: © Tony Freeman/Photo Edit, p. 137 © Mark Ahn, p. 140: © Ken Akers/First Image West

Concept 10

CO10: © David Stocklein/Ad Stock, p. 147: © Corel

Concept 11

CO11: © Mark Ahn, p. 171: © Sue Benett/Ad Stock, p. 175 © Mark Ahn, p. 178: © Mark Ahn, p. 186: © David Stocklein/ Ad Stock, p. 198: © Charles B. Corbin

Concept 12

CO12: © Mark Ahn, p. 210: © Charles B. Corbin, p. 222: © Charles B. Corbin

Concept 13

CO13: James W. Kay/Ad Stock, p. 233 © Mark Ahn

Concept 14

CO14: Corel, p. 251, 253: © Tony Freeman/Photo Edit, p. 255: © Charles B. Corbin, p. 258 Corel

Concept 15

CO15: © Charles B. Corbin, p. 277 © Charles B. Corbin, p. 278: © David R. Laurie, p. 281: © Bob Daemmrich/Stock Boston

Concept 16

CO16: © Novastock/Photo Edit, p. 312 Corbis Royalty-free Images, p. 314: © John Coletti/Stock Boston, p. 318 Corel, p. 319 Joanne Scott/Greg Kidd, p. 322 © David R. Frazier Photolibrary

Concept 17

CO17: © Mark Ahn, p. 336: © Mark Ahn, p. 337: © Cindy Charles/Photo Edit

Concept 18

CO18: © Brian Bailey/Tony Stone Images, p. 350: Corbis Royalty-free Images, p. 352: Roswell Angier/Stock Boston

Concept 19

CO19: © David Stocklein/Ad Stock, p. 366: © Gary A. Conner/Photo Edit, p. 367: © Michael Newman/Photo Edit

Concept 20

CO20: © David R. Laurie, p. 387: © Charles B. Corbin, p. 389: © B. Bachmann/Image Works, p. 391, 392: © Mark Ahn

Concept 21

CO21: © Myrleen Furgeson/Photo Edit, p. 406: David R. Frazier Photolibrary

Index

C

D

E

F

Q

R

S

Laboratory Worksheets